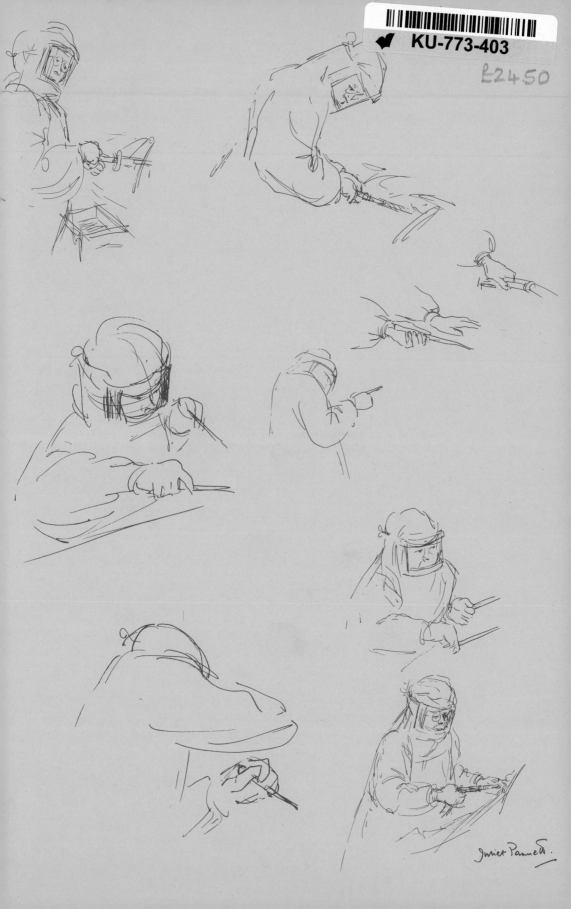

Juliet Pannett.

Steve Sturdy

Wellcome Unit for the
History of Medicine
Manchester University
January 1994.

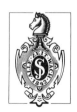

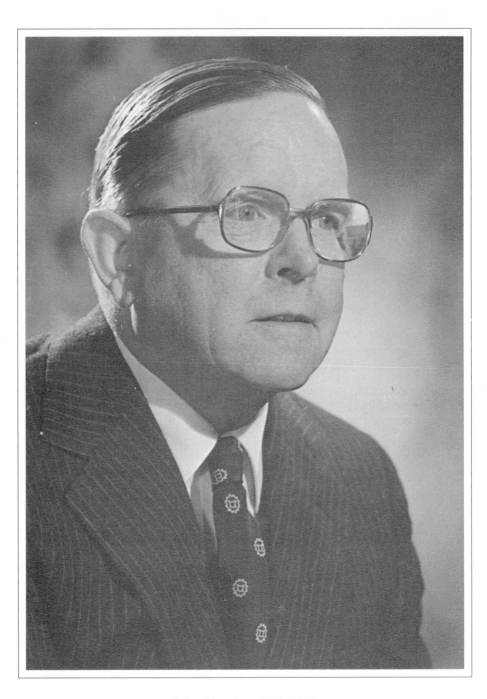

*John Charnley, 1911–1982*

# JOHN CHARNLEY

## The Man and the Hip

William Waugh

Springer-Verlag
London Berlin Heidelberg New York
Paris Tokyo Hong Kong

William Waugh, MChir, FRCS

Emeritus Professor of Orthopaedic and Accident Surgery,
University of Nottingham, and Emeritus Consultant Orthopaedic
Surgeon, Harlow Wood Orthopaedic Hospital, near Mansfield, UK

2 Mill Lane, Wadenhoe, Nr Oundle, Peterborough PE8 5ST, UK

ISBN 3-540-19587-4 Springer-Verlag Berlin Heidelberg New York
ISBN 0-387-19587-4 Springer-Verlag New York Berlin Heidelberg

British Library Cataloguing in Publication Data
Waugh, W.
  John Charnley.
  1. England. Medicine. Orthapaedics. Charnley. John
  I. Title
  617'.3'00924
  ISBN 3-540-19587-4

Library of Congress Cataloging-in-Publication Data
Waugh, W. (William), 1945–
  John Charnley: the man and the hip/by William Waugh.
  p.  cm.
  Includes bibliographicai references.
  1. Charnley, John.  2. Orthopedists—Great Britain—Biography.
  3. Artificial hip joints—Great Britain—History.  I. Title.
    [DNLM: 1. Surgery—biography.  WZ 100 C4827W]
  RD728.C48W38  1990
  617.5'81059'092—dc20
  [B]
  DNLM/DLC
  for Library of Congress                                    89–21895
                                                                 CIP

© Springer-Verlag London Limited 1990
Printed in Great Britain

Filmset by Photo·graphics, Honiton, Devon
Printed by The Alden Press, Oxford

2128/3916–5432    Printed on acid-free paper

# PREFACE

Hip replacement operations have become commonplace during the past ten years, but none the less it is well to remember the struggle to overcome the initial difficulties before the achievement of the successful results which are confidently expected today. Certainly, in the 1950s attempts to relieve pain and restore movement to an arthritic hip frequently failed. Such operations which were practised often involved a prolonged period of immobilisation which would now not be tolerated. For progress to be made orthopaedic surgeons had to rely on the loyalty and stoicism of their patients who allowed untried procedures to be carried out on themselves, often without appreciating the possible outcome. These surgical experiments resulted in progress being made, and the failures led to a greater understanding of the problems involved. The importance of collaboration with bio-engineers was also recognised, and the search began for suitable materials with which to make an artificial joint.

Progress was made in many centres throughout the world, and surgeons in the United Kingdom were at the forefront in devising original techniques. Although others also produced new models, John Charnley was a pioneer and an innovator who influenced the development of hip relacement more than any other individual. In telling the story of his life this book is inevitably also the story of the operation, but it is not intended to be a scientific evaluation of his work.

A biography of this nature is difficult to write chronologically, although I have written the first part in this way. The second part is approached differently in that various topics are taken separately, but the emphasis remains with biography rather than surgery.

At this stage, I should declare my own interest. In 1956, when I was working at what was then the Wingfield-Morris Orthopaedic Hospital (now the Nuffield Orthopaedic Centre) in Oxford, I wrote to ask Charnley if I could visit him in Manchester to learn about the operation for stabilisation of the hip joint which he had devised at that time. He took me out to dinner and I well remember going with him to his laboratory at the Medical School later that evening. There he had an ankle joint swinging in a pendulum apparatus which was part of his investigation into the lubrication of joints and which led to his original concept of his low friction arthroplasty. The next day he demonstrated the stabilisation operation; this was an arthrodesis to stiffen the hip, rather than an arthroplasty to restore movement. Back at Oxford, Professor Trueta, whose assistant I was, allowed me to follow Charnley's technique. I had some difficulty (I cannot now remember precisely what) so I wrote to ask his advice. What I do remember is that I received, within a day or two, a long handwritten letter (with diagrams) which explained precisely what to do. Unfortunately, this correspondence is lost, but the impression created endured; it seemed remarkable that he was prepared to go to so much trouble to ensure that a junior colleague should understand exactly what he thought should be done.

From then on, I followed his work with great interest and we often talked at orthopaedic meetings. It was not, however, until March 1969 that I visited the Centre of Hip Surgery at Wrightington Hospital with two of my colleagues from Harlow Wood Orthopaedic Hospital. We saw the new operation, as well as visiting the wards and a clinic; and, most important, the biomechanical laboratory. We were 'approved' and our hospital was allowed to purchase the prostheses. The operation at first seemed complicated, but we knew that it had to be carried out correctly and we persevered with his instructions. Those familiar with hip replacement today may find it difficult to appreciate how exciting an innovation this was. When we had trouble with infection, Charnley was sympathetic and helpful. At a visit to discuss the problem in 1971 I remember his school-boyish delight at wearing his 'space suit' for the first time. His enthusiasm was encouraging, and his attention to detail and his single-minded dedication were impressive. I remained convinced that Charnley's arthroplasty was the best, both in materials and method, and every assistant who worked with me during the next fifteen years always visited Wrightington to learn the technique at first hand.

Two coincidental personal connections interested me as I began work on the book. First, I found that Charnley's research in London was done with my father-in-law, Professor R.J.S. McDowall who was professor of physiology at King's College, London. Second, my teacher in orthopaedics at King's College Hospital, Mr St.J.D. Buxton, had left his war diaries to the Royal College of Surgeons in London: these made it clear that Buxton, who was then consultant orthopaedic surgeon to the Middle East Forces, had picked out Charnley to be in charge of a newly formed appliance workshop in Cairo in 1941. It is acknowledged that Sir Harry Platt played a critical part in Charnley's orthopaedic career, but there is no doubt that Buxton recognised his ability very early on and ensured that he had facilities to pursue his mechanical and engineering interests.

Towards the end of his life Charnley kept a record of his thoughts and activities, but his journal petered out after three months under pressure of other work which he must have considered to be of greater importance. However, he left a large number of published papers in orthopaedic and other journals, and at times these reveal glimpses of his personal opinions. I have quoted from his writing frequently; not to advance his scientific views, but rather to give an insight into his character. The library of the Medical School in Nottingham went to endless trouble to find and produce all (except two) of his publications. A certain amount of personal correspondence was kept by his secretary and has provided a core of information illuminating events in his life which have not been previously recorded.

What is now fashionably called oral history has formed a most valuable source. His widow, Lady Charnley entered into the project with enthusiasm and without her help the biography would not have been possible. I cannot recall how many hours we spent discussing John, but she never failed to provide whatever help I needed. Her two children were equally willing to answer my questions, and a Sunday morning spent on the floor with a large box of unsorted family photographs produced a great deal of laughter and many of the illustrations for the book. For all this, I am very grateful.

Another pleasure was tracking down (with Lady Charnley's help) and talking to John's surviving contemporaries and friends from his days as a medical student and young surgeon in Manchester and in the Army. They were all kind and hospitable, providing more photographs and answering more questions by letter. Some of them read the first draft of the early chapters and made constructive suggestions; in particular David Lloyd Griffiths and Norman Nisbet (not a contemporary, but co-author of the Royal Society's biographical memoir) acted as my 'intimate and judicious friends' as advocated by Dean Swift in his *Letter to a Young Clergyman* written in 1720. For the benefit of those unfamiliar with his advice, which applies equally well to writing as to lecturing, or giving sermons, the quotation is appended as a footnote*.

Many, many other people helped as well; beginning with the man who taught John physics at Bury Grammar School and was aged 97 years when I talked to him, and continuing to the surgeons who are now working at Wrightington Hospital. The list of names is so long that I have decided to take the unusual step of making acknowledgements chapter by chapter which has the merit of indicating the source of the information therein. These are listed, as are the references, at the end of the book. It is difficult to express adequately my gratitude to all these people.

Springer-Verlag published Charnley's last book, *Low Friction Arthroplasty of the Hip. Theory and Practice*; he was delighted with them and they appreciated working with him. It therefore is entirely appropriate that they should also be the publishers of his biography. Michael Jackson has given me encouragement at all stages, and his production team have literally smoothed the pages before publication. In particular, I am grateful to Howard Farrell who has not only dotted the 'i's and crossed the 't's, but has politely put me right about many other matters.

I hope that Charnley's life will be of interest not only to orthopaedic surgeons, but also to others who are curious about the man responsible for one of the greatest surgical advances taking place in the 1960s and 1970s (perhaps because they have benefited from it). Furthermore, the dogged determination shown by John Charnley in overcoming numerous difficulties (not least medical prejudice and Health Service bureaucracy) should be an inspiration to young men and women embarking on a medical career. Certainly his single-minded dedication resulted in an outstanding contribution to the relief of human suffering.

---

* And you will do well if you can prevail on some intimate and judicious friend to be your constant Hearer, and allow him the utmost Freedom to give you notice of whatsoever he shall find amiss either in your Voice or Gesture; for want of which early Warning many Clergymen continue defective, and sometimes ridiculous, to the end of their lives.

Jonathan Swift 1667–1745

*Author's Note*

The author wishes to thank the following journals and publishers who have given permission for substantial quotations to be taken from Charnley's writings: *Journal of Bone and Joint Surgery, British Journal of Hospital Medicine, British Journal of Surgery, British Medical Journal, Clinical Orthopaedics, The Lancet,* Churchill Livingstone, Butterworth and Co., Manchester University Press and C. V. Mosby. In particular, both Springer-Verlag and Churchill Livingstone gave me carte blanche to reproduce illustrations from Charnley's books. References and other acknowledgements are all given at the end of this book.

One special acknowledgement remains: Mrs Juliet Pannett, FRSA, a well-known portrait painter, made drawings of Charnley operating at Midhurst in 1978. The endpapers, and a page in Chapter 15, have been compiled from her sketch-books which she most generously made available.

Wadenhoe, 1989                                           William Waugh

# CONTENTS

# LIST OF ILLUSTRATIONS

# SOME IMPORTANT DATES IN CHARNLEY'S LIFE

1911   Born Bury, Lancashire

1919   Went to Bury Grammar School

1929   Entered Medical School of Victoria University of Manchester

1935   Graduated MB, BCh, and qualified as a doctor

1936   Fellow of the Royal College of Surgeons, England

1937   Resident surgical officer, Salford Royal Hospital

1938   Research at Kings College, London

1939   Resident casualty officer, Manchester Royal Infirmary

1940   Royal Army Medical Corps
      Involved in Dunkirk evacuation

1941   63rd British Military Hospital, Cairo

1944   Shaftesbury Military Hospital

1946   Demobilised
      Returned to Manchester as lecturer in orthopaedic surgery

1947   Honorary assistant surgeon, Manchester Royal Infirmary

1948   Consultant orthopaedic surgeon, Manchester Royal Infirmary and also to
      Park Hospital, Davyhulme and Wrightington Hospital

1950   *Closed Treatment of Common Fractures* published

1953   *Compression Arthodesis* published

1956   First PTFE (Teflon) arthroplasty

1957   Married Jill Heaver
      Moved to 'Naemoor', Hale, Cheshire

1958   Began development at Wrightington Hospital
       Started using cement (Nu-Life)

1959   Tristram born

1960   Henrietta born

1961   Biomechanical workshop opened at Wrightington
       First clean air enclosure ('the greenhouse')

1962   The Centre for Hip Surgery opened at Wrightington
       PTFE (Teflon) failures began to occur
       First polyethylene (HMWP) sockets used

1964   Doctor of Science, University of Manchester

1966   First 'permanent' clean air enclosure at Wrightington
       CMW cement introduced and marketed

1969   Began operating at Midhurst Hospital, Sussex

1970   Companion of the British Empire
       Results of the low friction arthroplasty first published
       *Acrylic Cement in Orthopaedic Surgery* published

1971   Moved to 'Birchwood', near Knutsford, Cheshire

1972   Professor of orthopaedic surgery, University of Manchester
          (personal chair)

1974   Granted the Freedom of the Borough of Bury

1975   Fellow of the Royal Society, London
       Retired from the National Health Service

1977   Knight Bachelor

1979   *Low Friction Arthroplasty of the Hip* published

1982   Died

1984   John Charnley Trust set up

*Chapter 1*

# GROWING UP IN BURY

## 1911–1929

*I wish either my father or mother. . .had minded what they were*
*about when they begot me; had they duly considered how much*
*depended upon what they were then doing;–that not only the*
*production of a rational Being was concerned in it, but that*
*possibly . . . his genius and the very cast of his mind . . .*

Laurence Sterne, *The Life and Opinions of Tristram Shandy,*
*Gent.*, published 1760

JOHN CHARNLEY was born in Bury, an industrial town in Lancashire, England, on 29 August 1911.

Little is known about his family, and the first record of his father, Arthur Walker Charnley, is in the electoral register of Bury in 1905. He then lived in South Bank Road and had a Chemist's shop at 25 Princess Street. The family moved house several times, presumably as their fortunes improved, and were at 100 Heywood Street when John was born. Much of the information which follows comes from the few people alive today who remember John in his school-days, or is deduced from faded snapshots in a family album.

Certainly the family had moved to 12 Heywood Street by the early 1920s. The street still exists and was clearly a respectable residential area for the stolid middle-class citizens of Bury. A former resident of the town remembers the street as:

> a small island of respectability which was close to factories and warehouses at one end, with some terrible slums at the other. But it was wide and lined by trees . . .

Number 12 is still there: a semi-detached Victorian villa with a lower floor baywindow, and a front door embellished with columns and decorative capitals. The house was close to the road, but there was a small back garden with a lawn over which John's father is shown pushing a lawnmower in one photograph in the family album, and relaxing in a deckchair in another.

1

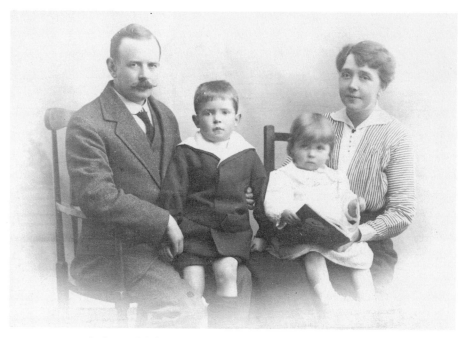

*Arthur and Lily Charnley with their children, John and Mary.*

Arthur Charnley appears as a well-built man with a waxed moustache, and in a formal portrait he is proudly wearing a Masonic badge. He seems to have stayed in the same chemist's shop in the centre of Bury all his working life. Princess Street was one of the main shopping streets and, in 1924, Arthur Charnley's immediate neighbours were a tripe dresser, a restaurant, a fruiterers, a confectioner, a boot and shoe dealer, a draper and a baker. In a photograph, the Charnley shop looks prosperous enough and is remembered by Mr Fred Campbell who has written about the recent history of Bury.[2] Mr Charnley used to do some dentistry at the back of his premises, and Fred Campbell went to him with raging toothache. This was in the 1920s when Fred was 13 or 14 years old. He only had a shilling, so he asked how much it would be to have a tooth out, and was told 'two shillings and sixpence'. 'How much will it be for cold steel?' (meaning with no anaesthetic). 'A shilling, but it'll hurt' Mr Charnley replied. Fred remembers that it did hurt, but that he was glad to be rid of the toothache. He recalls Mr Charnley as 'a neatly dressed man with a well-clipped sandy moustache, and a cheerful disposition – even when he was hurting you'. John at the time was 'a typical boy with short trousers and bare knees, and a Bury Grammar School cap; he always seemed to be running wherever he was going'. This characteristic will not surprise anyone who knew John Charnley later in life. His father's dentistry, however limited, must have had an influence because John initially intended to be a dentist, but was persuaded by his headmaster to go into medicine instead.

John rarely talked about his family to his friends in later life, and indeed he was always more interested in the future than the past. He was, however, known to say he did not have much in common with his father and that he had found him rather a 'dull' man.

Very little has come to light about the shop itself, but one of Mr Charnley's rivals in nearby Market Street advertised selling 'Holiday and toilet goods, Photographic requisites, and *Everything* of a Household Nature'. Charley Dean, who owned this shop and called himself Chemist and Optician (but not a dentist), was celebrating his 30th Free Gift Anniversary and was giving a Tablet of Perfumed Toilet Soap (originally priced at 10½d) to everyone spending one shilling and sixpence or more. Competition was clearly important among the chemists of Bury.

John's mother, Lily, had trained as a nurse at Crumpsall Hospital, in Manchester,[3] and looks to be in her late twenties in a photograph when John looks about six years old – pleasant, placid, slightly plump, she could perhaps be described as a comfortable-looking young woman. She was deeply religious and the family went regularly to the Union Street Methodist Church, always sitting in the same place. The Charnley family walking to church in their 'Sunday-best' were a familiar sight in the early 1920s. Lily Charnley was a society class leader in the church, and one surviving member of her class remembers her clearly. She was also active in the Girls' Friendly Society. Fond of reading, she encouraged her children to enjoy the English classics, which may explain John's enthusiasm for *Tristram Shandy*. This eighteenth century novel by the Reverend Laurence Sterne does not find much favour nowadays, but John continued to appreciate its robust humour and named his own son Tristram. None the less it hardly seems the sort of book which his mother would have enjoyed. The children were undoubtedly brought up in an atmosphere of moral rectitude, but the influence of a Christian upbringing was not to last in John's case; although both literature and religion continued to play an important part in his sister's life.

Mary Clare was a few years younger than John and in the family album they appear together as an affectionate brother and sister. She was very shortsighted and wore thick spectacles from the age of eight or nine years.

Snapshots show the family on holiday at Blackpool, Lancashire and Rhyl, Aberystwyth and Colwyn Bay in Wales, and Port Erin in the Isle of Man (which was perhaps as far overseas as they ventured in the 1920s); no doubt they also went to other seaside resorts favoured by the English middle-classes at the time. However much he may have enjoyed himself paddling and climbing rocks, John had no aspirations to sporting or social activities. Fred Campbell remembers that he did not play football and that he was not in the local troop of Boy Scouts. He was already showing signs of being 'good with his hands' and he is known to have made a model sailing yacht – not in the conventional way, but a true replica with timbers and planks. Splendid as this undoubtedly was, he did not realise what would happen when a boat of this construction was launched; it sank forthwith in the local pond where the family were on holiday. John, using the resource which became valuable to him later in life, got hold of a donkey and retrieved the boat without getting his feet wet.

Bury, where John lived for the early part of his life, was a product of the Industrial Revolution, and in the 1930s had a population of about fifty thousand. It was a thriving town, but small enough, as Pevsner wrote in 1979 in his *South Lancashire*, 'for the country and nearby hills to play a part in the visual scene'.[4] John's upbringing was entirely urban, and there is nothing to suggest that he had any interest in country pursuits.

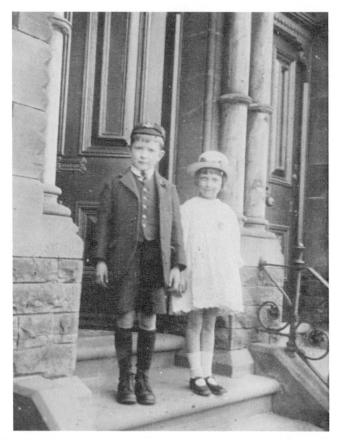

*John and Mary on the steps of their home at 12 Heywood Street, Bury.*

Local industry was based on cotton, wool, engineering and papermaking, and these are all depicted on the town's coat of arms; but there were also felt manufacture, calico printing, bleaching and dyeing, and a number of other industries. This diversity probably explains the relative prosperity which Mr Frank Ibbotson remembers in the 1920s and 1930s which were years of economic depression in many other industrial towns in Lancashire.

John went to the Bury Grammar Junior School in 1919, moving on to the Senior School in 1922. The school is an old foundation dating from the early seventeenth century. None of the original buildings remain, and the school was rebuilt at the beginning of this century through the generosity of the Hulme Trust, Lord Derby and other benefactors.

English education was, and still is, a complicated system; suffice it to say that Bury Grammar School provided a first-class education for the children of the citizens of Bury. It was a 'public' school (perversely a 'private' institution and not a state school); but since it took only day pupils, it might not have had quite the same status in some people's eyes as the prestigious boarding schools – the fees, for example, would have been a good deal less.

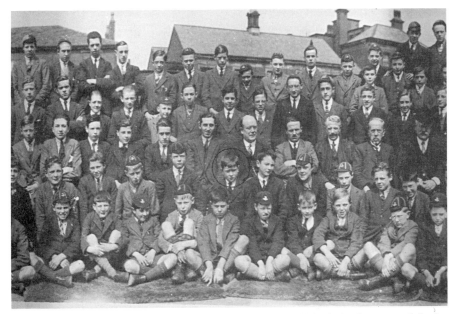

*Part of a Bury Grammar School photograph taken in 1925. John is in the centre of the boys who are kneeling.*


Bury Grammar School educated both boys and girls, but in John's day the sexes were strictly segregated, although they occupied the same building in the middle of which was the Assembly Hall. This was used first by the boys, say for morning prayers, and when they left the girls moved in. The building is a solid piece of Edwardian architecture; it is now occupied exclusively by the girls, and the boys are taught in modern buildings on a new site across the road.

John seems to have been reasonably happy and was one of a group of friends who called themselves the Musketeers. The three boys were all small for their age and were described by a contemporary as 'needing to stand on tuppence to see over thruppence'. John did not like games, such as football and cricket, and since these were not compulsory he was able to avoid taking part during his later years at school. He is known to have enjoyed playing chess. He was not a member of the Officers' Training Corps, but he was selected to represent the school at a Duke of York's summer camp in Kent – these camps were made up of 200 boys selected from public schools and 200 boys from working-class homes.

The junior boys all had lessons in woodwork, but there was no metal workshop and it seems unlikely that John could have learnt to use a lathe at school, or at home, although his father may have had a small workshop. John is remembered as being rather shy, although he had a keen sense of humour and was a 'great joker'. In spite of this, he could occasionally be rather abrupt; he might 'say something biting, but he would put it right in the next sentence'. This characteristic remained with him throughout his life. A school photograph taken in 1925 included about 290 boys (and their masters) and the section of it which is illustrated here shows him looking unusually serious.

Later in life John always said that he had not done well at school; he claimed to have failed matriculation, which was a general university entrance examination, but there is a paradox here. The school does not have his name on their list of those with matriculation certificates; but he himself wrote, in an application for a job in 1952, that he had gained matriculation in 1927. He should have studied Greek which he disliked; but fortunately he was allowed, with one of his friends (Fred Taylor Monks), to take chemistry and physics instead. This was exceptional at the time and, since they had very good teachers, they were both able to obtain the necessary university requirements in these subjects. It is said that his headmaster, Mr L.R. Strangeways, recognised John's potential and encouraged him to study medicine, rather than following in his father's footsteps as a dentist as was originally intended.[3]

The records show that he had an undistinguished career in the lower school and he was usually in the middle of the ranking order of his form. Frank Ibbotson, who taught John physics remembered quite precisely that:

> at the age of 10 or 11 John wrote perfect English, in a very good hand, and was able to express exactly what was in his mind.

Although his early achievements might not have been out of the ordinary, he certainly did much better after he reached the upper fifth form in 1926, when he was 15 years old. From then on, as he progressed into the sixth form, his scientific ability was considered by the school to have been 'outstanding'. He took the Northern Universities School Certificate in 1927 with distinctions in physics and chemistry. He became a member of the Library Committee and was secretary of the Roger Kay Society, which was a literary and debating society. He gained Letters of Success in Higher School Certificate in English literature, physics, chemistry and mathematics in 1928, and he obtained a distinction in chemistry the following year. Nowadays it is not easy to know how distinguished this really was. About 12 boys would have been entered for the examination in 1929 and, of the seven who passed, three (including John) obtained distinctions. In his final year in the sixth form, he won the form prize and was made a school prefect.

One other achievement remains to be mentioned: John was awarded the Henry Webb Memorial Prize for Science in three successive years. The prize was shared each year between two or three pupils and the name of Charnley is the only one which appears more than once in the years which he won it. His school record seems to demonstrate more than average academic ability and shows evidence of interest, and some degree of prowess, in science.

Mary, John's sister, was also educated at Bury Grammar School where she must have been a hard-working and diligent pupil. She won a scholarship to Girton College, Cambridge, where she obtained a 'double first' in English literature, which is a high award in the University degree examinations. She then became a schoolteacher and photographs taken during the second world war show her, without her spectacles, as an attractive young woman – and obviously taking pride in her appearance. She worked for some time in West Africa and then settled in London. She never married, but she was a very successful teacher, becoming the assistant head of a comprehensive school in the 1960s. She was always fond of people, and was an inspiration to her pupils, who adored her.

John is said to have resented his sister's academic success. He felt that he was considered not good enough by the school to enter for admission to the universities of Cambridge or Oxford, whereas Mary was able to go to Cambridge. He also thought that she did not make as much use of her opportunities as she might have done. They drifted apart after the war, but became reconciled and reunited after John was married. In the late 1970s, Mary had an operation for a spinal tumour (which John had diagnosed) and although she recovered, her health gradually deteriorated; so sadly it has not been possible for her to contribute personally to this book. She did, however, keep the small family photograph album, the brief captions in which are in her own neat handwriting. She had, of course, discussed these early days with Lady Charnley and some of the facts recorded here originate from her. Mary died in 1988.

A final, but vivid, glimpse of family life at Heywood Street in the middle 1930s is given by a cousin who now lives in Eire:

> Going to Bury was something that usually happened on wet or foggy Saturday afternoons. I simply cannot remember a summer visit. Uncle Arthur (J and M's father) had a chemist's shop, and I think of him as H. G. Wells. He is not in the least vivid, unfortunately, but that is the image that sticks. Aunt Mary, now J and M's mother, I liked. . . I remember her as having a sort of helmet of thick dark-brown hair. . . she was pale, and had glasses and a kindly look. She was quiet, and quiet-spoken, but made me, as a child, feel all right. It was not a bad sort of room, dark brown or green, inevitably, but with lots of books. The great thrill was encountering John and Mary. I remember going in on a dark afternoon, after the lamps were lit; a good Northern fire on the hearth, a sofa at right angles to it on the right, a lamp on the table behind, and John and Mary sitting there, smiling and laughing so well together, a skull on the cushion between them. [John had just become a medical student.] They enjoyed our reactions. But they were both splendid to me; although their own lives were proceeding brilliantly, they turned their attention on this timid inarticulate young girl – perhaps because they were fond of my mother. They fascinated me – they were so easy and friendly and I forgot to be afraid of their appalling cleverness. . .

The Charnley chemist's shop has been swept away by post-war 'improvements' in Bury. Princess Street is no longer recognisable and in its place is Princess Parade which is a functional, but not very attractive, shopping precinct. On the other hand, while Heywood Street is little changed structurally, it is no longer the type of respectable middle-class residential area which it must have been in the 1920s. Other remnants of Bury's past can be found: the most distinguished of these is the Art Gallery and Library, an exuberant expression of the town's prosperity at the end of the Victorian era.

Bury's two most famous citizens are John Kay and Robert Peel, both of whose families were involved in the textile industry. Kay invented the fly shuttle in 1733, a revolutionary step forward in cotton spinning which allowed a single worker to manage a hand-loom, and so doubled the quantity of cloth which could be woven in one day. Sir Robert Peel was prime minister in 1834, and again in 1841. His grandfather had founded a calico-printing firm in Bury which was built up by his father to become the most prosperous textile business in the world. Peel was a great reformer, and his Police Bill of 1829 established the Metropolitan police force whose members were nicknamed 'peelers' or 'bobbies' after him. Kay and Peel are both honoured by statues in the centre of the town, one in Market Street and the other in Market Place.

Not far away, in front of the modern Town Hall, but separated from it by a railway line, is a handsome stone clock-tower erected in 1914 as a memorial to Professor Walter Whitehead, a Manchester surgeon. Whitehead had been born just outside Bury in 1873 and was a direct descendant of John Kay. He worked for a time in his father's dyeing business, but then took up medicine and qualified in 1864, after being apprenticed to a local practitioner in Bury. He became a surgeon and was elected to the staff of the Manchester Royal Infirmary in 1873, becoming professor of clinical surgery at Owens College in 1891. He was a skilful, but adventurous, operator using scissors whenever possible; for example, to remove the tongue for cancer and the pile-bearing area to cure haemorrhoids – both procedures for which he was well known. He regarded a knowledge of anatomy to be a great drawback to a surgeon: 'it makes him timid'.[1]

It is encouraging that a town should recognise the surgical skill of its sons, and Bury did so again when it conferred the Freedom of the Borough on W.R. Douglas. He was a successful general surgeon and a good teacher who was on the staff of the Manchester Royal Infirmary from 1922 to 1945.

Professor Sir John Charnley's contribution to surgery was acknowledged in the same way when the Freedom of the Borough was conferred on him in 1973, an honour which he much appreciated. He was accompanied by his wife to the celebratory dinner; his contemporary at school, Fred Taylor Monks, who had become a dental surgeon, and his old physics teacher Frank Ibbotson sat, with their wives, near to him.

Although Bury was able to honour Sir John Charnley by making him a freeman, changing attitudes are such that it is unlikely that a memorial to him will be erected in his home town, as was done for Professor Whitehead. There is, however, no doubt that Charnley's work resulted in more relief of human suffering than that achieved by his distinguished predecessor.

*Chapter 2*

# TRAINING FOR SURGERY
## 1929–1940

*He was very bright, very clever and very good company. . .*
Alan Nicholson remembers John Charnley in 1939

HAVING SUCCEEDED in gaining his right to university admission, John Charnley entered the Medical School of the Victoria University of Manchester in the autumn of 1929.

Manchester was a prosperous city which had flourished as the centre of the cotton trade. An account in Chambers' Edinburgh Journal of 1858 gives a memorable description:

> Manchester streets may be irregular, and its trading inscriptions pretentious, its smoke may be dense, and its mud ultra-muddy, but not any or all of these things can prevent the image of a great city rising before us as the very symbol of civilisation, foremost in the march of improvement, a grand incarnation of progress.

This is quoted by Asa Briggs in *Victorian Cities* at the head of his chapter *Manchester, Symbol of a New Age.*[1] Many unfavourable words have also been written, but Manchester has always had something rather special about it. The population in the 1920s was almost three-quarters of a million, but by then its greatest days were over, although the aura of the past remained.

The Medical School was founded in 1824 and became the first complete medical school in England outside London. John Owens had left the bulk of his fortune to found a university college, which opened in 1851, and it acquired what had by then become the Royal Medical School in 1872. When the Victoria University was founded in 1880, Owens was the sole college. This university became the Victoria University of Manchester after the university colleges of Leeds and Liverpool, which had previously joined Manchester, became separate universities in 1903.

9

Bury lies only ten miles north-west of Manchester and was connected by an electric railway on which John Charnley travelled daily into the city when he was a medical student. He was only just over 18 years of age when he enrolled, with 55 new students, for the medical course. The ultimate aim was the degree of MB, ChB (Bachelor of Medicine, Bachelor of Surgery) of the University of Manchester and there were numerous examinations over the next six years. The first two terms were spent doing physics, chemistry, botany and zoology (lst MB); then came anatomy and physiology with a very important examination (2nd MB) in March of the third year – 1932 in Charnley's case. He worked hard, as indeed he did throughout his life, but his natural ability meant that the course did not tax him unduly.

By all accounts, he led the typical life of a medical student. He became one of a group of men who enjoyed each other's company and regularly sat together (usually in the back row) at lectures. His particular friends were Eric Greenhalgh and Frank Firth, who later became general practitioners in the Manchester area; Geoffrey Rhodes who joined the Royal Navy, and William Kershaw who specialised in tropical medicine after the war and later became professor of biology at Salford University. Charnley is remembered for his boyish sense of eagerness and the way in which his approach to learning was motivated by natural curiosity; he absorbed facts intelligently, rather than by rote.

He began by taking class medals in anatomy (junior and senior), physiology (theoretical) and histology in his first two years. During this period he also won various scholarships and prizes. He was awarded the Dauntesey medical junior scholarship (£50) on the basis of his results in the lst MB examination in the subjects of botany and zoology.

At the end of the second year (in September 1931), about a dozen of the most promising students were invited to work for a BSc (Bachelor of Science) degree, in addition to their work for the 2nd MB. This ordinary degree could be obtained after the student had done a statutory three years at the university. Charnley undertook this additional course, consisting mainly of lectures in anatomy and physiology; in addition two theses had to be written. His subjects were 'a study by dissection of the tracts in relation to the corpus trapezium of the brain stem' and, in physiology, 'the concentration of simple constituents of the urine following diuresis induced by the ingestion of large quantities of water'. The former was illustrated by the kind of careful drawings which were a feature of so much of his later work. Although the subjects seem somewhat esoteric and detached from practical application, Charnley did enough to gain his degree. Next came the Professor Tom Jones exhibition in anatomy at the end of the Lent (spring) term examinations in 1931 – and he acted as prosector in the department during the following year.

He did equally well in physiology winning the Sidney Renshaw prize after the 2nd MB examinations. In the same year, 1932, he also won the Dauntesey medical senior scholarship (£100) as a result of the recommendations of the professors of anatomy and physiology on the results of the 2nd MB examination. There was an element of caution on the part of the authorities because only half the sum was paid initially; the remainder was to be given in the following Michaelmas (autumn) term 'only if the work and conduct of the Scholar have been satisfactory' – there is no reason to doubt that Charnley fulfilled this condition.

His interest in anatomy and physiology led to his taking another step which his Manchester contemporaries regarded as exceptional (although it was not so unusual in London medical schools). Regulations of the Fellowship of the Royal College of Surgeons of England then allowed its primary examination, which was in these two subjects, to be taken at the end of the pre-clinical years. He was encouraged to do this by the head of the anatomy department, Professor Stopford (later Lord Stopford and vice-chancellor of the university) whose advice turned out to be correct: John passed without difficulty – taking it in his stride without apparent effort, as one of his friends remembers. Later, this gave him an advantage because he was able to become a Fellow of the Royal College of Surgeons at a very early age.

An early sign of Charnley's inventiveness is illustrated by his approach to histological work in the laboratory. He regarded staining sections for the microscope as a tedious waste of time, so he built a machine out of wood to automate the process. However, it was driven by water, and when someone turned the tap on too strongly, the pressure caused a burst so that he and others were spattered with indelible stain.

Although many medical students find the first part of their course a tedious interlude which they have to put up with before they can begin working in hospital, Charnley had done so well that it is reasonable to suppose that he must have enjoyed his pre-clinical work. However, he would have been as delighted as everyone else to start at the Manchester Royal Infirmary in July 1932.

Nearly all clinical teaching was at this hospital, itself a great deal older than the university, having been founded in 1752. It was established first in Garden Street, but moved in 1755 to a site near Piccadilly in the centre of the city. An attempt was made to move to a bigger and better site in 1875, but this was turned down by the General Board of Trustees. The question was raised again at the turn of the century and, although once more there was considerable controversy, a decision was finally reached – not to re-build the hospital on the existing site, but to move to Stanley Grove, Oxford Road (about half a mile from Owens College). The old hospital was purchased by the City Corporation and the land for the new hospital was provided by Owens College. After an architectural competition, construction went ahead and the result was a massive building enterprise in the most stylish Edwardian baroque. There were separate blocks based on a pavilion system with units of 50 medical and 60 surgical beds, with a total of about 500 beds in the first instance. The opening by the King and Queen took place in July, 1909.[2]

The instruction of medical undergraduates in the United Kingdom has always been based on patients in wards and clinics; students were assigned to individual physicians and surgeons in groups of not more than ten. The senior teachers were 'honoraries', and although this appointment was unpaid, it provided an essential introduction to general practitioners in the neighbourhood, and hence to private patients. The paid teachers were mostly part-time and on the staff of other hospitals, though the most junior were full-time at the Manchester Royal Infirmary (with salaries of about £100 a year).

Two attachments of three months each were allocated to medicine with the same to surgery. Students were expected to examine patients and write up their case histories, which they would then present on ward rounds. A fifth period of three months was spent, mostly in the post-mortem room, learning pathology.

The special subjects, such as ophthalmology, diseases of the ear, nose and throat, and dermatology were covered more briefly and two months were set aside for obstetrics, which was usually studied either at the nearby St Mary's Hospital or in London or Dublin. Orthopaedics was covered by twelve lectures from general surgeons, but there were also twelve lecture-demonstrations by Mr H. Platt or Mr. H.O. Clarke at the Manchester Royal Infirmary and Mr. R. Ollerenshaw at the Salford Royal Hospital. There were many brilliant medical teachers in Manchester at the time and Platt is remembered as being 'a marvellous stimulus' by one student. He often entertained groups of students at his home, and he might well have known Charnley at this time although there is no evidence to confirm this.

Charnley continued to do well in his clinical work, gaining the class medal in operative surgery in 1934/35, and he won the John Henry Agnew prize in diseases of children and the Dumville surgical prize. There were two awards of the latter prize, worth £100, each year, based on the results of the final MB examination. Charnley spent part of his £100 on a Leica camera which he kept and used throughout his life – always being proud of its superb optical system. Finally, after an essay and a difficult clinical examination, he was awarded the Bradley memorial scholarship on the recommendation of the medical board of Manchester Royal Infirmary.

He graduated MB, ChB Manchester in 1935 and also took the diploma of MRCS (member of the Royal College of Surgeons of England), and LRCP (licentiate of the Royal College of Physicians of London). The latter qualifications, although sounding very grand, were considered to be relatively easy examinations, and students often took them as a 'safety-net' in case they failed their MB degree; more importantly, the possession of the diploma allowed a candidate to sit for the Final Fellowship two years earlier than would otherwise have been possible.

Charnley had been an outstanding student and showed an early, and successful, interest in both anatomy and surgery. His life was always centred on his work; but in his student days he took part in various extra-curricular activities and he enjoyed his holidays.

His first venture abroad was in 1931 when he went with a group of fellow students to Germany for a month, staying in youth hostels – there was then a mutual arrangement between the Youth Hostel Associations of Britain and Germany. Greenhalgh was in the party and still has photographs taken during the holiday. An article, *Ambulamus Apud Germanos*, written by Charnley (but signed only JC) was published in the Manchester University Medical Gazette in October, 1931 describing his travels in Germany. After train journeys to Cologne and then Gottingen, the party walked to Bad Harzburg and on to climb the Brocken mountain in the Harz. Two paragraphs show the style of the first of his many published works:

> "To travel hopefully is better than to arrive" says R. L. Stevenson, and the profound significance of the adverb was revealed to me in a Continental railway carriage. . . there should be displayed, in addition to those notices imploring him to refrain from expectoration and other less mentionable habits, a placard bearing the legend "Abandon hope all ye who enter here!"

And the last paragraph:

> In the hall of the Youth Hostel (in Cologne) the letter rack was displayed in full view of the public. Imagine, then, my horror on seeing a letter there

facetiously addressed to me as Prof ―― ――. For some time I dare not claim it. Then, making sure that no Englishmen stood in the group around the rack, I stretched forth my hand and snatched the offending object from its place. Feeling many eyes upon it I prepared to ignore lewd grins and sniggers – but none came. Instead, the group had fallen back and made way for me with every appearance of respect. Such is the Prussian attitude to a title.

He also wrote *Meditations on the Wasserman* in the Gazette in 1933 which was a light-hearted account of a test for syphilis. The article is short and witty, with rather obscure literary references to Ambroise Paré, Catherine de Medici, Alexander Dumas and ancient Scottish customs.

Another enjoyable holiday was taken with a group of friends on the Shropshire Union Canal in an old Mersey salvage boat which they had hired; their adventures sounding reminiscent of *Three Men in a Boat* by Jerome K. Jerome. Drinking beer in the pubs by the canal was clearly an important part of the exercise.

Fell-walking and rock-climbing (in that order of preference) were activities which Charnley pursued energetically as a medical student and a newly qualified doctor. He joined the University Mountaineering Club and met Arthur Bullough who was a year senior to him in medical school (and who later became a general surgeon). They were to become life-long friends and as students frequently went climbing or walking together at weekends and on holidays. They would go to the mountains of North Wales, which are only about 90 miles from Manchester, as well as to Derbyshire, the Lake District and Scotland.

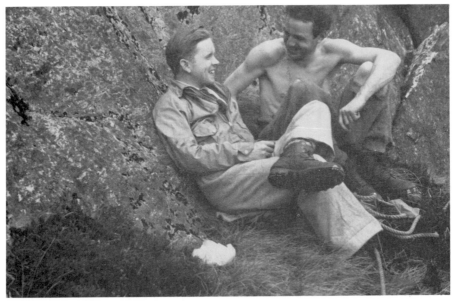

*Charnley resting after climbing with Arthur Bullough in North Wales, probably in 1936.*

One very cold February in 1932, they were staying with a group of medical students in a youth hostel in Cwm Idwal. Part of their climb involved jumping across the gap between two large rocks, called Adam and Eve, on the summit of Tryfan. The rocks are about fifteen feet high and three feet apart. It was wet and slippery, but all the party negotiated the leap successfully until it came to the last man. He was John Scully, who was rather older than the others, and he was very reluctant to attempt the jump. When he eventually was persuaded to do so, he slipped and hurt his leg as he fell. He was examined by all the students who, thinking he had not damaged himself seriously, left him behind. He stuggled down the mountain and made his own way back to Manchester where he was found to have a fracture of his leg. This caused a great deal of embarrassment to the rest of the party and the story was much later told against Charnley. The point becomes rather lost when it is appreciated that this was almost certainly a minor fracture of the fibula – and probably the type of injury which Charnley later came to believe did not need treatment in plaster of Paris. Nevertheless a little more sympathy for poor Scully from his fellow medical students would not have been out of place.

During the summer vacations of 1933 and 1934, Arthur Bullough and John Charnley went together on climbing holidays on Wester Ross and Skye in Scotland. Bullough took an old portable wind-up gramophone with them and they enjoyed listening to classical music, particularly Mozart and Beethoven, in the evenings.

Eric Greenhalgh and William Kershaw were keen athletes, and Charnley took up fencing, which he did with some enthusiasm, although he did not persist with it for long. However, a decrepit ex-police car, bought for £14, demanded a great deal of his time and effort to get it in working order, and car maintenance continued to be a hobby. He, and his friends, also attempted to construct a glider; but, perhaps fortunately for their safety, this had to be abandoned before they could fly in it.

After six years in medical school, the time had come to start work in hospital or general practice; in 1935 there were no regulations stipulating that there should be a pre-registration period under supervision, so young doctors were allowed to begin practising straightaway after qualification. It was considered highly desirable to work in your own teaching hospital and Charnley was appointed house surgeon from August 15, 1935. At first, he was at the Royal Infirmary's Central Branch in Roby Street where Frank Nicholson, another life-long friend, was the resident surgical officer.

The Central Branch had been built after the Infirmary had moved two miles out to Oxford Road in 1909 (and then almost in the country) in order to serve the needs of those who 'resided too far to attend conveniently at the new hospital'.[2] Completed in 1914, the unit had an out-patient department and an accident room with four observation beds, also an operating theatre and an X-ray room. On the first floor, there were four wards with ten beds in each which were used mainly for surgical cases. The unit was busy, with plenty of work for the resident surgical officer and the two newly qualified house officers. The Central Branch closed in 1943 apparently because it was not possible to 'obtain sufficient protective material to allow of its use as an in-patient hospital' (presumably sandbags and the like against blast from German bombs).

After three months, Charnley went to the main Infirmary where he completed his year as house surgeon to Professor Telford, and his assistants, Mr Buckley and Mr Bryce. Telford had become professor of systematic surgery in 1922 and occupied the chair until 1941. He was a general surgeon in the old-fashioned sense; he was against specialisation, and regarded orthopaedics (which he practised as well as everything else) as a branch of general surgery. He was a good teacher with the great ability of making surgery seem simple; he was also a very conservative surgeon, who tended to be rather behind the times (apart from sympathectomy). Telford was an excellent chief, who had a great sense of responsibility to his juniors, and he thought very highly of Charnley.

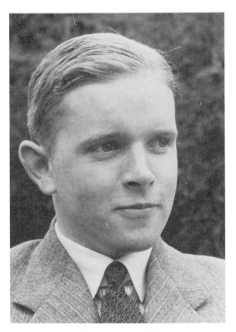

*Charnley in 1936.*

David Lloyd Griffiths, who was three years senior to John Charnley, but had met him when Charnley was a student, was resident casualty officer at this time and was responsible for the daily fracture clinic. The two men became friends and after the war they were consultant colleagues in Manchester. Lloyd Griffiths remembers that John Charnley seriously considered the possibility of going into cancer research, but Telford persuaded him that this would be a waste of time and he abandoned the idea. In many ways it was fortunate that he did not falter in his surgical career because his early start enabled him to go ahead very quickly. Although he had sufficient vision and intellectual ability to pursue an academic career, he was always best at the practical application of his many original ideas.

He wisely decided that he would go ahead and take the Final Fellowship examination as soon as possible. Time had to be found for reading surgical textbooks and to achieve this he spent part of the summer working as a locum at Withington and Cheadle Royal Hospitals. The latter was a private mental institution where the house physicians had plenty of time to study and where the accommodation and food were particularly good. He then attended, with Arthur Bullough, the Fellowship course at Guy's Hospital in London in the autumn of 1936. Immediately the course ended, he sat the examination and was admitted to the Fellowship on 10 December. He had passed the examination at his first attempt – many surgeons have had to face the examiners two, three, or even more, times. This also was the earliest that he could have been awarded the Fellowship because the lowest age allowable was 25 years – which he had reached only four months previously.

Charnley was now in a position to plan his future surgical career. There was no vacancy at his teaching hospital so he obtained the post of resident surgical officer at Salford Royal Hospital, starting on January 1, 1937. He worked mainly with Mr Garnett Wright, who was well respected as 'a surgeon's surgeon'. Charnley was fascinated by general surgery and, in particular, he enjoyed the challenge and excitement of dealing with the 'acute abdomen'; no thought of orthopaedics had entered his mind. Mr D. Poole-Wilson was a young consultant at the hospital and remembers Charnley as a 'happy young man with a very active independent mind and a bright outlook'. He looked so young that when he was called to the accident room, the patients thought that the 'boy' had been sent for, not the resident surgical officer. If anyone wanted any special piece of apparatus or instrument, he would make it in Bury where Poole-Wilson believes he had access to a lathe.

An indication of the quality of the work at the hospital was given at the memorial service for Charnley by Sir Harry Platt:

These resident surgical posts were a characteristic of the major teaching, and non-teaching, hospitals in the North of England. Their holders were not attached to any one chief, but were available to assist in difficult operations, and they were in full delegated charge of the emergency practice of their hospitals. Their experience was unique, both in acquiring diagnostic judgement, and in operative skills. The young men who after such experience, ultimately entered any one of the divisions of surgery – the so-called specialities – carried the hall-mark of the generalist throughout their active surgical lives. This was especially true of John Charnley. His roots in the principles and unity of surgery were deep and lasting.[4]

There could be no greater retrospective recommendation.

Arthur Bullough remembers having many discussions with John Charnley at about this time and they always concerned broad principles (the need for gentleness, asepsis and the importance of stopping bleeding), rather than the minutiae of surgical technique. Undoubtedly he gained considerable experience during his time at Salford and later, when writing an application for a job, he said that he had done 'over 300 major surgical operations, mainly on emergency cases' during the 21 months he was there.

He next applied for the post of resident surgical officer at the Manchester Royal Infirmary, but was not appointed, so he had to make other plans. He had wanted to gain experience of laboratory research and he took advice from Professor Raper, the professor of physiology in Manchester, who suggested that he should go to London to work with Professor R.J.S. McDowall at King's College. He was appointed as a demonstrator in physiology in October, 1938. He set out on a project designed to extend previous work on experimental shock,

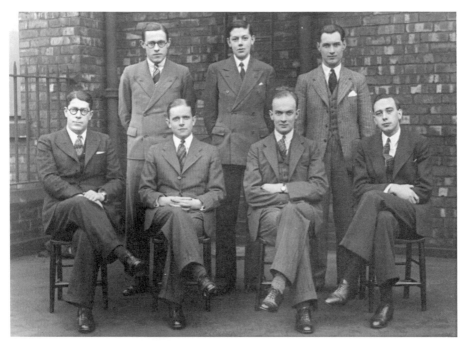

*Residents at Salford Royal Hospital in 1938. Charnley, who was the resident surgical officer, is seated and second from the left. (By courtesy of Salford Health Authority.)*

but encountered difficulties because a new technique of photo-electric colorimetry, which he wanted to use, did not give consistent results.

Quite suddenly the opportunity arose for him to go back to Manchester, and he gave his notice to King's on March 22, 1939. His research was abandoned and it seemed as though nothing had come of his six months in London. In fact, he published a paper in the *British Medical Journal* in 1944 on *Experimental traumatic shock* which described the work which he had done in McDowall's laboratory in 1939.[3] To understand the reason for the delay it is necessary to look forwards: Charnley joined the Army in 1940 and it was not until he returned to England from Egypt that he was able to publish his results.

His paper was on a slightly different aspect of his work from that which he had originally planned; it represented his first serious laboratory research, and indeed it was the only animal work which he ever published. He described it as an 'old experiment presented in a new light' and sought to answer the question 'why does an animal pass into surgical shock when severe mechanical trauma is applied to the lower limb'. Experiments were carried out on more than thirty cats and the results threw some light on the physiology of shock, and contributed to knowledge of this difficult subject.

Even if Charnley later belittled the value of this contribution, it had given him some experience of the discipline of scientific methods, which cannot have been harmful to him. No doubt life in London also had other benefits and one thing he did during this period was to try to learn to play the piano. He went about this methodically (as was his nature), and numbered the notes in the music and the individual keys so that he knew which to strike – an indication of his lack of natural musical ability.

The reason for his return to Manchester in April, 1939, was that the resident casualty officer (RCO) at the Royal Infirmary had been granted leave of absence; and this news must have reached Charnley in London. He applied for the post, which was an important step on the hospital ladder, and was appointed, without salary at first, but later receiving £12 10s a month.

The RCO was really the assistant resident surgical officer (ARSO) and so had a very active job: in the mornings he had to deal with casualties and out-patient fractures, and on alternate afternoons and nights he acted as resident surgical officer (RSO). He would probably have to see and treat about five emergencies each night he was on duty; these would include acute abdomens, head and limb injuries, cut throats and so on. At busy times, he might well be operating all night.

The element of fractures in this job brought Charnley into contact with orthopaedics for the first time since he had qualified as a doctor, and a digression is needed to explain the status of orthopaedic surgery in the United Kingdom before the Second World War. The speciality had become well established as a result of the great efforts of Sir Robert Jones: first, through his organisation of a casualty service for the workers on the Manchester Ship Canal in 1888 and his work for the Army in the First World War; and, second, he had set up a country-wide service to care for crippled children immediately the conflict was over. It might be imagined that, with this background, orthopaedic surgeons would have been appointed to all major hospitals in the United Kingdom in the 1930s. This unfortunately was not the case, largely because general surgeons were a powerful caucus who wished to continue to do a little orthopaedics as well as their general surgery. They also wanted to treat fractures, although it is difficult to see why, unless it was a matter of prestige. None the less, changes were occurring slowly, and Manchester was in the forefront.

Harry Platt (1886–1986) was a Lancastrian who graduated in medicine at Manchester and then trained in orthopaedic surgery at the Royal National Orthopaedic Hospital in London, and in the United States at the Massachusets General Hospital and the Boston Childrens' Hospital. He returned to England in 1914 and was appointed as an honorary consultant surgeon to the Ancoats Hospital in the centre of Manchester. He was able to devote himself to orthopaedics and, with the support of his colleagues (notably John Morley, later professor of surgery, and W.R. Douglas), he started the first segregated fracture clinic in the United Kingdom. Platt was appointed to the staff of the Manchester Royal Infirmary in 1932, and was invited to attend the hospital to advise about 'special cases'. He did not, however, leave Ancoats until a new orthopaedic department was set up at the Infirmary in 1934. He brought with him H.O. Clarke as his chief assistant. The orthopaedic department was expanding and a new block was built for it, including a physiotherapy department which was opened in January, 1939. Platt was appointed to a personal chair in the university and became the first professor of orthopaedic surgery in Manchester later in the same year.

The resident casualty officer at the Royal Infirmary was responsible for the daily fracture clinic; this consisted of minor fractures, that is patients with fratures who were treated throughout as out-patients. During this time Charnley's work would frequently be interrupted when he was called to the accident room by the house surgeon on duty to see serious injuries. Patients who had been admitted for the treatment of their fractures would subsequently be seen as out-patients at the major fracture clinics which were held by the chief assistant and the resident casualty officer on two mornings a week.

The unit was supervised by Platt and he had appropriate help. Clarke had been promoted to clinical tutor in orthopaedics; a post he retained until he joined the Royal Air Force after the outbreak of war, when Roland Barnes became chief assistant. Lloyd Griffiths, who had been resident surgical officer in 1937, succeeded Barnes who left in 1939.

Platt (later Sir Harry) and Clarke (later Sir Henry Osmond-Clarke), not only influenced Charnley's orthopaedic career, but were always greatly respected by him. They, in turn, supported him in many ways. They also both influenced the development of orthopaedic surgery not only in Manchester, but throughout the whole country and, indeed, the world.

During this early period, Charnley again showed signs of his inventiveness when he designed something which he called a 'clavicle cuirass'. This was a well-moulded, unpadded plaster shell which was used to treat fractures of the clavicle. It was applied to the front of the patient's chest while he lay recumbent, after the fracture had been reduced. The method was an impractical and an unnecessary form of treatment; fortunately he was persuaded not to publish it.

A house surgeon at the Manchester Royal Infirmary remembers Charnley's kindness when he helped him do his first appendix operation. He also recalls the riotous parties which were part of a junior doctor's hospital life. On one such occasion, nearly naked and clasping a Ewbank carpet sweeper, Charnley rushed down the corridor claiming loudly to be Cupid.

In June 1935, just after he had qualified as a doctor, he had an experience which must have affected him deeply. The University Mountaineering Club had a meet at Wasdale Head in the Lake District, and two members were undertaking the north climb on the Pillar Rock. Both men were experienced and this was a well-known climb, but when they came to the Nose, Frank Roberts (a senior lecturer in electrical engineering) mistakenly attempted the difficult pitch of the Savage Gully when he slipped and fell. He was badly injured and could not move from the narrow ledge where he had landed. His colleague returned as fast as he could to the valley and rallied the other members of the party to help with the rescue. Organisation for this kind of emergency was not as good as it would be today: not enough people were available and the stretcher they had was much too heavy. When they reached the top, John Charnley (who had the merit of being small and a doctor – just) was lowered to the ledge where Roberts was lying with a fractured femur. Charnley managed to apply a Thomas' splint and they both were pulled up to the top of the crag. By now night had fallen and it was impossible to carry the injured man down the mountain. Charnley stayed with him, but Roberts, who was severely shocked, died during the night. It has been suggested that this incident may have stimulated Charnley's interest in orthopaedics. This may or may not be the case, but it is interesting to speculate whether his climbing experience in general may have been reflected in his attitude to his work. In this hazardous pastime every step assumes the greatest importance if difficult passages are to be negotiated safely. Those who indulge in it have to be painstakingly careful and disciplined if they are to survive. Charnley certainly showed a meticulous attention to detail in his surgery which may be related to his climbing experiences. It would be equally easy to argue that those who climb have this particular trait as part of their inborn make-up – but either way Charnley showed many of the characteristics of a good climber in his approach to orthopaedics. He once said to a colleague that there was 'something wonderful about climbing, if you were frightened and if you got there'.

There was still time for active holidays; climbing with Arthur Bullough and fell-walking with Frank Nicholson. A trip to the Pyrenees in May 1936 with Nicholson took them by train through Lourdes. Charnley was horrified by the sight of the discarded callipers and crutches, but it seems unlikely that this inspired him to take up orthopaedics.

The following year he had a more adventurous holiday with William Kershaw driving through Europe to Italy in Kershaw's Austin car. They were somewhat impecunious but, as they enjoyed the pleasures of life, they compromised by sleeping either in sumptuous hotels or by the roadside in hay-stacks or quarries. Kershaw remembers that they were impressed by Milan Cathedral and a spectacular thunderstorm over Lake Como. At one point they struck a cow and its horn penetrated the car's radiator; they had to plug the leak temporarily with soap and fill up with water from a spring. In Germany, they gave a lift to two brown-shirted and leather-belted young men, and became aware of the menace of the Nazi party.

A final glimpse of Charnley in peacetime remains in a black and white cine-film taken in Snowdonia fifty years ago by Alan Nicholson (not related to Frank Nicholson) who was resident surgical officer at the Manchester Royal Infirmary in 1939, while Charnley was resident casualty officer. He appears smiling, if not grinning, eating a sandwich, and smoking a pipe. Nicholson remembers that he was 'very bright, very clever and very good company'.

# Chapter 3

# WAR SERVICE

## 1940–1946

*I have worked hard and created quite a local reputation here –*
*perhaps for mechanical eccentricity more than anything else.*

John Charnley in Cairo, 1942

BY THE END of 1939, John Charnley had been doing surgery for almost four years, but any plans he may have had for his future career were shattered by the outbreak of war on 3 September 1939.

Like many of his friends, he volunteered for service in the armed forces as soon as he could, enlisting with an emergency commission as a lieutenant in the Royal Army Medical Corps (RAMC) on May 1, 1940. His first posting was to the depot at Crookham, near Aldershot, for induction training which usually lasted two or three weeks.

In April 1940, the Germans had invaded Norway and Denmark, and then they attacked and overran Holland and Belgium in a matter of weeks. The Maginot Line was turned on May 10 and Paris entered on June 14. The British Expeditionary Force in France fought a rearguard action and withdrew to the coast.

Although there is a gap in Charnley's official army record at this point, he was posted to Dover as a regimental medical officer during this terrible period. He was there when the evacuation of British troops from Dunkirk, and the neighbouring beaches, began on May 29, 1940, and he remained there at least until the operation finished on June 3. It seems more than likely that in the flurry of events, he was sent straight from Crookham to Dover during the last week in May.

He probably made five or six trips across the Channel to help with the wounded who were being picked up from Dunkirk harbour and the nearby beaches. He thoughtfully sited his first aid post over the depth charges, taking the view that if he was going to be killed, he might as well avoid half measures. By a strange

21

chance, he met his old friend William Kershaw who was in the medical branch
of the Royal Naval Volunteer Reserve and was serving in HMS Harvester (an
H-class fleet destroyer). Charnley was posted to Kershaw's ship and they made
one or two crossings together. Kershaw has written:

> . . . to my astonishment and delight I found that the one (medical officer)
> appointed to HMS Harvester was my old friend and colleague John
> Charnley. . . He went with us to the beaches on the second trip. . . We
> went to Dunkirk port, where a ship was moored ahead of us. It was full
> of soldiers and either a small bomb or shell had dropped through it,
> although it did not stop her from getting away. John went to deal with the
> casualties which, though few, were beyond his aid.

After this they parted company and did not meet again until after the end of the
war.

Charnley had some exciting moments: he reflected afterwards on the hazards
of crossing a narrow gangplank 30 or 40 feet above the water when carrying a
wounded soldier. He told this story to his son many years later; none of his
friends, or his wife, were aware of it.

The naval evacuation, in which 370 000 troops were brought off during the
course of a week with the loss of 6 destroyers and 24 smaller ships, had been
nothing short of miraculous. But a very black time lay ahead with the German
Army poised on the coast of France. Later in 1940 the Battle of Britain was won
in the air and the threat of invasion receded.

Charnley rarely spoke about his experiences at Dunkirk, either during the war
or later; but when he visited the Manchester Royal Infirmary in June 1940, one
of his friends remembers that he was very subdued, and sat in the surgeon's
room saying little and without his usual laugh. There is no doubt that the
experience affected him deeply and he was depressed for a time. He recovered,
feeling that life did have a purpose, and that he had a contribution to make; he
later told his wife that the episode was a turning point in his life.

His next posting, on June 10, was to 31st General Hospital at Hellingly, East
Sussex, for general surgical duties and he stayed there for two months. He was
already being considered for specialist grading and it was noted that he had done
over 600 laparotomies before joining the Army, so 'he would be most useful in
a Casualty Clearing Station'.

There is another hiatus in his Army record which does not mention that he
was sent to Northern Ireland at about this time. Charnley, in a television
broadcast recorded just before he died, recalled that he was sitting in a tent near
Carrickfergus when he heard he was being posted to the military hospital at
Davyhulme in the outskirts of Manchester. He attributed this move to Platt's
influence.

Urgent representations had certainly been made for an orthopaedic surgeon at
Davyhulme, and 'information stated we have two psychiatrists, but they are not
much good at treating fractures'. After the war this hospital became Park Hospital
where Charnley worked between 1946 and 1962. His official posting was dated
August 7, 1940, and now his interest in orthopaedics was revived; Platt coming
to the hospital every Thursday morning to supervise his work. Charnley was
known 'to be willing to take a class or two on orthopaedics' at Davyhulme; one
medical student, who had just come from Cambridge to Manchester, remembers
'being very impressed with his very lucid explanation of how a knee joint worked'.

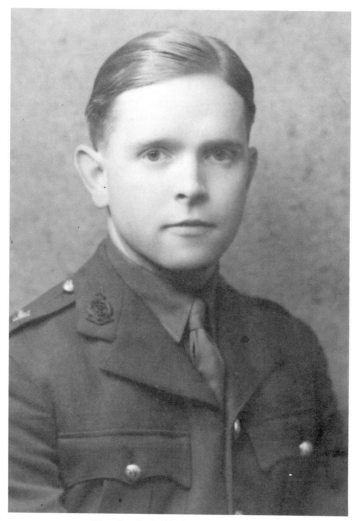

*Charnley in RAMC uniform, 1940.*

This welcome respite lasted for six months, after which he was sent to 3rd General Hospital at Garrioch School, Glasgow in February, 1941. The hospital was preparing to go to the Middle East, and here he met Frank Nicholson, who had been resident surgical officer at Roby Street, Manchester when Charnley was a junior house surgeon, and who was now a graded surgeon in the RAMC. They embarked on March 19, 1941, and may well have been glad to get away; Glasgow had been very severely bombed on March 13 and 14, with more than 1000 people killed. Their troopship was SS Otranto, an Orient Line ship, and they were in a convoy of about 19 merchant vessels escorted by two battleships, two cruisers and several destroyers. The voyage around the Cape of Good Hope was uneventful and took about two months. After disembarking at Suez on May 14, the 3rd

General Hospital was set up in tents at Buseili, near Rosetta – a waste area 35 miles east of Alexandria.

Charnley was in the Middle East from 1941 to 1944 during a critical phase of the war. Although Egypt (previously a British protectorate) had become a sovereign state in 1922, the Anglo-Egyptian Treaty of 1936 pledged mutual aid in time of war. Libya, Egypt's western neighbour, had been annexed by Italy in 1911; and when Mussolini declared war on the Allies in June 1940, Italian troops were at the Egyptian border, prepared to invade. The War Cabinet in London was determined to defend Egypt at all costs, and the British Armies under General Wavell were soon able to take the initiative, driving the Italians out of Cyrenaica (the north-west province of Libya) and capturing Benghazi by early February 1941. German forces now landed in western Libya to reinforce the Italians and General Rommel's Afrika Korps drove the Allies back to the Egyptian border by the end of April 1941. Wavell's counter-offensive failed and he was replaced by General Auchinleck in June 1941. Again the battle swung and the Allies pressed forward. Tobruk was relieved (for the first time) in December and most of Cyrenaica was reoccupied. After a lull of four months, Rommel broke out, his armour capturing Tobruk in June 1942, and penetrating even farther into Egypt before being finally checked in July at El Alamein, about 80 miles from Cairo. The situation was desperate; Winston Churchill flew to Cairo in August 1942. General Alexander replaced Auchinleck as Commander-in-Chief Middle East Forces, and General Montgomery took command of the 8th Army. Success followed rapidly. Rommel was defeated at the battle of El Alamein in October 1942 and the Allied Forces swept along the coast. Shortly after, the Anglo-American armies landed in French North Africa. Tunis was occupied in May 1943 and the fighting in this theatre was virtually over. This was a turning point of the war: Churchill is quoted as saying 'Before Alamein we never had won a battle, after Alamein we never had a defeat'.

Charnley had been posted to 63rd General Hospital near Cairo as surgical team officer and from there went to 12th General Hospital at Sarafand, near Tel Aviv, in Palestine for a short time. His senior colleague was Major Clifford Brewer who was then an orthopaedic surgeon in charge of No. 5 Orthopaedic Unit in Sarafand (he became a general surgeon in Liverpool after the war). He remembers Charnley well and they shared a large American car between them. Charnley spent a great deal of his time in a workshop making foot supports for flat-footed soldiers, apparently doing so very well.

The consultant orthopaedic surgeon to the Middle East Forces was Brigadier St. J. Dudley Buxton, who had been a consultant orthopaedic surgeon at King's College Hospital, London, before the war. He was responsible for organising orthopaedic services in the Middle East and, in May 1941, proposed that there should be a number of orthopaedic centres in military hospitals. These were set up as follows:

No. 1 Orthopaedic Centre in 15th BGH* (Scottish), Cairo

No. 2 Orthopaedic Centre in 63rd BGH, Cairo

No. 3 Orthopaedic Centre in 106th BGH (South African), Canal Zone

---

(*BGH = British General Hospital)

No. 4 Orthopaedic Centre in 64th BGH, Alexandria

No. 5 Orthopaedic Centre in 12th BHG, Palestine

Buxton met Charnley at Sarafand and was greatly impressed by him. He arranged for his posting back to No. 2 Orthopaedic Centre in the 63rd General Hospital. After Buxton retired in 1952, he deposited his war diaries at the library of the Royal College of Surgeons and they contain some brief, but interesting, references to Charnley. There are daily entries which provide good evidence for dates. It is, however, difficult to know exactly when Charnley started working at the 63rd General Hospital. His army postings (which do not mention Sarafand) have recorded the date as November 1, 1941; but the diaries suggest that he must have been back there by September, if not earlier.

Buxton had put Major Ewan Jack in charge of No. 2 Orthopaedic Centre. Jack was from Edinburgh and he returned there as a consultant orthopaedic surgeon after the war; he died in 1953, aged 48 years. He was joined by Charnley, who had been promoted Captain in May 1941 and became his second-in-command, and by Captain Brian Thomas. Thomas, a Welshman who had trained at St Thomas' Hospital, London, was a very able surgeon and became a very close friend of Charnley's while they were together in Egypt, and for the remainder of their lives.

An entry in Buxton's diary dated August 5, 1941, referred to the 'opening of an orthopaedic workshop at No. 4 BOW' (Base Ordnance Workshop) and goes on 'I shall put Charnley in charge'. A typewritten order is attached to the diary and reads:

> recommended that Captain Charnley (63 BGH, Cairo) visit appliance factory at 4 BOW once a week or as often as appears to him to be necessary.

There are three more relevant entries:

> 1.9.41 Charnley doing good work at the factory
>
> 4.10.41 Charnley has made a good transfixion apparatus. . . He is a good lad
>
> 25.10.41 To 4 BOW. Charnley has moved into new shops and has eight men working hard. Design of calliper not quite correct. Leatherwork too loose – scrap being largely used. Good retractor and re-dresseur nearly finished. Excellent work. [Later the same day]. . . Charnley in good form.

These brief comments raise several points. It is clear that the idea of an appliance workshop was initiated by Buxton and that he was responsible for Charnley working there. Charnley got the workshop going remarkably quickly and made it a success. He not only designed a walking calliper and a modified Thomas' splint, but he devised various surgical instruments – all within three or four months. The calliper was called the British Army Adjustable Calliper and it had an oval, rather than a round, ring. Its main merit was that its adjustable ring made it easier to fit and supply quickly to individual soldiers.

It is possible that Charnley could already use a lathe, but the workshop was a unit of the Royal Electrical and Mechanical Engineers and there would have been skilled craftsmen available to help him develop his natural mechanical skill.

Although Platt had a great influence in Charnley's advancement in orthopaedics, Buxton should be given credit for recognising his ability very early on and for

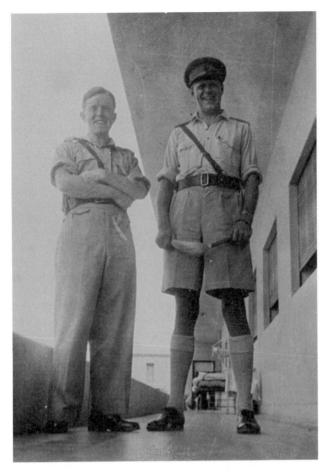

*Charnley with Colonel 'Tiny' Holt in Cairo, 1941.*

giving him support and encouragement. Charnley's enthusiasm and ingenuity come out very clearly in Buxton's words.

The 63rd General Hospital was at Helmieh, near Heliopolis in the northern outskirts of Cairo, and occupied an old Egyptian Army barracks. There were about 1000 beds housed in brick buildings with verandahs; the staff quarters were in army huts. The officer-in-charge of the Surgical Division was Lieutenant-Colonel Robert Holt of Manchester; he was succeeded by Lieutenant-Colonel Michael Boyd who became professor of surgery at Manchester University after the war. Holt and Charnley are seen together in a contemporary photograph: Holt, who was nicknamed 'Tiny' because of his great bulk and height, is wearing shorts, but Charnley has long trousers; it is said that he disliked shorts because they made him look too 'juvenile' (or perhaps he just wanted to avoid getting his knees sunburnt).

Boyd was a brilliant, though eccentric, man and it is said that he may have been 'over-awed by John's questing approach and uninhibited search for the truth'. He was prone to refer to 'scientific John, with just a hint of sarcasm', but the two were good friends.

The orthopaedic unit had two of the most modern wards in the hospital, with easy access to the operating theatre and plaster rooms. There were large numbers of men with limb injuries to be treated, particularly when the fighting was in an active phase. During the two occasions when the Axis troops reached the Egyptian frontier in April 1941 and in July 1942, the hospital was within 80 or 100 miles of the front line, and so received casualties soon after wounding.

Major G.A.G. Mitchell, who became professor of anatomy in Manchester after the war, had been asked by Buxton to form No. 1 Orthopaedic Centre in the 15th (Scottish) General Hospital, in Gezira, near the centre of Cairo. He and Jack visited each other's units whenever possible. On Mitchell's first visit Jack introduced him to his second-in-command – 'a very youthful-looking John Charnley'. Mitchell continues:

> However Jack had warned me not to be misled by appearances and he said that Charnley was mature, well informed, competent, dexterous and brimful of ideas.

The standard of treatment was acknowledged to be high. Mr. Watson-Jones, who was then civilian consultant orthopaedic surgeon to the Royal Air Force, visited the unit and is quoted as saying:

> I find it ridiculous for me to have only one day to inspect a show like this; I would still be learning new things if I were here for a month.

There is also the story of how John Charnley made an uncomplimentary remark when Watson-Jones appeared wearing a fez and Charnley failed to recognise him. Watson-Jones' approval of Charnley's work should be noted at this stage – they later crossed swords over various orthopaedic issues.

Charnley applied to become an orthopaedic specialist in 1942 and received very strong support from his senior officers. He was graded and promoted Acting Major on September 2, becoming Temporary Major on December 2, 1942.

Shortly after his promotion, Charnley wrote to his sister Mary to tell her the news and this is the only surviving letter from him during the war. Brother and sister were clearly on affectionate terms:

> It was good to get your letter – short tho' it was. Why do you expect me to write before I can provoke a letter from you? or have I got it the wrong way round! Funny how I have to urge myself to start writing tho' I never mind when I start. I can't write home try as I will – everything I say seems so dull and stupid that I can never bear to pen it out.

He writes about a girl-friend he left behind in England, saying that he had volunteered for the Middle East in order to escape from her, and he includes a short poem, composed in 'a fit of alcoholic despond', for Mary's criticism. The last few lines are:

> But Time's blunt wedge can deep affection split
> more wide than leagues of desert sand;
> and solitude impediments can raise
> which Reason once dispelled.
> His love – his fear, that blindness it might prove
> and dissipated, leave him lifeless aim.

'Personally', he comments, 'I rather like that last bit – "lifeless aim" for what more can devotion to pure science be'.

He obviously was enjoying Egypt:

> . . . I have worked hard and created quite a local reputation here – perhaps for mechanical eccentricity more than anything else.

He ends

> My dear, I am very happy here. . . The winter is coming, the climate is lovely – the war may soon be over. . .

But he was too optimistic; in spite of recent victories in the desert, he was to stay in Cairo for another 18 months.

Major Bernard Williams, who had been in a field surgical unit in the Western Desert, returned to the 63rd General Hospital in April 1943 after the battle of Mareth. He had been at Cambridge and St Thomas' Hospital with Brian Thomas, and through him got to known John Charnley very well. A note which he wrote gives such a clear impression that it is quoted in full:

> John in those days had the appearance of a cherubic teenager, but it did not take us long to realise that we had a young genius in our midst. He had an astonishing gift of being able to strip any clinical problem down to its bare essentials without being in any way blinded by traditional teaching. He also had a very sound knowledge of general surgery; so much so that I often sought his advice on clinical problems in my department. I was never disappointed. His opinion was always a monument of good sense, arrived at by step-by-step reasoning. Throughout the eighteen months that we were colleagues together, my respect for his extraordinary mind steadily increased. He had a dynamic energy, and no sooner had he finished one project he was on to the next. His humour was impish, while Brian's tended to be somewhat Rabelaisian. Together they were great company, blending laughter and learning in an unforgettable way.

Not everyone was quite so impressed. One of his old Manchester friends felt he had been treated in rather an off-hand manner, and was critical of Charnley's lack of respect for senior officers when he had them as patients. None the less, Charnley was well liked and respected by most of his colleagues, both junior and senior; but there must have been times when he did not attempt to disguise his feelings.

Charnley wrote two papers about the work he did at No. 2 Orthopaedic Centre. The first was on *The two-stage amputation* and was written jointly with Jack and published in the *British Medical Journal* in July, 1943.[1] Having described the disastrous consequences of sepsis after primary closure of a formal amputation, Jack and Charnley advocated a two-stage procedure. After amputation, the flaps were loosely sutured over a large, dry gauze pad impregnated with sulphonamide powder. Four or five days later, the pack was removed, and the flaps were trimmed and sutured over drains. The procedure had been carried out in 26 patients with only two cases of infection. The vital principle of secondary wound closure, which has had to be re-learnt in many modern wars, was emphasised; and it proved life-saving in practice.

The second paper, published in *The Lancet* in February 1944, was by Charnley alone and described the mechanics of reduction and fixation of fractures of the

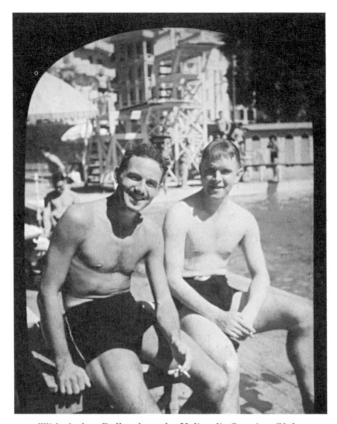

*With Arthur Bullough at the Heliopolis Sporting Club.*

femoral shaft.[2] His analysis of the use of traction on a Thomas' splint to control such fractures was based on 130 cases which passed through the unit between November 1941 and May 1943. Logical argument, illustrated by simple analogies, was used to emphasise the main points. A number of gadgets to attach to the splint, and which Charnley had made in the workshop, were described. Sufficient detail was given so that anyone could easily follow the method in practice.

It is said that he did some experimental work on bone-grafting in goats, but unfortunately there is no record of the outcome. The suggestion is plausible because this was a subject in which he was interested, and indeed he had an experimental bone graft done on his own leg after the war (Chapter 4).

There was also time in Cairo for pleasure. Charnley was able to swim on most days in the pool at the Heliopolis Sporting Club which was near the hospital. Photographs show him enjoying parties in the Officers' Mess, and in the Officers' and Sisters' Club. He had a horse, Sandy, which he kept in stables on the edge of the desert and rode whenever he was able to spare the time. Brian Thomas held a pilot's licence, and John Charnley was keen to learn. On one occasion, his Egyptian flying instructor was scared stiff by his manoeuvres and called out in mid-air 'Major – you will kill us both'. They both survived, but Charnley

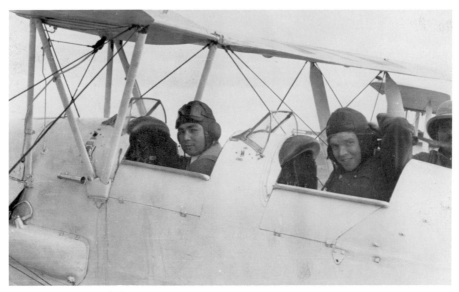

*Learning to fly in Egypt. Charnley is in the rear cockpit behind the instructor.*

never flew as a pilot in peacetime. On a less exciting level, he took lessons in conversational French from a local family.

An idiosyncrasy, which persisted throughout his life and which gave rise to a number of stories, became evident to his friends at this time. He never could put up with extraneous noise and could not stand hearing anyone snore. The partition walls of the officers' quarters were very thin at the 63rd General and he was subjected to loud snores from his next-door neighbour. Unable to stand what to him was a persistent irritation, he drilled a Steinmann's nail through the wall close to the sleeping body in order to disturb the offender in a way he would most certainly remember.

As the campaign in North Africa drew to a close, the casualties decreased and there was less work to do. Many of Charnley's friends departed to follow the fighting through Sicily and Italy, going on to France after the Normandy landings. Repatriation was based on a scheme called PYTHON, those left behind consoled themselves with LOLLIPOP – Lots Of Local Leave In Place Of Python. Charnley remained in Cairo until May 1944; the homeward journey was quicker than the outward because it was now possible for Allied convoys to sail through the Straits of Gibraltar. His overseas service was officially recorded as three years, two months and twelve days.

His next posting was to the military hospital in Shaftesbury, where Major Philip Newman (later consultant orthopaedic surgeon to the Middlesex Hospital and the Royal National Orthopaedic Hospital) had been the orthopaedic surgeon. Newman left just before D-Day which was on June 6, 1944, and Charnley arrived to replace him on June 22. He was the only orthopaedic surgeon to cover all the army personnel on Salisbury Plain, which was a very active military area. There were 40 acute beds and three convalescent units to be looked after. He continued to design, and make, new splints and instruments.

A smart, black MG sports car was his pride and joy. He maintained it himself and frequently took the engine to pieces in attempts to improve its performance.

Lieutenant-colonel Arthur Eyre-Brook (later consultant orthopaedic surgeon to the Bristol Royal Infirmary and Winford Orthopaedic Hospital), became officer-in-charge of the surgical division at Shaftesbury after the German surrender on May 7, 1945. He was there with Charnley for about two months which he found 'a very stimulating and enjoyable time'. The two men had bedrooms next to each other and in his room Charnley had an electric drill and an oxyacetylene blowlamp. Eyre-Brook was interested in recurrent dislocation of the shoulder and needed a special instrument. Between them they fashioned a Steinmann nail into a strong hook with a flattened end and a hole to take a suture; so making a simple, but very useful, instrument. Eyre-Brook writes 'everyone recognised that, in Charnley, we had something special'.

Charnley had been elected an associate member of the British Orthopaedic Association at a meeting in London in October, 1943. This is surprising because he was still in Egypt, but perhaps is explained because Buxton was just about to become president, and it is more than likely that he put Charnley's name forward. Charnley made the first of his many contributions to the Association in December 1944 when he described the calliper he had made in Egypt. The following extract is from the proceedings which were reported in the British volume of the *Journal of Bone and Joint Surgery* in 1945:

> Major John Charnley, RAMC, demonstrated an adjustable weight-bearing calliper, designed on the Thomas principle, but suitable for mass production in a variety of sizes, which is adjustable within limits for different thigh circumferences, and with upright irons adjustable for length by a screw-fitting extension. Supplying the appliance took only an hour or two provided the parts were available, instead of the usual two or three weeks.[3]

Charnley was demobilised into civilian life in February, 1946; he did not relinquish his commission until 1956 when he was granted the honorary rank of Major, but he saw no further service after 1946. In many ways he had been fortunate in the war. After Dunkirk, he was not involved in any front-line activity and he spent almost three years in one hospital in Cairo. Here he gained valuable orthopaedic experience, particularly of the treatment of fractures, and was able to learn from his very able senior colleagues. This initially was to form the basis of his orthopaedic practice in peacetime. He also was able to make the best of the opportunity when he was put in charge of a workshop where he made and modified the appliances and instruments which he needed.

Charnley had kept in touch with Lloyd Griffiths when he was in Egypt and Griffiths was stationed at Aldershot. They met in London in 1945 and had an enjoyable lunch together at Hatchetts in the West End. No doubt the future, and what might lie in store for them on their return to Manchester after the war, was a major topic for discussion.

# Chapter 4

# BACK TO MANCHESTER

## 1946–1960

*. . . after that year, nothing about the brilliance of Charnley's
subsequent rise to fame was any surprise to me.*

John Fairbank after spending 1946 in Manchester

PROFESSOR HARRY PLATT had been based in Manchester during the war because
his stiff knee, caused by tuberculous arthritis in childhood, made him unfit for
military service. He had, however, been extremely busy as consultant orthopaedic
adviser to the Emergency Medical Service and deputy to Sir Thomas Fairbank.
He spent a great deal of time travelling around the country on these duties,
returning to Manchester to see patients and operate at the Royal Infirmary and
the Private Patients Home. Clearly he had great influence in orthopaedics both
locally and nationally; and Lloyd Griffiths and John Charnley depended on him
finding suitable posts for them when the war was over. Charnley returned to
Manchester immediately after he was demobilised in February 1946 and Lloyd
Griffiths a few months later.

Although Charnley had become a competent fracture surgeon, he had had
relatively little experience of elective orthopaedics. In the 1940s and 1950s, bone
and joint tuberculosis was still prevalent and every orthopaedic surgeon was
expected to work in a 'country' hospital to learn about the long-term management
of this and other chronic orthopaedic conditions. And long-term management it
certainly was: the basic treatment for tuberculosis was still fresh air and prolonged
bed-rest on suitable splints and frames, so that many patients stayed in hospital
for two or three years, or even longer. Poliomyelitis was still endemic in the
country and there was much reconstructive surgery to be done. These two
diseases formed the bulk of orthopaedic practice in the country hospitals.

Sir Robert Jones was responsible (together with G.R. Girdlestone of Oxford) for
introducing a National Scheme for the Cure of Crippled Children which was
published in the British Medical Journal in 1919.[8] The outcome was the creation,
from the 1920s onwards, of open-air country orthopaedic hospitals (and their

peripheral clinics) throughout the United Kingdom where children and adults with tuberculosis and other crippling disorders could receive appropriate treatment not available in the town hospitals. The foremost of these special hospitals was at Gobowen, near Oswestry, in Shropshire. It was founded by Agnes Hunt and Robert Jones and was called the Shropshire Orthopaedic Hospital, but the name was changed to the Robert Jones and Agnes Hunt Orthopaedic Hospital in 1933 – an appropriate honour for the two people who had made the hospital what it was. But the new name was rather too long for colloquial use, and the hospital is usually spoken of, simply, as Oswestry; and by the local inhabitants as The Orthopaedic.

This, then, was the hospital where Platt decided that Charnley should go to learn what was then called 'cold' orthopaedics. An odd-sounding descriptive term which has been superseded by 'elective', but in either case what was meant was the kind of orthopaedics carried out away from the rush of fractures and other emergency work. Charnley was resident in the hospital for six months in 1946 and enjoyed himself there. He was one of a group of surgeons from the services, which included Edgar Somerville and his friend from Cairo days, Brian Thomas. They both apparently spent a good deal of time making and flying model aeroplanes. Somerville remembers Charnley returning from Manchester in a furious temper. He had stopped for refreshment but the barmaid had refused to serve him because she would not believe that he was over eighteen years of age, so youthful was his appearance.

An episode during this period demonstrated that Charnley was prepared to experiment on himself when he wanted to try out one of his ideas. He had become very interested in bone grafting and, in order to satisfy his curiosity about the part played by the periosteum in bony union, he persuaded one of his junior colleagues to operate on his leg. Discussion amongst the more senior staff as to whether this was a sensible scheme led to the conclusion that 'if he is foolish enough to want to have it done, and anyone is foolish enough to do it, then let them get on with it'. A piece of cancellous bone was removed from the upper end of his tibia and divided into two pieces: one was re-implanted under, and the other outside, the periosteum. His leg was put in plaster of Paris, but he insisted having the cast removed after a short time. One of his non-orthopaedic friends remembers that he and his wife took John to see Julius Caesar at the Shakespeare Theatre in Stratford-on-Avon a few days later. They could not get seats and, at the interval, his leg had become so swollen and painful that he could hardly walk – fortunately they then found somewhere for him to sit. He returned to Oswestry and it was clear that the wound had become infected. This, of course, not only jeopardised his experiment but also caused him to develop osteomyelitis, and Brian Thomas had to operate on him. Fortunately, all went well in the end, although he was left with an ugly scar. Many years later, in 1958, he developed osteomyelitis of his scapula, an unusual condition (especially in an adult) which might possibly have been associated with the previous osteomyelitis of his tibia. Fortunately this time the condition, which he asked Lloyd Griffiths to treat, settled down with antibiotics and without the need for an operation.

One colleague remembers that Charnley was not impressed by the work at Oswestry; indeed he must always have been difficult to impress in this regard. Another has said that he did not do much work while he was there. None the less, he always remained very faithful to the hospital, and in future years he went there regularly to demonstrate the various operations which he devised. He was a member of the Old Oswestrians (the club for past and present members of the medical staff) and gave their Gold Medal lecture. He was also president of the Club in 1973, and this was one of the very few presidencies which he accepted. When the hip courses began in Oswestry in 1979, he took part in every one up until his death. The hospital recognised his contribution when they named the clinical laboratories in their Institute of Orthopaedics after him.

When Charnley returned to Manchester, he lived for a time in High Street, and later shared lodgings with Arthur Bryson and Jose del Sel in Victoria Park, both were 'observers' in the orthopaedic department at the Manchester Royal Infirmary at the time. For a few months Charnley was acting chief assistant, but he then replaced Miss Willis who had been full-time lecturer in the department during the war.

Professor del Sel (as he later became), a British Council scholar from Argentina, was in Manchester in 1946 learning othopaedics. He made many subsequent visits and remembers his time there with great pleasure and that he was at once impressed by Charnley. He found him an excellent surgeon and meticulous in writing the patients' hospital records. The two men became close friends and used to lunch together in the university refectory. Charnley would always choose a table with someone he was interested in talking to – 'it might be the professor of physics, a neurosurgeon or the man in charge of the dental school laboratory'. He would also take del Sel to the Salford Royal Hospital to watch Sayle Creer, whom he considered to be a good technician, operate. They visited Norwich to see H.A. Brittain carry out his method of arthrodesis of the shoulder, a method which Charnley used later in Manchester.

Two aphorisms remain in del Sel's mind. Charnley always acknowledged the importance of serendipity, saying 'you have got to be able to see where others do not appreciate the importance of fortuitous facts'. The other concerned operating on the back: 'we must never explore a spine in the hope of finding a disc protrusion, one must always be absolutely certain before one starts'.

By 1946 Platt was at the peak of his activity, claiming to work never less than 26 hours a day, and he had brought together a group of very bright young men at the Royal Infirmary: Lloyd Griffiths and John Charnley; John Fairbank was chief assistant with Tony Ratliff and Tony Quinlan as junior residents. A particular feature of their work at this time was the Sunday morning ward round (the three junior members of the team were not expected to take weekends off): after the patients had been seen, everybody sat over coffee while the Professor reminisced, often about his experiences in the United States before World War One. He would range widely – music, cricket and current affairs might be discussed. He and Charnley would often talk about the treatment of fractures and hip surgery, and about plans for the future. It was apparent to those present that the two men had great friendship and respect for each other. There were many brilliant people in the Infirmary at the time: Geoffrey Jefferson was professor of neurosurgery, Michael Boyd professor of surgery and Robert Platt (later Lord Platt) was professor of medicine. Fairbank found his stay in Manchester very stimulating and writes:

after that year, nothing about the brilliance of Charnley's subsequent rise to fame was any surprise to me.

Charnley was awarded a Hunterian professorship at the Royal College of Surgeons of England in 1946. This is in no sense a conventional university chair, but the title professor is conferred on those who deliver Hunterian lectures at the College. The lectures were originally given on comparative anatomy and were illustrated by preparations from the Hunterian collection. For many years, however, they had been regarded as an opportunity for the lecturer to report current research. Charnley's lecture, given on May 23, 1946 in London, was on 'The conservative treatment of fractures of the femoral shaft' and formed the substance of a paper published under a different title in the *Journal of Bone and Joint Surgery* in 1947 (Chapter 6).

The normal age for retirement at the Manchester Royal Infirmary was 60, which Platt reached in October 1946. Not surprisingly, he wished to continue and in 1947 his appointment was extended for a further four years. Lloyd Griffiths and John Charnley were both offered posts as joint honorary assistant orthopaedic surgeons. After some hesitation they accepted and were appointed in July 1947. The rather long title meant in practice that both men were still acting as Professor Platt's assistants and had no beds under their own care. After more discussions, this difficulty was resolved and the minutes of the Medical Board record that

> Beds in the Orthopaedic Department shall in general be held in a common pool out of which three shall be allocated to each of the Joint Honorary Assistant Orthopaedic Surgeons. (10.11.47)

Behind these words is an indication of the struggle the two junior men had to achieve clinical independence. At the same time, they both became part-time, rather than full-time, lecturers in orthopaedic surgery.

These, of course, were the days before the National Health Service when the major hospitals were called 'voluntary' in that they were supported by voluntary subscriptions and endowments. Most senior doctors working in them were only paid a very small salary (if any at all) and were called 'honoraries' for this reason. Their income was largely derived from private practice.

Lloyd Griffiths and John Charnley both had a relatively small commitment at the Manchester Royal Infirmary and so they needed additional hospital appointments. Platt arranged for Charnley to become visiting orthopaedic surgeon at Park Hospital, Davyhulme (which was a general hospital in Manchester) in 1947, and a similar post at Wrightington Hospital in 1949. Wrightington was near Wigan and about 25 miles from Manchester. The hospital belonged to the Lancashire County Council and was used for patients with tuberculosis. Meanwhile, Lloyd Griffiths was appointed to Crumpsall and Ancoats Hospitals and to Booth Hall Children's Hospital, all in Manchester.

An important orthopaedic event in Manchester in 1947 was a meeting of the British Orthopaedic Association; this was a modest affair compared with today's gatherings. Charnley's contribution was on 'The three-point action of splints'. The report of the proceedings which were published in the *Journal of Bone and Joint Surgery* was:

> Mr Charnley illustrated by ingenious models the methods he used in instructing students as to the basic mechanical principles of fracture treatment. The principles were well known: they were being taught in every Medical School in the country. Nevertheless the audience were spell-bound.

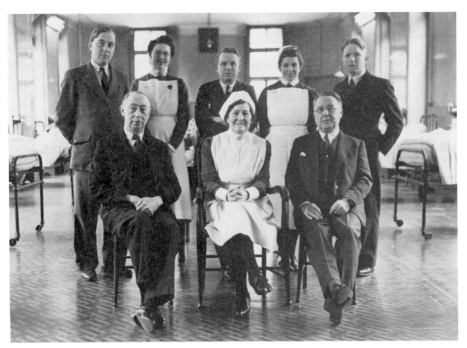

*Ward group at the Manchester Royal Infirmary in 1948 on the occasion of Sister Adams' retirement. Sitting (left to right): Geoffrey Jefferson, Sister Mary Adams, Harry Platt. Standing: Richard Johnson, Sister Potter, Lloyd Griffiths, Sister Davidson, John Charnley.*

The writers of proceedings were not given to hyperbole, so the use of the word 'spell-bound' is remarkable. Charnley clearly had the ability to hold the attention of an audience from the outset of his career, in spite of his confessed lack of self-confidence in speaking in public. He also appeared to be showing an interest in teaching medical students.

At the same meeting, Charnley demonstrated cases of compression arthrodesis by Key's method and of spinal fusion after operations for lower lumbar disc protrusion.

Harry Platt was created a Knight Bachelor in the New Year's Honours List of 1948 for services to the Emergency Medical Service during the war: 'he was the able lieutenant of Sir Thomas Fairbank in moulding and developing orthopaedic units in the service and assisting to plan future regional orthopaedic developments'.[7] He was also chairman of the newly formed British volume of the *Journal of Bone and Joint Surgery*. In 1958, when he was president of the Royal College of Surgeons, a baronetcy was conferred on him.

The introduction of the National Health Service on July 5, 1948, transformed British hospitals. They were now administered by the Department of Health through regional health authorities, or boards of governors in the case of teaching hospitals. Doctors were paid reasonable salaries, and all those of appropriate seniority in the hospital service were made consultants – all with equal status, at least in theory. This, of course, included Lloyd Griffiths and John Charnley.

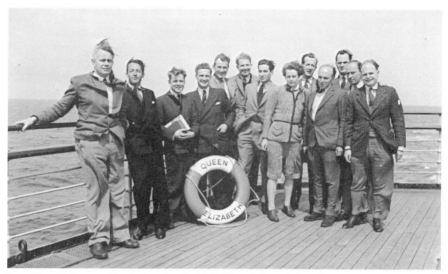

*Travelling Fellows to North America in 1948 (from left to right): James Patrick, James Ellis, John Charnley, St.Clair Strange, Philip Newman, Freddie Durbin, John Adams, Marion Pearson, John Fairbank, Ian Smillie, James Wishart, Cecil Langton and Edgar Somerville. (By permission of the Editor of the Journal of Bone and Joint Surgery.)*

Institutions like Wrightington were transferred from the local authority to the Health Service.

In the midst of this major upheaval of medical organisation in the United Kingdom, Charnley was about to embark on his first trip across the Atlantic. He had been selected as one of a group of 17 young orthopaedic surgeons to visit orthopaedic centres in North America and Canada. These were the Nuffield and Travelling Fellows,[5] and they were the pick of the new post-war generation of orthopaedic surgeons. They were the predecessors of the Travelling Fellows who take part in a regular exchange of orthopaedic surgeons between English-speaking countries.

The party sailed on May 12, 1948 on the liner Queen Elizabeth for a tour lasting six weeks, with twelve centres in the United States and Canada to visit. They were also guests at a combined meeting of the American, Canadian and British Orthopaedic Associations which was held in Montreal, and where John Charnley read a paper on 'Positive Pressure in Arthrodesis of the Knee'. This supported the work of J. Albert Key, a distinguished orthopaedic surgeon from St Louis, and was very well received. He made a notable impression on the Americans and from then on his name was well established with their orthopaedic hierarchy, many of whom were there. For his part, he was very impressed by what he saw during the trip. He wrote to a friend afterwards:

> I picked up a large number of technical aids in which the Americans delight . . . we saw the general attitude which a high pressure economy has on the treatment of fractures and general orthopaedic conditions. Radical early surgery for tuberculosis was a shock to us and we had to review our standards of prolonged splintage and bed rest.

At one time Charnley thought seriously about going to the United States permanently in order to get better facilities for his work, and when Dr Blalock, an eminent cardiac surgeon, visited Manchester he tried to persuade him to take a post in his university. But Charnley knew that any advances he might be able to make in orthopaedic surgery were likely to involve testing his ideas on human beings rather than on animals. He was aware that the North American patient did not have the same uncomplaining stoicism as his British counterpart; so he wisely, from this point of view, decided to stay in his native Manchester, where his patients were likely to be grateful for whatever he did for them. Today, this kind of acquiescence no longer exists, but in the 1950s and 1960s there were no ethical committees and surgeons were able to introduce new procedures in a way which would now not be possible. The situation should not be misinterpreted, and it is important to understand that the implicit trust between doctor and patient could mean that results were obtained much more quickly than would otherwise be possible. There might be misfortunes to be overcome before success of new techniques was achieved, but this was regarded as a necessary price which had to be paid. The way Charnley dealt with the problem will become clear when the development of hip replacement is considered later in the book. In spite of his wish to make progress, he always maintained the highest ethical standards according to his considered judgement.

There is no doubt that in the late 1940s Charnley was thoroughly enjoying orthopaedics in Manchester. Tony Ratliff, who subsequently became a consultant in Bristol, remembers:

> John was tremendously effervescent, tremendously happy with life . . . and it was all fun . . . he had the happy facility of doing any operation at three times the speed of anyone else . . . he was a superb spontaneous, but thoughtful, postgraduate teacher and was full of new ideas which he would try out on us . . . He was very sociable, easy to talk to, and he loved the residents' parties.

These words, in part paraphrased, provide a good picture of Charnley at this period.

Charnley was now running the orthopaedic department at the Manchester Royal Infirmary; Sir Harry had many other commitments and Lloyd Griffiths was doing virtually all his work at Crumpsall Hospital.

In 1951, Sir Harry reached the age of 65 years, and became due for retirement (for the second time), but he continued working at the hospital for as long as he could. Late in the year, he was made professor emeritus and consulting orthopaedic surgeon to the Manchester Royal Infirmary. There was some delay before the decision was reached to appoint a new professor, and Lloyd Griffiths and John Charnley were invited to attend an interview. Both men had received letters from the vice-chancellor and believed that an appointment was going to be made. They did not know that some members of the University's Senate were opposing such an appointment, or that potential candidates outside Manchester had been approached. Furthermore, neither was aware that the other was going to be interviewed, and so they did not discuss between themselves what line they should take. The unfortunate outcome was that at the beginning of 1952 it was decided not to make an appointment. Although Charnley was awarded a personal chair in 1972, the University of Manchester did not have an established chair of orthopaedics until 1976.

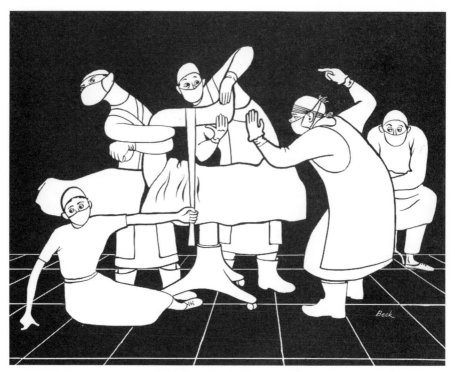

*This cartoon, drawn at Manchester Royal Infirmary, shows Charnley engaged in aligning a fracture of the tibia which is being put into a plaster cast.*

The next step, after the failure to appoint a professor, was the advertisement for a consultant orthopaedic surgeon to be in charge of the University Department of Orthopaedics in place of Sir Harry Platt. Four candidates were interviewed, including Lloyd Griffiths and John Charnley. Lloyd Griffiths was appointed and took up his duties in September, 1952. He recalls receiving a charming letter from Charnley congratulating him and ensuring him of his co-operation. Lloyd Griffiths now had eight sessions (half-days) at the Royal Infirmary. Charnley, having been an honorary assistant orthopaedic surgeon at the Infirmary in 1947, had been made a consultant at the hospital in 1948 (under the National Health Service regulations), and he now continued with four sessions there.

The timetables of orthopaedic consultants in all the teaching hospitals in the United Kingdom were published in the *British Journal of Bone and Joint Surgery* in 1952 and Charnley's programme was given.[9] There was a staff round at the Infirmary on Tuesday morning, and he had an operating session there on Wednesday morning, with out-patients on Tuesday afternoon and a fracture clinic on Thursday morning. He shared an operating list with Mr Cullen on Monday afternoons at Wrightington. At Park Hospital he did a ward round on Thursday afternoon and an operating list on Friday afternoon (the day of his out-patient clinic was not given).

Operative surgery came easily to Charnley; indeed, it has been said that he was a better surgeon than he was a doctor. This may or may not be true, but he clearly liked getting on with things and would not waste time on side issues. He was a swift operator, but he was always prepared to explain exactly what he was doing. He did not, however, stop in order to talk; and he never made superfluous movements or gestures. It would probably be fair to say that he was an effective rather than an elegant operator. In the face of serious difficulties, he remained calm and could extricate himself from awkward corners with aplomb.

His desire to make any operation as simple as possible led him to design and make his own instruments. In the past, many an orthopaedic surgeon has struggled with inappropriate instruments, and put up with them. Many of Charnley's inventions were effective and helped a great many surgeons. Nothing he ever made was ever ill-thought out or shoddy.

As far as his patients were concerned, he was quite unable to cope with those he considered to be hypochondriacs, and, as he was by no means always tactful in this situation, some found it difficult to accept the way he explained that there was really nothing wrong with them. On the other hand, he went to untold trouble to help those who presented a challenging clinical problem. None the less most of his patients thought the world of him.

He recognised his own ability and he was not bashful. Lloyd Griffiths remembers an occasion when Charnley told him he had given up travel saying 'if the disciples want to learn any more they can come to Nazareth, I'm not going to them'. This prompted Lloyd Griffiths to ask what he thought the initials J.C. stood for – which was taken in good part.

Towards the end of 1947, John Charnley had succeeded in getting a bachelor service-flat in Rusholme Gardens in the south of Manchester. The flat was in a block in which a number of senior doctors from the Infirmary lived; the Platts and Sir William Fletcher Shaw were there at this time, as was Dr Reginald Luxton, a physician, and two gynaecologists Mr J.W. Hunter and Mr. C.E.B. (Tex) Rickards who were bachelors. He did not have to do much cooking for himself as there was a restaurant in the building, so he was able to turn his kitchen into a small laboratory which del Sel remembers seeing when he visited the apartment in 1951. This was the year they travelled together to an international orthopaedic meeting in Sweden where Charnley read a paper, on the imbibation of fluid by the lumbar intervertebral discs, which was based on experiments done in his kitchen.[3]

Although he could not be said to be domesticated, Charnley always took an interest in the surroundings in which he lived. At one time, he had a room decorated with wallpaper which was a high-powered magnification of cancellous bone – an attractive idea and one which was entirely appropriate for him.

In another room stereophonic loudspeakers were installed to produce the best possible sound from his gramophone which he stabilised in concrete and, to reduce extraneous noise, the walls were curtained from floor to ceiling. It may be that he was more interested in the quality of sound reproduction than the music itself. He rarely went to concerts, partly because he found any coughing or noise from the audience very irritating.

A wise, and ultimately profitable, acquisition was a painting by L.S. Lowry (1887–1976). Lowry was born in Lancashire; and his pictures of the local urban and industrial landscape had not then achieved their later popularity or value.

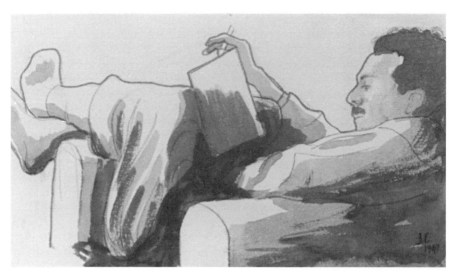

*A sketch of Arthur Bullough by John Charnley. Isle of Skye, 1947.*

The picture had been exhibited in a Manchester art gallery at a price of £35, but while Charnley was making up his mind whether or not he could afford it, it was sent to a gallery in London. Once he had decided that he wanted the picture, he determined to get it – and he did, for £36. When valued in the 1980s, it was worth about 1000 times that amount, so he had acquired a splendid work of art, which is still owned by his widow, and an inflation-proof investment. He also bought two Augustus John drawings and some good watercolours around this period.

For some years after the war, he took up drawing and painting with great enthusiasm and had lessons. In 1946, he had produced his own Christmas card: a linocut which seems to be showing a surgeon doing something to a bone, exactly what is not quite clear. A pencil sketch of Arthur Bullough, drawn when they were on holiday together on the Isle of Skye in 1947, shows his skill. An oil-painting of the wife of a friend is in existence; it is competent and a fair likeness. He was very demanding of his sitter for this portrait, and in no circumstances would he allow her to move, even to go to her screaming baby. His interest in sketching for pleasure gradually diminished, but the skill that he learnt was very valuable to him as he was always able to illustrate his ideas graphically on paper or on a blackboard. He produced his own diagrams for many of his early publications; these, and the operative drawings in his last book (Chapter 16) demonstrate the value of this skill, which persisted throughout his life.

Rock-climbing with Arthur Bullough resumed in 1947; and although they went together on climbing weekends in Wales during 1948, Charnley's enthusiasm faded saying 'one's ideas change, Arthur'.

Skiing replaced climbing as regular holiday activity. He first went in 1947 with Brian Thomas and Edgar Somerville, and for many years they went to Zürs. He never performed elegantly on skis, although his style never lacked verve or

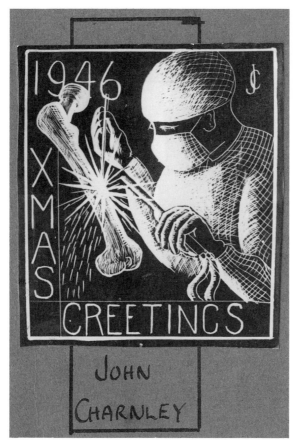

*Christmas card drawn by John Charnley in 1946.*

courage. Every year he used to return to the slopes with a new theory about how to overcome his various skiing problems and improve his technique. On one occasion he took a cine-camera with him, and Brian Thomas was instructed to photograph him doing various turns. This was studied carefully later, and the following year he was quite sure that he knew what he had been doing wrong and was going to triumph at last. It seems he never did; but his technique became adequate, and he continued to ski adventurously and with abundant enthusiasm. An injured knee was a setback in the early 1960s; Somerville was with him and remembers how his knee 'went sideways' when he held his leg up afterwards. He had ruptured his medial ligament, his leg was put into plaster at the local hospital and conservative treatment was continued in Manchester by Lloyd Griffiths.

Motor cars and their maintenance were another form of relaxation. The black MG which he had at Shaftesbury was replaced after the war by a Sunbeam, and later he acquired an Aston Martin, a British car of some distinction. One of his great pleasures in these early days was to try to reach 100 mph along the Chester

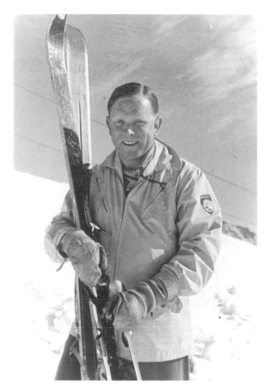

*Charnley skiing in Switzerland. (From Mrs Brian Thomas.)*

road on Sunday mornings. He was by nature a fast driver, but he tended to be somewhat erratic because his thoughts were often on other matters. He had one or two accidents, but his competence is shown by the fact that he kept the car on the road after striking a sheep at high speed in Scotland. He continued to do his own repairs for a number of years. An engineer, with whom he was collaborating on joint lubrication, remembers that he carried out the maintenance on the steering king-pins in two hours while his car was parked outside the Medical School. He regarded this as a good instance of Charnley's 'extraordinary manual dexterity'. Charnley had the car for many years and was very fond of it, but it was written off after an accident in which he was fortunately not hurt.

He rarely returned to his family home in Bury where he found little to interest him. There were cousins with whom he kept in touch, one of whom was married to a general practitioner in Blackburn. They provided moral support in emotional crises, such as after a broken engagement, and there were times when he wrote anguished letters to them. Personal relationships were hard for him to maintain, at least with the opposite sex, as he once explained:

> I am primarily interested in ideas and things and only in people in so far as they are necessary for supplying those ideas and things. I love my Aston Martin more intensely than any woman – it is as near a perfect solution to an intellectual problem as one can imagine at the present moment. . .

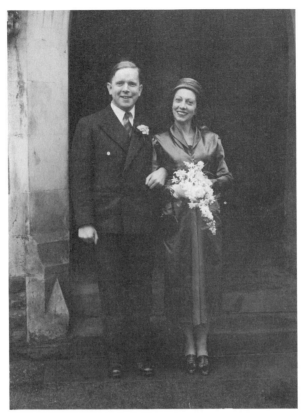

*Anna Bullough 'given away' at her wedding by John Charnley 'in loco parentis', 1951.*

He was worried by his neglect of the 'principle of family' and he was made aware of what he was missing when visiting one of his godchildren; he recognised the 'intense warmth of love inside that family'. In one respect he fulfilled family obligations; he was godfather to the children of three of his old friends.

Charnley regularly visited Frank Nicholson (whom he had known since before the war) and his family in Hale, just south of Manchester, where he was always popular with the children. He used to take their son, Roger, for a ride in his Aston Martin; and once they went together for a five shilling flight during an air-show at Ringway Airport. Their daughter, Jane, was one of his godchildren; but he only accepted the responsibility after he had examined her, paying particular attention to her hips.

When Arthur Bullough was going to marry Anna, whom he had met in Italy during the war, Charnley carried out the somewhat unusual task of acting in loco parentis, in the absence of her father, and gave her away at the ceremony in Manchester. There is a charming photograph, taken after the wedding, with Charnley looking very happy and quite ridiculously young.

Young doctors at the Royal Infirmary found him easy to talk to. He enjoyed parties in the residents' mess at the hospital where he found no difficulty in relaxing in congenial company. When he entertained his friends at Rusholme Gardens, his absorbing interest in orthopaedics was frequently evident. He is remembered standing with a bottle of wine in one hand and a human femur in the other expounding his ideas about the hip joint – he was quite unconcerned about his guests' need for food.

To turn to some of John Charnley's characteristics as they are recalled by his friends: he had straight fair hair, a round face with blue eyes and an engaging chuckle. Physically he looked younger than his years and he was always young in spirit. He was highly intelligent and questioned everything he read or heard. At the same time, he had a very practical approach to problems. He was good with his hands and he always wanted to know how things worked, even quite trivial things like children's toys and domestic appliances. Whatever he turned his mind to, he thought about thoroughly and if he undertook anything he would always do it with efficiency and skill.

One friend was impressed that he never reacted aggressively to any intellectual challenge. 'If you said something that he disagreed with, he would not only not react aggressively, but he would never give an absolute rebuttal – even if he felt very strongly about the subject. He would purse his lips and say very slowly "w-e-ll", with a smile. He would then pause for thought and very patiently, and most tentatively, would refute clearly and in detail what you had said.' An approach which was much more likely to engage and convert his listeners than a more vigorous and damning response.

A junior colleague at Oswestry writes: 'he always listened to what you had to say, and he always made it seem as if the methods he was criticising were just another way of doing things'. But not everyone met such a reasoned response, as a comment from a very old friend, who became a paediatrician, indicates: 'on surgical questions he could be receptive and constructive, but he could be very intolerant and argumentative; he had a fierce temper on occasion'.

He often seemed not to brook opposition against his firmly held ideas with a single-minded determination: 'behind his magnificent charm and smile, which could be devastating, there was an element of toughness'. Stupidity and idleness he could not tolerate and those who exhibited these failings in front of him were likely to feel the lash of his tongue. It was not that he did not suffer fools gladly, he did not suffer them at all.

During this time Charnley had been pursuing the work on bone healing and the treatment of fractures which he had begun as soon as he returned to Manchester. He wanted to do experimental work on animals, and Platt suggested that G.A.G. Mitchell, who had become the professor of anatomy in 1946, might be able to provide facilities. Mitchell and Charnley had, of course, met when Mitchell was in charge of No. 1 Orthopaedic Centre in Cairo. Mitchell was in the process of converting empty rooms in his department in the medical school into animal houses. He readily agreed to Charnley's request to be allowed to start a programme of work to investigate fracture healing and joint lubrication. Charnley obtained a Home Office licence to allow him to carry out animal experiments in 1949. Although he had the support and encouragement of the Professor, he planned and carried out all the experiments himself. A senior technician was available to help with histology, and there was an old (ex-Army) X-ray machine which he could use. The experimental work on fracture healing did not lead to any publications.

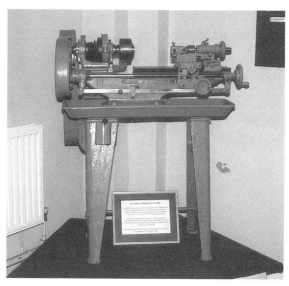

*The original lathe bought by Charnley in 1946. (By courtesy of Chas. F. Thackray Ltd, Leeds.)*

The other bonus which Charnley gained from his association with the anatomy department was the use of room in their cellar as a workshop where he installed the lathe which he had bought in 1946, and where he made prototypes of appliances and surgical instruments. There is no doubt that he was skilled in this field, and throughout his life he was able to 'mock-up' any surgical device in his workshop, and try it out himself before having it manufactured. The story of the purchase of tools for his lathe has been published by Hardinge who recounted verbatim the words of Mr Harry Boulton:

> In 1948 I was technical sales engineer with E.C. Hopkins, 229 Deansgate, Manchester. About July or August, Mr Charnley visited the showroom requiring a machine to make stainless steel screws. These were not available commercially. After some discussion he purchased a $\frac{1}{2}$hp flexible shaft machine, a tool post grinder and grinding wheels. These used in conjunction with a lathe would meet his requirements. Payment was made by a personal cheque and at this point he said "I hope I'll get repaid by the Hospital, but I can't wait to go through all the procedure". It was only after further discussion that he revealed that he was not an engineer but a surgeon . . .
>
> Out of curiosity, I delivered the machine to his workshop under the Medical School in a basement. This turned out to be a well-equipped engineer's workshop with the added aspect of a number of hip bones . . .[6]

About this time Charnley was developing a cannulated coarse-threaded screw for the fixation of fractures of the neck of the femur.[2] His compression screw came later.[4] He kept and used the lathe all his life and it was given to Chas. F. Thackray Ltd by Lady Charnley after his death; it is now displayed in the seminar room at their Beeston works in Leeds.

At a later date, Charnley moved from the department of anatomy, and Professor Walter Schlapp, who was professor of physiology, provided him with a workshop in an old fodder store in the basement of the medical school. These events have not been recorded, and there is an element of uncertainty as to exactly where Charnley did his work in the early 1950s. Dr F.B. Beswick, who was a lecturer in experimental physiology at the time, remembers helping to empty the fodder store. Whatever the details, there seems little doubt that Charnley had to struggle to find the accommodation he needed. In 1956 he wrote that 'he had carried out a number of experiments, through the courtesy of Professor A.M. Boyd, in the Department of Surgery'. He clearly had to obtain laboratory facilities wherever he could find them.

Two basic orthopaedic problems engaged his interest: the first concerned the effect of compression on the healing of cancellous bone; the second, which came rather later, was the lubrication of joints which had far-reaching implications because it led ultimately to his design for a hip replacement. Collaboration with other scientists, particularly engineers, was imperative for him to be able to make progress.

It should be made clear at this point that Charnley never had any formal training in any kind of engineering. This may surprise some orthopaedic surgeons because his knowledge of the subject may have led to the belief that he had a degree in it; but this was not so. He did, however, have a remarkable ability to grasp the fundamentals of any problem he was interested in. He quickly realised the importance of working closely with engineers, and was one of the first surgeons to appreciate the significance of the new, somewhat hybrid, subject of bio-engineering. Indeed, he showed the way in this, and demonstrated that progress in orthopaedic surgery can only be made with the collaboration of other medical scientists and engineers.

His first adviser in this field in the early 1950s was Professor Louis Matheson, who then held the Beyer Chair of Engineering at Manchester University. Charnley was working out his method of compression arthrodesis and wanted to measure the force with which the cut surfaces were being clamped together by his apparatus. The method they devised and their results were included in Charnley's book on *Compression Arthrodesis* (Chapter 6). In the course of this study he needed help with the histology of bone and he was fortunate in being able to collaborate with Professor S.L. Baker, an authority on the pathology of bone, whose help as his teacher he readily acknowledged.

Professor Sir Louis Matheson, who is now living in Australia, writes:

> John had an intuitive feel for mechanisms and mechanical devices and he certainly was a gifted craftsman. The spherical joints that he made . . . were beautifully done, but he was understandably light on theory . . . While I would hesitate to describe him as an engineer, at least in the Continental sense, he was certainly a fine craftsman.

Sir Louis gives the German interpretation of an engineer as a 'highly trained and qualified professional engineer graduating from a technical university'. This, as he says, is something which Charnley was not.

When he came to realize the importance of lubrication in joints, he needed more help and he went to Professor Diamond, who had succeeded Matheson as head of the department of mechanical engineering. Again he learnt quickly, although there apparently were times when his somewhat superficial knowledge was an embarrassment when he was talking to engineers; however, his knowledge of engineering never failed to impress most orthopaedic surgeons (engineers might say that this would not be difficult). He was always full of ideas, some of them considered to be outrageous by those advising him – and they often found it difficult to change his views.

Charnley was always prepared to seek advice and he was fortunate that people of the calibre he needed were accessible in Manchester. Those to whom he went for help seem to have been delighted to work with him which is a tribute to his personality. Professor Tanner, now also in Australia, regarded him as 'an excellent collaborator'.

The following two chapters will review Charnley's publications in the 1950s which give a good indication of the clinical work and research he was doing in Manchester. One of his major interests, which was to investigate mechanisms of joint lubrication, will wait till Chapter 9 where it forms an introduction to his evolution of arthroplasty of the hip.

*Chapter 5*

# AN EXACT MAN
## 1945–1960

*Reading maketh a full man; conference a ready man and writing an exact man.*

Francis Bacon

CHARNLEY BEGAN writing early in his career, as his student and wartime articles have shown. Between 1945 and 1960 he published papers on a variety of subjects which indicated the breadth of his interest and the contribution which he made to the speciality before he became totally involved with arthroplasty of the hip joint. The period chosen is not entirely arbitrary and is appropriate because from 1960 onwards he wrote only ten papers on general orthopaedic subjects; these are included in this chapter because they can be regarded as left over from his 'pre-arthroplasty' era.

He published an average of two or three papers a year, less than might be expected from an academic scientist, but a remarkable achievement for a man engaged in active surgical practice, and incomparably more than the average orthopaedic surgeon would produce. His contributions over this fifteen-year period may well be regarded as the preparation for his life's work on the hip joint.

Charnley's main publications will be reviewed subject by subject; the aim being not so much to describe their orthopaedic content, but rather to illustrate his approach and attitude to the matters he chose to write about. His letters to medical journals will be included where they are relevant. In this, and in the following chapter (which will be concerned with his first two books), his words will frequently be quoted so that the reader will be able to appreciate the flavour of his literary style. I am grateful for permission to make these extracts and there is a full list of references (in chronological order) at the end of the chapter. Not all his papers are mentioned, but those which are have been given a reference number in the list and a corresponding number in the text. Charnley's contributions at various meetings, the proceedings of which have been recorded

51

in the British volume of the *Journal of Bone and Joint Surgery*, are recorded and indicate his involvement in both national and international orthopaedics. Finally, a list of book reviews which he wrote in this journal is appended.

During the war, large numbers of meniscectomies were carried out in servicemen, and no doubt this accounted for Charnley's interest in the subject. *The exposure of the posterior horn of the medial meniscus* was a short paper published in *The Lancet* in December, 1945.[1] It was thought necessary by many surgeons at this time to remove the whole meniscus (not just the torn part), and if symptoms continued as they often did in soldiers, then it was the practice to remove the posterior part if it had been left behind. The paper describes a simple way of doing this, and the attention to minor details is characteristic of Charnley's descriptions of operative techniques.

A point of semantics needs to be explained here concerning the term 'medial meniscus'. In the past, the term meniscus was used interchangeably with semilunar cartilage to indicate the same structure within the knee joint. Without labouring the matter, it should be said that meniscus is nowadays considered correct in order to avoid confusion with articular cartilage.

*The horizontal approach to the medial semilunar cartilage* was published in the British volume of the *Journal of Bone and Joint Surgery* in 1948.[6] Charnley must have seen Platt using a horizontal incision, but he modified the technique by opening the joint beneath the meniscus; the scar in the synovial membrane thus lay against the head of the tibia, and so would not rub on the femoral condyle. The idea was to avoid what Charnley called the 'scar-friction' which occurred after the standard incisions. He believed that recovery was quicker in the 105 cases in his series, but the late results were no better than those reported with other incisions. A particular feature of this paper was the excellent operative photographs which are difficult to produce in this kind of keyhole surgery. His method did not become widely used by other surgeons, many of whom preferred one of the more traditional approaches.

Another paper resulting from his wartime experiences was *The walking calliper* published in *The Lancet* in 1947.[2] This described the Thomas' calliper and various modifications which had been made to it. The adjustable calliper, which had been designed by Charnley in Cairo, was included. He noted that 'experimental work [on the adjustable calliper] was done with the generous facilities of the Royal Electrical and Mechanical Engineers of the Middle East Force' at 4 Base Ordnance Workshop.

Although Charnley designed many new appliances and instruments, his publications about them were relatively few. In 1945, a *New dissecting forceps for no-touch technique* was described in the *British Medical Journal* – a useful instrument for the orthopaedic surgeon who had to tie knots without touching the suture material, as was the practice at the time.[25] The forceps were manufactured by Down Bros. Ltd, of London. The next instruments he described were *Retractors for operations on the nucleus pulposus* which greatly helped exposure of the lower lumbar discs and nerve roots – also made by Down Bros.[26]

The British volume of the *Journal of Bone and Joint Surgery* had always been reluctant to accept articles on gadgets, but they published four contributions from Charnley which came into this category. The first, in 1950, was *A method of inserting the Smith-Peterson guide wire* which described instruments used for

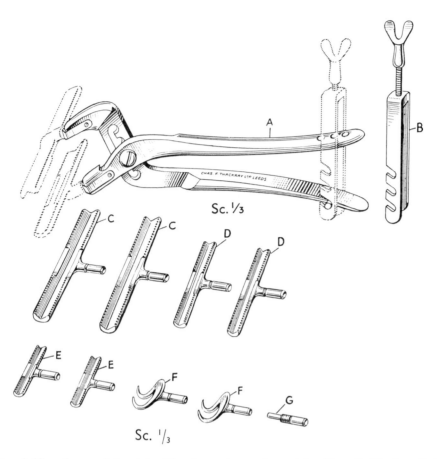

Sc. ⅓

Sc. ⅓

*Bone-holding forceps designed by Charnley and manufactured by Chas. F. Thackray Ltd, Leeds. (By courtesy of Chas. F. Thackray Ltd.)*

fixing a fracture of the neck of the femur.[8] These were made by Messrs Chas. F. Thackray Ltd of Leeds, and this is the earliest recorded instance of his long association with the firm which made both the instruments and the prostheses for his arthroplasty of the hip. In 1951, he described *A new walking aid for spastic paralysis* and *A spring exerciser for arthroplasty of the hip joint*.[27,28] The walking aid was of a type familiar today and consisted of 'a tubular frame with four legs which can be made to creep forward by alternately raising and depressing the handles'. This had been invented by the father of a spastic child, but no doubt Charnley had a hand in its design. The spring exerciser was to be used after the cup arthroplasty operation. In the early 1950s the leg was immobilised on a Thomas' splint for three weeks after this procedure, and the exerciser was then used. *The new pattern of bone-holding forceps* was an extremely effective instrument designed to hold the fragments of bone while a screw was inserted or a plate and screws applied during the internal fixation of a fracture.[29] This was also manufactured by Chas. F. Thackray Ltd.

*Intramedullary nailing of fractures* was a letter in the British volume of the *Journal of Bone and Joint Surgery* describing a 'useful trick' of interlocking two of the clover pattern of intramedullary nails in order to fill an exceptionally wide bony canal.[35]

For completeness, two more publications in *The Lancet* of 1965 are included in this section: *A drilling jig for intertrochanteric osteotomy* and an *Improved short hip spica cast* – the latter was a plaster cast which extended from the trunk over the medial side of the knee, with the idea of protecting the hip and allowing mobilisation of the knee.[30,31] Within a year or two, both these devices became obsolete in Charnley's practice as arthroplasty became virtually the only operation which he carried out on the hip.

Biomechanicalorthopaedicengineeringung sounds like a joke, but it was the title of an article written by Charnley for the Manchester University Medical School Gazette in 1949.[7] It was unearthed by Mr L. Turner, a Manchester surgeon, when he was writing a biographical note on John Charnley for the *Lives of Fellows* published by the Royal College of Surgeons of England.[60] *Biomechanicalorthopaedicengineeringung* was recently reprinted and circulated to members of the Charnley Low Friction Society by Lady Charnley (Chapter 10).

Maybe Charnley had his tongue in his cheek when he invented the title:

I have selected for my contribution to the Medical School Gazette a subject which I hope will be quite useless for the Final Examination; hence, biomechanicalorthopaedicengineeringung. . . But let me not delude the reader that there is no purpose in my effort; I would like to try and show in the least didactic manner possible how and why the student must face an orthopaedic problem and solve it by using his wits rather than by trying to seek the answer in the remembered pages of a book.

He goes on to contrast the rather limited field of general surgery compared with the much wider scope of orthopaedic surgery:

The orthopaedic surgeon's faculties must be adaptable to a wide compass; the delicacy of a neurosurgeon, required in nerve and tendon surgery; the power and accuracy of a sculptor wielding the osteotome and heavy mallet; the engineering skill of a fitter, in using precision tools in bone grafting and internal fixation; the indefinable art of closed reduction, in manipulating a fracture with the touch and craft of a bone-setter; pleasure in perfect dissection under a tourniquet, and satisfaction in the carnage of a hindquarter amputation.

Many of his colleagues must have had similar thoughts about their speciality, but few have written them down so graphically and with such conviction. He then reveals his very early interest in the hip joint:

This attitude of mind and hand is one which the student of orthopaedics must train himself; no rules can be given. Many of the successful results of orthopaedic surgery will be original creations stemming from a mind exercised by thinking on analogous problems.

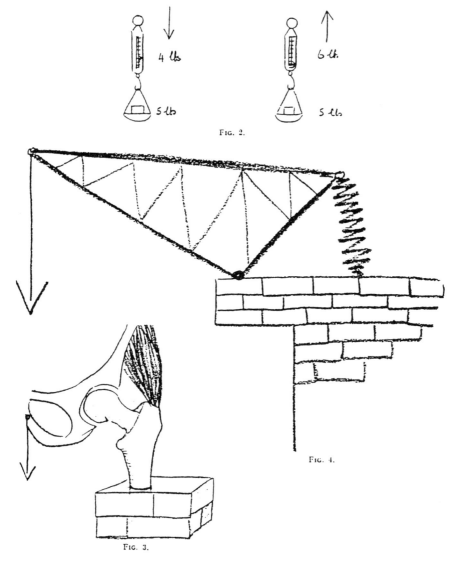

FIG. 2.

FIG. 4.

FIG. 3.

*Charnley's sketches used to illustrate an article in the Manchester University Medical School Gazette. This page is demonstrating a mechanical analogy to explain the action of the gluteus medius muscle.*

To illustrate this approach I have chosen examples from the function and dys-function of the most fascinating of all the great articulations – the hip joint.

The article continued with a very clear analysis of why a patient may limp, with particular reference to the importance of the gluteus medius muscle. Operations for the treatment of a limp caused by an old congenital dislocation of the hip, or nonunion of a fracture of the femoral neck, are explained. The text was written in a manner which could be easily understood by medical students and was illustrated by line drawings by the author.

Charnley was invited to take part in a discussion on fractures of the femoral shaft at a meeting of the British Orthopaedic Association in London in October, 1945. He described his method of treatment of these fractures using a special apparatus he had designed for skeletal traction with a pin through the tibia. Lateral deformity was controlled by pads which were screwed to adjustable attachments on the side bars of the Thomas' splint.[41] The other orthopaedic surgeons speaking on this occasion were R. G. Pulvertaft, G. R. Fisk and V. H. Ellis.

*Knee movement following fractures of the femoral shaft* was published by Charnley in the *Journal of Bone and Joint Surgery* in 1947[3] – an American journal which became the American volume of the *Journal of Bone and Joint Surgery* when the British volume began publication in 1948. The paper was based on Charnley's Hunterian lecture 'The Conservative Treatment of Fractures of the Femoral Shaft' given at the Royal College of Surgeons in 1946. Charnley demonstrated that the most important cause of restriction of movement of the knee was adhesions in the quadriceps muscle which occurred as the fracture healed. He went on to postulate that scar tissue would be minimal if the fracture united quickly, which was best achieved by immobilisation with fixed traction on a Thomas' splint. If knee movement was started early, union would be delayed, scar tissue would persist and the knee would be stiff. He had two comparable groups of patients: 20 had fractures which united before eight weeks and 12 in whom union took longer. The first group regained a greater range of flexion at the end of six months, compared with the second group. The evidence seemed convincing, but this was in the days before statistical analysis was mandatory in medical papers. However, analysis today confirms that the correlation between time of union and the recovery of knee movement is significant.

Three papers by Charnley appeared in *Practitioner*, a journal as its name implies for general practitioners, and were presumably written by invitation. The first, in 1948, was on *Amputations*[4] and no doubt was asked for because of his 1943 paper on the subject (Chapter 3). The other two were published in 1950: *Sprains and dislocations*[9] and *Injuries of the spine and pelvis*[12]. There is nothing remarkable in these papers, but they show that Charnley was prepared to write for the purpose of teaching others, apart from orthopaedic surgeons, and did so very well. Another contribution which comes into this category, but in a different area of orthopaedics, is *Peri-arthritis of the shoulder* published in the *Postgraduate Medical Journal*.[19]

An article by Sir Reginald Watson-Jones and others in the British volume of the *Journal of Bone and Joint Surgery* in 1950 on the intramedullary nailing of fractures had suggested that credit for the introduction of this idea should be given to an English surgeon, Hey-Groves, rather than the German, Küntscher, who had popularised the technique during the war.[61] Charnley wrote to the journal challenging this idea.[36] The merits of the argument need not concern us here, but having boldly stated that the article 'was spoiled by an element of propaganda unworthy of a scientific journal', he went on to make an observation about innovators in general:

> in attributing credit for technological advance the conception of an idea is frequently the least inspired part of the research . . . The credit for evolving

a successful technique should go to the worker who has the vision to see the solution of a modern problem in an old and discredited method; whose imagination and intuition is of such an order that he can retain, undimmed, his faith in the value of the idea through the long months of technical disappointment and until success is finally achieved.

Charnley took part in a debate during an 'orthopaedic day' in Liverpool in 1952.[45] The proposition was that 'modern advances in internal fixation will render obsolete the use of splints in the treatment of fractured bones' and was clearly intended to arouse dispute. His colleague, Lloyd Griffiths opened, and Charnley's contribution was summarised thus in the proceedings reported in the *Journal of Bone and Joint Surgery*:

> Charnley claimed that bone, being largely dead, could be treated with scant courtesy, but periosteum which was very much alive should be handled with reverence. He was developing his thesis in a strong speech for the motion, but in the end his cheek could no longer contain his tongue.

His contribution to another debate held at a meeting of the British Orthopaedic Association in Liverpool in 1955 is worth quoting. This time the motion was 'That Lucas Championnière was right'.[48] Championnière had used massage and early movement in the treatment of fractures. Mr Robert Roaf said that the Frenchman 'was an arrogant writer but no true scientist, a believer in "all-or-nothing", a surgical Karl Marx.' Mr Philip Wiles pointed out that bone needed rest and the soft parts needed mobilisation so a compromise was needed. This was the account of Charnley's contribution.

> The middle course, as advocated by Mr Wiles, was dangerous. The motion was either right or wrong; he felt that massage was the real basis of Championnière's theme. There were three possible causes of failure to unite: (1) the callus never crossed the gap; (2) the callus succeeded in crossing the gap, but was too fragile, broke down and reverted to (1); and (3) the callus would cross the gap successfully if only it were immobile. If a bone were plated, only (3) could be relevant because immobility was far greater than could be achieved by any other method. He ventured a Law of Conservative Treatment: full mobility could be restored if the bones and joints were fixed for no longer than the physiological maximum of eight weeks. If union were delayed and longer fixation were required, joint stiffness would follow. But prolonged splintage alone was not the cause; there was some other factor.

Charnley continued to be sought after as a speaker; and he was invited to take part in two symposia of the orthopaedic section of the Royal Society of Medicine in London; his contributions being published in the Proceedings of the Society. The first was held in May, 1957, and the subject was 'The Use of Metal in Bone Surgery'.[15] The opening speaker was G. K. McKee of Norwich who began by discussing corrosion testing of metals used for internal fixation and went on to describe his own early models of an artificial hip joint. He was followed by Charnley who concentrated on the reaction of bone to metal in both the short and long term.

The second occasion was on 2 December, 1958 when the symposium was on 'The Treatment of Fractures of the Shafts of the Long Bones' and William Gissane, of the Birmingham Accident Hospital, began the discussion.[18] As we shall see in the next chapter, Gissane had reviewed the first and second editions of *The Closed Treatment of Common Fractures* by Charnley (Chapter 6) and the two men had somewhat different views. Gissane admitted that if his practice were restricted to one or other method of treatment, he would unhesitatingly choose closed manipulation for early treatment. Since he 'happily' was not so restricted, he went on to make a very strong case for early open reduction and rigid metal fixation of the more severe types of both open and closed fractures of long bones. Charnley, to the contrary, eloquently exposed what he called the 'three fallacies': the fallacy of accurate reduction: the fallacy of defective osteogenesis and the fallacy of absolute fixation. He concluded this part of his talk by saying that the most important feature in the union of a fracture is the extent to which the soft parts are torn at the time of injury. This rather fatalistic approach led him to suggest that the good results of internal fixation will be precisely in those fractures which would unite well by conservative means.

Some time before this, Charnley had set out to devise a method of obtaining union in fractures of the neck of the femur. This common fracture, which occurs in old people, has always had a bad reputation for the incidence of nonunion. The bone has a poor blood supply and is porotic so that standard methods of internal fixation, such as the Smith-Petersen nail, often failed. Charnley wished to apply compression to the cancellous bone at the fracture site, in line with his work on compression arthrodesis, and he devised an ingenious spring-loaded screw to do this. He published the method in the British *Journal of Bone and Joint Surgery* of February, 1957.[16] His fellow authors, N. J. Blockey and D. W. Purser, were both registrars in Manchester. This was a long paper (20 pages) reporting the results of 34 operations. Charnley reviewed the whole subject in *Acta Scandinavica Orthopaedica* in 1960 when he had added a further 15 cases to his series.[22] The compression screw did not, however, gain wide acceptance. By 1957 Charnley was well on the way to giving up fracture work in order to concentrate on arthroplasty of the hip joint. Whether he would have managed to convert more surgeons to his method had he continued with it himself is a matter for speculation.

Charnley was a member of the editorial board of the British *Journal of Bone and Joint Surgery* from 1959 to 1963. It is said that he was proposed by Watson-Jones, who was editor, on the grounds that 'John has been such a stern critic of the Journal'. He was an efficient member and regularly attended the meetings, held every two months in London. On one occasion the board had accepted a paper on experimental fractures in rats by two Canadian surgeons.[57] The board were anxious that publication should not be mistaken as their approval for a clinical trial of the technique on human subjects. Accordingly, Charnley was asked to write an editorial.[21] He welcomed the authors' emphasis on the biological approach to osseous union as opposed to a purely mechanical attitude. None the less, he put forward reasons why their operation might not be effective in human fractures.

*Delayed operation in the open reduction of fractures of long bones* was published in 1961 and written, jointly with an Egyptian assistant, J. Guindy, from Park Hospital, Davyhulme.[23] This concerned the observation, which another orthopaedic surgeon had made, that fractures of the forearm bones united more quickly when operation was delayed. Charnley and Guindy demonstrated that this was also true for intramedullary nailing of fractures of the femoral shaft.

Their series of 38 cases was too small to offer conclusive proof, but it was suggested that this was an important idea which ought to be investigated by many more observers.

In 1966 Charnley reviewed the book *Technique of Internal Fixation of Fractures* by M. E. Müller and other members of the AO group – Charnley avoided the long German word and interpreted AO as the 'Association for Osteosynthesis'. He took a traditional British view:

> In a subject which is so fundamentally controversial as the operative treatment of fractures, there will be many critics; many [of the] illustrations . . . could be used to support the view that this book will do more harm than good, as for instance the treatment meted out to the patient in figure 157 . . .[51]

The figure reproduced in the review, which was in the British volume of the *Journal of Bone and Joint Surgery*, showed a comminuted supracondylar fracture of the femur which had been immaculately fixed with two plates and many screws. He continued:

> . . . even though this result was perfect . . . the book is not intended for persons without experience, but surgeons who have the judgement to select and reject will find a real thrill in their first reading . . .

Charnley had made important practical contributions to the treatment of fractures which remain of value to this day. His basic observations on the healing of bone, particularly under compression, have also made a permanent addition to the corpus of knowledge about the process of union.

Although Charnley claimed to dislike coping with the large numbers of patients with backache who came to his clinic at Park Hospital, he wrote papers and letters on the subject in 1947 and 1958. He was probably like many orthopaedic surgeons who are quite happy dealing with backache when they have a patient with physical signs, in whom a diagnosis could be made and useful treatment prescribed. The unfortunate sufferers, who have nothing to show to explain their symptoms and in whom orthopaedic intervention is unlikely to be helpful, are those who strained his patience.

In 1947, he wrote to *The Lancet* criticising diagrams which B. H. Burns and R. H. Young (from St George's Hospital, London) had used to illustrate their paper on *Backache*, and which he considered did not give an accurate representation of the discs he had seen at operation.[32,53] In the next year, he took part in a symposium on the 'backache–sciatica syndrome' which was held jointly by the Manchester Medical Society and the Liverpool Medical Institution. The main speakers were Sir Harry Platt and Sir Geoffrey Jefferson. Charnley is recorded as 'strongly supporting radical measures'.[42]

His hackles were raised in 1949 by correspondence in *The Lancet* about 'Osteopathy' and he was vitriolic in his castigation of osteopaths:

> . . . two factors have made it possible for osteopathy to have survived, and even flourished, in the face of rational criticism: firstly the personality of the successful operator, and secondly the absence of a genuine follow-up system for late results.[33]

He was particularly incensed by previous correspondents who suggested that osteopathy would be acceptable if it were carried out by doctors:

> But it is the general conclusion that osteopathy would be permissible if the practitioner were medically qualified which . . . is pure cant. If a doctor, after years of training in pathology and allied subjects, decides to abandon the scientific method and forget all the facts that its application to medicine has revealed since the days of Harvey and Hunter, then there would seem to be only two explanations for such conduct: either he possesses a paranoid mental state and prefers to follow a systematised delusion rather than rational thought, or he is guilty of wilfully suppressing evidence. The only grace for the osteopath is that he should remain non-medical and therefore unable to be intellectually dishonest.

He wrote again on a more serious note to *The Lancet* in response to an article by a patient in a series on 'Disabilities'.[34,55] He considered that the writer, who had suffered from backache and sciatica, had been deprived of the benefits of surgery through three, or even four, errors of surgical judgement. The first error which had been made in this case was 'to explore the lumbar discs in a case of lumbago when spinal fusion might have been the correct treatment – if the symptoms were severe enough to warrant surgery'. He continued in this vein and concluded that the operative removal of a disc protrusion, which is causing sciatica, is one of the most gratifying procedures in surgery.

These expressions of his views indicate his interest and led to serious work on the subject. *Orthopaedic signs in the diagnosis of disc protrusion* was published in *The Lancet* in 1951.[10] It was the result of four years' work in the orthopaedic department of the Manchester Royal Infirmary and carried out with the encouragement of Sir Harry Platt. The aim was to correlate the various signs of deformity and limited mobility with the operative findings in 88 cases. The most important outcome was the demonstration that a disc protrusion was always found if there was severe restriction of straight-leg raising. Although this may seem a relatively simple conclusion, it needed to be confirmed by clinical observation, and those surgeons who accepted the findings were able to avoid frustrating operations when they would fail to find a protrusion (and the patient would be no better).

This clinical study was followed by an account of some basic experimental work which was carried out at the same time. *Fluid imbibition as a cause of herniation of the nucleus pulposus* was given as a paper at the Fifth International Congress of Orthopaedic Surgery and Traumatology (SICOT are the initials of the French name of this organisation) at Stockholm in 1951 and published in *The Lancet* in 1952.[11,44] The experiment was carried out on cadaveric specimens of the lumbar spine and Charnley demonstrated that the discs would swell when immersed in saline. Pressure measurements were also made with an adapted plethysmograph and levels of 150–200 mmHg were often reached. He postulated that under 'certain' conditions a disc would imbibe fluid and that the sudden episode of hypertension within the disc would produce an acute attack of lumbago. Once the pressure had risen, a spontaneous protrusion might start, and thereafter some slight injury would finally complete the bursting of the annulus.

In January, 1955, he took issue with L. S. Calvert who had written to the *British Medical Journal* late in the previous year.[54] Calvert had suggested that orthopaedic surgeons were failing in their responsibility to deal with backache and that departments of physical medicine should be enlarged to treat patients with the condition. What follows is part of Charnley's response:

> If the taxpayer is to foot the bill for the treatment of the backaches of his fellow citizens, he is surely justified in expecting the medical profession to be unanimous on three points: (1) that in the majority of cases there is a significant organic cause; (2) that the rationale of treatment is scientifically sound; and (3) that the results of treatment are worth the financial outlay, either in the terms of crude economics or as a gift to human happiness. . .
>
> If orthopaedic surgeons were to relax their grip on ad lib physiotherapy . . . the backache problem would become totally unmanageable. Physical medicine can never cure low backache, and if pampered the first time the majority of these patients will be back again . . .

This robust attitude would have been accepted by most of his orthopaedic colleagues and he was expressing a commonly held view at the time. He concluded his letter with a hope which has unfortunately never been fulfilled:

> There is hope that in the near future pain arising in 'collagen degeneration' may be brought under control, which research is common ground for rheumatology, physical medicine and orthopaedic surgeons. Until this happy day dawns, I believe the majority of orthopaedic surgeons show a very highly developed sense of perspective in regard to pain and the public purse.[38]

Charnley had contributed a paper on *Acute lumbago and sciatica* in the *British Medical Journal* in February, 1955, as part of a series on emergencies in general practice.[13] This was a splendidly clear account, with simple diagrams showing the sequence of events which occur in the course of a disc protrusion. Any general practitioner reading the article would gain a helpful understanding of the cause of lumbago and sciatica. The conclusion gave an insight into Charnley's thinking about patients with backache:

> The importance of a cheerful and even a light-hearted approach by the physician cannot be too strongly emphasised. It is much healthier for the patient's attitude to future back trouble, which in some measurement is

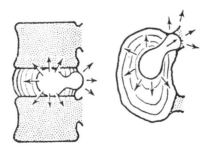

*Diagram in Charnley's article on acute lumbago and sciatica in the British Medical Journal in 1955. (By permission of the Editor.) A true disc protrusion is shown which is likely to cause pressure on a nerve root and thus sciatic pain.*

almost certain to recur from time to time, to try to regard lumbago as the sort of music-hall joke it used to be ten or twenty years ago. This does not mean that the practitioner need be insensitive and heartless, but that well-meaning but over-conscientious worry about "slipped discs" does not help the patient in the early stages of an acute attack.

These passages show Charnley's attitude to the difficult problem of backache. The paper stimulated a vigorous response from its readers, as twenty letters followed over the ensuing five weeks in the correspondence columns.

Finally, he wrote to *The Lancet* in 1958 about the *Physical changes in the prolapsed disc*.[39] He gave a simple explanation of the changes which take place in the discs with age and when a protrusion (or prolapse) occurs. This arose because a previous annotation in the journal had expressed difficulty in reconciling the theory that pain can be caused by swelling of the disc, yet at operation the material removed was stringy and dessicated.[52] Charnley believed it was important that general practitioners should be given a sound working hypothesis if they were to be able to reassure their patients confidently. He went on to describe the normal slow physico-chemical degenerative process, which is symptomless, and suggested that a disc which was the cause of acute lumbago in middle age might have undergone these changes in a matter of days or weeks. The disc then swelled and produced the characteristic pain and spasm. A 'sequestrum' was pushed out of the disc by an episode of raised internal tension affecting the mucoprotein which was as yet undegenerate.

Undoubtedly Charnley had a reputation for being unsympathetic to patients who had backache, and he is said on occasions to have stormed out of his clinic at Park Hospital when faced by large numbers of them. His writing shows that he had given the problem much thought, but some of his irritation became clear in part of the letter to *The Lancet* which has been referred to previously:

> It is the problem of reassurance which is the most important yet the least satisfactory, both to surgeon and patient. In the first place, one can only reassure an intelligent, decent, and sensible patient. Most of the patients to whom these adjectives apply have already been reassured by the first two doctors they have seen – that is, the general practitioner and the first health service consultant on the 'periphery'. This means that the teaching hospitals . . . accumulate an astonishing number of patients of a type impossible to reassure . . .
>
> . . . the process of attempting to reassure a patient by sympathetic explanation is extremely exhausting for a conscientious consultant . . .[34]

He was clearly expressing his profound frustration with some of his work in Manchester (and also what today would be called his élitist attitude). None the less, it should be appreciated that he had made a serious contribution to the understanding of the basic mechanisms of lumbar disc protrusions. His clinical judgement was sound, and he also carried out the necessary operations superbly well.

In the early 1960s, Jill Charnley developed backache and sciatica and she now recalls 'one thing John never wanted was a wife with backache'. In fact, he only took it at all seriously when he found out that she had consulted a chiropractor, without benefit. Operation, he considered, was needed and he decided to carry it out himself – telling his friends that he wanted to be sure that 'she had the best'. Most surgeons are reluctant to operate on members of their family and Charnley did not make his decision lightly. Everything went smoothly, the backache being completely cured without complications.

After the Second World War, many orthopaedic surgeons used an arthrodesis to relieve pain in joints affected by osteoarthritis, at the expense of complete loss of movement. The handicap produced by this restriction could partly be overcome by compensatory movement in neighbouring joints, particularly in younger patients, and those who had severe pain were often prepared to pay this price when there was no alternative treatment. Certainly, a successful arthrodesis could be relied on to relieve pain completely, provided that sound bony fusion was achieved.

Various ingenious methods were devised to achieve bony union which could be applied to different joints in different circumstances. Charnley was aware that Dr J. Albert Key of St Louis, Missouri, had reported in 1932 that compressing together the two cut bony surfaces, when attempting to arthrodese a tuberculous knee joint, helped to promote union.[58] His claims were modest and a few years later, he described another method which did not involve compression.[59]

Charnley now improved the technique by passing Steinmann nails through the femur and tibia above and below the excised joint. Clamps were attached to the nails so that a compressive force could be exerted after the operation, while the leg was supported on a Thomas' splint. He always stressed that the compression was continuous because of the elasticity of the nails.

Mr A.H.C. Ratliff remembers what was an epoch-making moment in the story of arthrodesis after Charnley had started using compression. A patient, who had had the operation ten days previously, complained of severe pain. One of the nails had broken, and Charnley found to his surprise that the arthrodesis felt completely solid on clinical testing. He realised for the first time that compression speeded union in cancellous bone to a remarkable degree, and all his basic work on the subject followed from this simple observation.

He demonstrated cases at the Manchester meeting of the British Orthopaedic Association in 1947, and his first paper on *Positive pressure in arthrodesis of the knee joint* was published in the British volume of the *Journal of Bone and Joint Surgery* in 1948.[5] In the opening sentence he credits Key with first using compression. Nevertheless, it is clear that not only did Charnley popularise the method, but he produced a satisfactory technique for producing compression and rapid bony union. Moreover, his experience lead him to draw conclusions of fundamental significance about the mechanism of bony union. He published his results in the British volume of the *Journal of Bone and Joint Surgery* in 1958.[17] He also reviewed his experience of 171 cases in *Clinical Orthopaedics* in 1960, and commented that orthopaedic surgeons in England appeared to be less reluctant to fuse the knee for arthritic conditions than their colleagues in the United States.[20] He attributed this to the fact that patients in England would accept with equanimity the advice to have the knee 'stiffened' (his quotations). He also pointed out that when both knees were arthrodesed, the patient's main difficulty was to sit in a theatre or in public transport, but that the operation would never be contemplated if their disability had not prevented these activities previously. Another observation, which was beneficial to the result, was that when $\frac{3}{4}$–1 inch of bone was removed, the hamstrings were relatively lengthened so that it was easy for a patient to reach his foot. By this time, he had become adept at the operation which he said could usually be carried out in less than twenty minutes.

Charnley first spoke about his central dislocation technique for arthrodesis of the hip at a meeting of the British Orthopaedic Association in Belfast in 1948.[43] He reported six cases and the presentation apparently caused 'a little merriment in the audience because it was admitted that bony union had failed to occur, although excellent functional results were achieved in a remarkably short time, and with full knee movement'. This operation will be considered further in the next chapter when his book *Compression Arthrodesis* will be discussed.

He continued to give papers about the principles and technique of central dislocation arthrodesis of the hip on numerous occasions, including a meeting of the combined French and British Orthopaedic Associations in Paris in 1955;[47] a meeting of the South African Orthopaedic Association in Pretoria in 1956,[49] and at international congresses in Bern in 1954[46], and Barcelona in 1957.[50]

Charnley's basic views about arthrodesis of the hip were expressed in a letter to *The Lancet* in 1954 under the heading *Arthroplasty v arthrodesis*.[37] The correspondence followed an editorial[56] on the subject and was begun by Watson-Jones, who was an enthusiastic exponent of arthrodesis, but used a different method. Charnley responded:

> As one who believes ardently in arthrodesis of the hip joint, I am in complete agreement with Sir Reginald regarding the excellence of hip fusion in unilateral disease . . .
>
> But to suggest that the painful hip can quite easily be got into the idyllic state of osseous union is not the experience of most orthopaedic surgeons. If arthrodesis of the hip by standard methods were a trouble-free procedure, recent exponents of arthroplasty would have had to face much more serious competition than has been the case . . .
>
> The fact is that the patient with a failed arthrodesis (by orthodox techniques) is in almost as pitiful a state as one with a failed arthroplasty . . . A stiff hip and a stiff knee is a calamity. . .
>
> The technique of central dislocation which I advocate guarantees full knee movement because the knee is only fixed for four weeks. But even [then] . . . I have never evaded the frank admission that osseous union is possible only in about 75% of older patients with osteoarthritis. The almost uncanny feature of this operation, however, is that the ability to bear weight without pain is just as good when it is a fibrous ankylosis as when osseous. This is a statement which may appear exaggerated and irresponsible to surgeons accustomed to identifying fibrous ankylosis with failure.

Already, by 1955, Charnley was acknowledging that his method was failing to produce a reliable arthrodesis so that the title of his papers in Bern, Paris and Pretoria was *Stabilisation* [rather than arthrodesis] *of the hip by the technique of central dislocation*. The change was subtle, but honest. The operation is now outmoded, but the reasons for this was the development of a successful arthroplasty.

Charnley's last contribution to the subject of arthrodesis was a paper published in 1964 (with J. K. Houston) on his results of arthrodesis of the shoulder.[24]

Congenital pseudarthrosis of the tibia is a very rare condition in which a fracture occurs in the tibia of an infant as a result of a congenital abnormality in the bone itself. There are a number of variations, but union fails to occur. A pseudarthrosis (or false joint) develops and standard methods of bone grafting are invariably unsuccessful. Charnley treated two cases in Manchester in the late 1940s. He devised an operation in which he inserted an intramedullary nail through the heel and upwards across the ankle joint, and into the tibia so that it crossed the pseudarthrosis. He also applied thin osteoperiosteal grafts around the defect in the routine manner. He believed that the essential feature of his success in these two cases was mechanical: the angulatory strains being converted into longitudinal compression forces. He was encouraged by Professor Trueta, then Nuffield professor of orthopaedic surgery at Oxford, to use the method and was very disappointed when the paper was rejected by the editorial board of the British volume of the *Journal of Bone and Joint Surgery*. It was subsequently accepted by the American counterpart and published by them in 1956.[14] The technique aroused interest at the time, and is still used by some surgeons in certain situations.

Bedsores may seem an unsuitable subject with which to conclude this chapter, but a letter which Charnley wrote to *The Lancet* in 1959 illustrated the consideration which he was prepared to give to an important, but in a sense a minor, problem.[40] He drew attention to a type of sore over the sacrum which he described as an exquisitely painful blister (in contrast to the deep, painless decubitus ulcers which occur in patients prostrate with serious illness or old age). He suggested that the 'blister' was caused by the common nursing practice of using an impervious sheet of rubber or polyethylene with nothing other than a layer of cotton sheet to separate it from the skin. His solution was to use material commonly available in the packaging industry where wrappings for various products could be constructed which were totally impermeable to liquid water, yet at the same time porous to water vapour. He had slept at home on such a fabric, which was woven from nylon thread and impregnated with polyvynyl chloride, and found it much more comfortable than rubber sheeting which, in the interests of science, he had also tried. The new sheeting had been used in his hospital ward for four months and found satisfactory. He said he could not pursue the matter further, but hoped that others might be in a position to develop his idea.

*Chapter 6*

# BOOKS TO INSTRUCT
## 1950 and 1953

*Books we are told propose to instruct or amuse . . . All that is literature seeks to communicate power; all that is not literature, to communicate knowledge.*

Thomas de Quincy 1785–1859: *Letters to a Young Man* .

THE BOOKS which Charnley published in 1950 and 1953 are major works which make a significant contribution to orthopaedic surgery. The first was *The Closed Treatment of Common Fractures* (1950)[1] and the second *Compression Arthrodesis* (1953)[2], both published by E. & S. Livingstone Ltd (now Churchill Livingstone) of Edinburgh and London. These contain many of the ideas which were included in his papers, but the two books are important because they allowed Charnley space in which to expound his personal opinions.

Charnley became interested in the nature of bone healing and the mechanical problems of fracture treatment when he was in Cairo, and he maintained this interest when he returned to Manchester. He wrote *The Closed Treatment of Common Fractures* in a manner which would appeal to practising surgeons, and the preface of the first edition (1950) made it clear for whom the book was intended:

> This book is written primarily for the resident casualty surgeon [this was the post he had filled at the Manchester Royal Infirmary before the war]. In Britain this resident appointment is usually held by young men whose practical experience, for obvious reasons, cannot match their theoretical knowledge. It is possible for such casualty officers to be fully conversant with modern textbooks of fracture treatment and yet be unable with any degree of certainty to reduce many of the simple fractures. I believe that this follows from the fact that in many large textbooks the space devoted to the detailed description of technique in the treatment of common fractures is disproportionately small. An important step, on which might depend the

success of a reduction, can be overlooked if it is concealed within one sentence. The full significance of many sentences in standard textbooks is often only fully realised.on reading them again at a later date, when one has learned to reduce fractures by practical experience.

The essential difficulty . . . can usually be traced to the surgeon not having a clear mental picture of what he is trying to do. In these circumstances a series of manipulative movements is carried out as a ritual and an X-ray is then taken 'to see if it is reduced'. If then, the fracture is not reduced the operator is nonplussed; *he does not know what to do having learnt nothing from his previous attempt.* In the following chapters I have tried to create pictures for the surgeon to visualise in his mind's eye; it must be confessed that some of these mental pictures may be more symbolic than true representations of the facts, but this approach has helped me to improve my own results, and those who attempt to follow can make their own images starting from this groundwork.

It should be the aim of the good manipulative surgeon to know that *a fracture has been reduced by his sense of touch without utter dependence on X-ray . . .*

During a recent visit to the United States he had become aware of an increasing interest in the operative treatment of fractures. Although he appreciated the economic advantages of operative treatment, he pointed out that good operative techniques were being unfairly contrasted with poor manipulative techniques.

But the appearance of scientific precision which is always associated with operative methods is only superficial; this apparent precision will not alter the convictions of the manipulative surgeon and will not blind him to the ill-effects of many operative interventions on the blood supply of the bone fragments and the process of normal callus formation. For this reason *an attempt is here made to re-emphasise the non-operative method, and to show that far from being a crude and uncertain art, the manipulative treatment of fractures can be resolved into something of a science.*

The book was dedicated to 'my teacher, Sir Harry Platt' who contributed a foreword in which he summed up the essence of the book.

In this most stimulating monograph Mr Charnley has sought to illuminate some of the obscurities of the mechanics of fracture treatment, and he has succeeded, in a most vivid fashion, in creating by means of text and illustration a series of mental pictures – a frame of reference so to say – whereby the young surgeon can get the feel of a fracture; first the anatomy of the displacement, and then that confident 'clinical sense' of precise correction of the deformity which follows a skilful manipulative act of reduction.

The first two chapters concerned the principles of conservative treatment and showed Charnley's original thinking about these basic aspects of fracture management. His ability to get to the root of the matter and his penetrating analysis of clinical problems was impressive. He never hesitated to question accepted dogma and to say exactly why he was doing so.

The rest of the book dealt with schemes of treatment for individual fractures and, although his methods were sometimes controversial, his arguments for closed

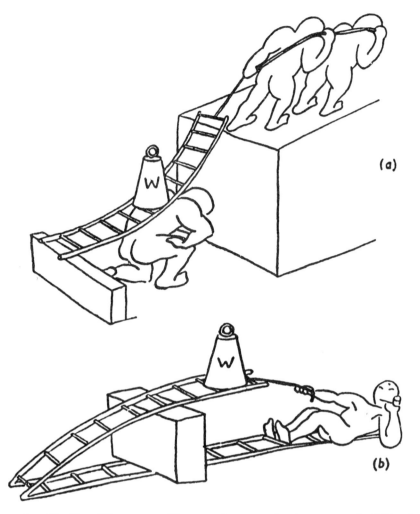

*Diagram from* The Closed Treatment of Common Fractures *showing an example of Charnley's simple line drawing to illustrate a principle of treatment. (By courtesy of Churchill Livingstone.)*

manipulation were sound. In particular, his description of the way in which plaster of Paris should be used to maintain the position of a fracture gave the reader a rational explanation of what might otherwise have been an unthinking routine.

The first edition was reviewed by William Gissane in the British volume of the *Journal of Bone and Joint Surgery*.[6] Gissane was a distinguished and outspoken Australian surgeon, who had created the Birmingham Accident Hospital, and whose ideas might well be expected to differ from Charnley's. And indeed they

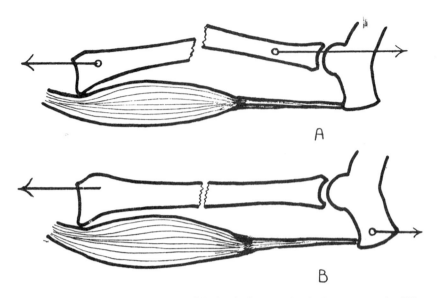

*Another example from* Closed Treatment. *This simple diagram clearly demonstrates the different consequences of applying traction through the lower end of the tibia or through the os calcis. (By courtesy of Churchill Livingstone.)*

did. Charnley's concepts of Colles' and Potts' fractures were criticised and the illustrations showing the intact periosteal hinge in these fractures were considered to be 'inaccurate oversimplifications'. The reviewer wrote 'my intention has not been to damn the book with faint praise' which presumably meant he felt that this was precisely what he might have done. He concluded 'the first edition has achieved a great deal that is very good; I hope and expect it to live through many more editions'. His prediction was correct.

The second edition was published in 1957 and again merited a full review in the *Journal of Bone and Joint Surgery* – again by Gissane[7], who began by gently chiding the author for 'belittling the importance of his achievement. He should not be so modest'. The new book was 73 pages longer and had 66 more illustrations than the previous edition; the price had increased to £2 10s. But 'as a better, a wiser and a beautifully produced book', the reviewer considered it to be well worth the additional fifteen shillings. Gissane still did not entirely agree with all Charnley's arguments. He maintained that, although closed methods were safer and resulted in a higher proportion of bone union, the functional results were not always satisfactory either for athletes or to meet the physical requirements of certain types of jobs. This argument continues today, but the review ended 'yet if my practice in the treatment of fractures was restricted to one or other method then I would join the "Charnley Camp"' – a considerable concession in the circumstances.

A third edition appeared in 1961 with a new preface which contains some fundamental thoughts from the author:

> I have persisted in my attempt to write a book . . . which at one and the same time would be a vade-mecum for the junior man and an interesting

treatise for the experienced surgeon. It might be considered that these two objectives might be incompatible, and that it would have been better to have written a simple text-book for the junior man and to have reserved my ponderings on the nature of fracture repair for a separate monograph. In the training of young surgeons I believe that the habit of making clinical observations and questioning accepted beliefs ought to start from the earliest moment. There is still a great deal of information concerning the healing of fractures waiting to be deduced, by the process of logic and close reasoning, from clinical facts collected in the operating theatre and out-patient department.

There is a tendency to imagine that serious research now-a-days can only come out of a laboratory, and that contributions from the pure act of thinking on clinical facts ended with the great clinicians of the past. The old clinicians had their faculties for observation by sight and touch heightened by the absence of X-rays and laboratory tests. But though the clinical acumen of the old observers was greater than ours, it was offset by a strain of credulity, which is apparent in a different form among clinicians today. In the past the clinical philosopher was credulous because he was the victim of inherited beliefs, but to-day our credulity lies in the accuracy which we attribute to our special research tools, such as the electron microscope. We must not forget that sight and touch together make the greatest clinical faculty of all, namely, commonsense. As an instance of this may I venture to suggest that the recent failure of 'bone glue' could have been predicted from the facts of blood supply in the process of fracture repair and that this conclusion could have been reached by arguments from the depths of an armchair without ever resorting to trials on the human subject.

Charnley was somewhat repetitious in his enthusiasm for the virtues and defects of the 'older clinicians', but his general sentiments would have appealed to most of his surgical colleagues. His support for 'pure reasoning' expressed the basic philosophy which informed his approach to every problem he tackled. Although he did not always follow scientific method in substantiating his theories, he did himself less than justice in suggesting that he solved problems 'from an armchair'. The more so because, although he thought deeply about problems, he was always quick to test his hypotheses in practice.

This edition was reviewed by Sir Reginald Watson-Jones[8] who was then editor of the British *Journal of Bone and Joint Surgery*. The two men had the kind of mutual respect for each other which can only be held by those with diametrically opposed views. We shall see in due course how Charnley devoted a whole chapter in his book on compression arthrodesis to refute Sir Reginald's arguments, which he described as 'archaic'. The review is brief and so entertaining that it is quoted in full:

Mr Charnley has honoured us by preparing a third edition of *The Closed Treatment of Common Fractures*. He is one of the most interesting, stimulating and enigmatic figures in British orthopaedic surgery. Perhaps it is because he is so enigmatic that he is so stimulating. At one moment you find yourself in complete agreement with his sound teaching and within seconds you are infuriated by his observation. This is the basis of good teaching. You are never allowed to go to sleep, changing only from warm approval when you want to clap aloud, to stern disapproval when you just frown. This is the calibre of his brilliant monograph which every orthopaedic surgeon should read, study and have in his library. I trust very much that they will regard as nonsense the idea that displacement of fractured bones should be increased before they can be reduced. Figure 105 on page 131, showing reduction of a Colles' fracture fills me with horror, and I am glad only that he does not now emphasise the same idea in treating supracondylar fractures of the humerus. But such criticism confirms the success of this stimulating monograph which is so rewarding and so exciting that every young surgeon should read it again and again.

What can the reader do but sit back and gasp at these verbal fireworks, which were a typical Watson-Jones polemic and, perhaps, reveal more about the writer than the book he was reviewing. Come what may, young surgeons did continue to read *Closed Treatment* and the third edition was reprinted in 1963, 1968, 1970, 1974, 1976, 1982, and is still in print. The first and second editions each sold just over 3000 copies; but the sales for the third have now reached 27 000 (just over 9000 being sold from 1976 to the present day).

An anecdote illustrates the wide circulation of the book and how much its teaching is still appreciated. Lady Charnley was travelling in Nepal on a plant collecting expedition after her husband had died. She became ill, probably as a result of altitude and spartan living conditions, and was taken to a mission hospital. When the American doctor treating her discovered her name, he did not respond by asking if her husband had anything to do with the Charnley who invented a hip operation. Rather he associated the name with a book on fractures which he had with him, and which he regarded as his bible – at least in the context of treating injuries.

Charnley's papers on compression arthrodesis were considered in the previous chapter, and we can now turn to his book of that title which was published in 1953. The subtitle 'including central dislocation as a principle in hip surgery' indicated the importance he attached to his efforts to produce an arthrodesis of the hip joint. The whole work was very much a collaborative effort and contained a chapter on mechanics by Professor J. A. L. Matheson, Beyer professor of engineering, University of Manchester. This was entered on the title page, as was the fact the book included histological observations by Professor S. L. Baker, Department of Rheumatism Research, University of Manchester. Charnley generously acknowledged those who had helped him and he thanked by name a further 19 people (technicians, radiographers, photographers, artists and orthopaedic surgeons). He used the first person plural throughout, so perhaps the circumstances justified this literary artifice.

The second paragraph of the preface transcended his usual scientific style:

The survival of a bone-graft, when used to induce arthrodesis, is not unlike the survival of a sailing ship on a long ocean passage. To lie idle during flat calm, to be powerless in the face of tempests, to take long and indirect routes against unfavourable winds, and, finally, after many vicissitudes, in most cases to reach harbour are all incidents which have their parallels in the vagaries of osseous union. How like the captain of a windjammer is an orthopaedic surgeon; daily he is pestered by his patients to say when they

might reasonably expect to arrive at their longed-for destination; how expert
he becomes at evading the question!

What a splendid description this was, and the final sentence hinted at the author's
approach to his patients. There was, in fact, much truth in what he said. The
kindest orthopaedic surgeons often seemed to find it hard to tell their patients
how long their treatment was to take, and the predicted days would run into
weeks, and weeks into months.

Charnley acknowledged that his theories were based on limited evidence:

> In venturing to make deductions from biopsy examinations in compression
> arthrodesis of the knee, I am well aware that the number of observations
> is small. The "crucial" experiment is itself restricted to one single
> observation. But, for obvious reasons, these observations cannot be repeated
> on the human subject as frequently as would be necessary to satisfy the
> demands of a controlled experiment; for the same reason, even a dozen
> similar observations would still not be free from carping and unimaginative
> criticism.
>
> A few observations on the human are often of more value than a large
> series of experiments on animals, especially if a few observations illuminate,
> and are consistent with, a considerable operative experience. It has rightly
> been said that every surgical operation is a biological experiment. Though
> the laboratory experiments are few I have not merely illustrated biopsy
> findings which favour the thesis and suppressed others which do not. The
> "crucial" experiment was an isolated observation and yet, because the result
> was so unequivocally in line with what had been predicted, it seems that
> this in some ways makes it all the more significant.

The first five chapters gave a detailed consideration of the effect of compression
on the healing of bone and were illustrated by radiographs, photomicrographs
and beautiful microradiographs. Much of the material came from specimens of
core biopsies taken with a trephine from the line of arthrodesis four weeks after
operation in seven patients. In the 'crucial' experiment, an arthrodesis was carried
out in a patient, but the femur was cut in such a way that there was only a
narrow area of contact with the flat cut surface of the tibia. This arrangement
inevitably allowed a few degrees of movement for some days after the operation.
The thickness and density of new bone formation was greater under these
circumstances than in the usual cases where compression had produced rigid
immobilisation. Charnley drew two conclusions from this: firstly, maximum bone
formation took place at the site of maximum pressure; and, secondly, new bone
produced was stronger when a high compression force was used than occurred
when there was immobilisation without compression.

Having established that compression applied through his arrangement of nails
and clamps promoted union, Charnley wanted to know the forces which were
being generated by his system and the next chapter was written by Professor
Matheson. There were difficulties in making calculations in patients and so a test
rig was set up. It was then possible to estimate the forces from the deflection of
the nails seen in radiographs taken after operation. The greater the load generated,
the more likely was the arthrodesis to be clinically solid at four weeks after
operation.

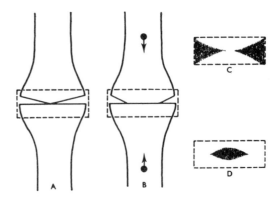

*Diagram of the 'crucial' experiment in arthrodesis of the knee. (From* Compression Arthrodesis *by courtesy of Churchill Livingstone.)*

Charnley devoted his next chapter to his personal argument with Watson-Jones, and he began:

> In the 1952 edition of his textbook [*Fractures and Joint Injuries*], Sir Reginald Watson-Jones, with all the eloquence of which he is a master devotes a chapter to an ardent denunciation of the use of mechanical compression in osseous union. Though at first rather disheartening, the attack has proved a blessing in disguise because, in the attempt to refute each detail of his argument, ideas were evoked and special observations made which otherwise might have passed unnoticed had the stimulus been lacking.
>
> In its construction Sir Reginald's argument is archaic; an attempt is made to substantiate opinions by miscellaneous instances apparently favourable to the argument, but ignoring others unfavourable, and all is reinforced by reference to authority reminiscent of Galen or Hippocrates. . .

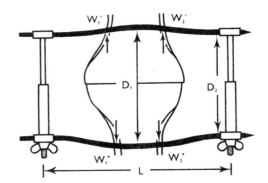

*Diagram showing bending of the nails in arthrodesis. (From* Compression Arthrodesis *by courtesy of Churchill Livingstone.)*

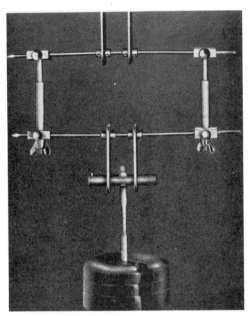

*The experimental rig used to reproduce bending of the nails as occurs after operation and allows calculation of the forces involved. (From* Compression Arthrodesis *by courtesy of Churchill Livingstone.)*

Nothing will be gained by resurrecting this acrimonious dispute, but Charnley stated his case with conviction, and whatever the rights or wrongs of the issue, one cannot but admire his courage in attacking his illustrious opponent.

After this interlude, the book continued on a more practical level and described, first the design of an ideal arthrodesis, and then the surgical application of this principle to various joints. The descriptions were absolutely precise and gave clear guidance to a surgeon embarking on any of the procedures. This was always a feature of Charnley's writing and was based on his firm belief in the importance of technical minutiae in operative surgery. He dealt with the knee, the shoulder, the ankle, the tarsal joints of the foot, the elbow and the finger-joints before reaching the hip.

The technical problems of arthrodesis of the hip clearly had a fascination for Charnley, as they did for many other orthopaedic surgeons. Watson-Jones was a great exponent of the operation and propounded its advantages (or perhaps the lack of disadvantages) with all the hyperbole and eloquence he could command. But the technique which Charnley first conceived, as early as 1946, was based on totally different principles. The head of the femur was shaped into a cone and was driven through a hole in the floor of the acetabulum which had been reamed to a corresponding section. Fixation was then obtained by a long screw. Charnley subsequently proceeded to carry out 44 operations with 'simple central dislocation, without any internal fixation, and with the deliberate object of getting a "sound" fibrous ankylosis'. He reported in the book that 'the results have been

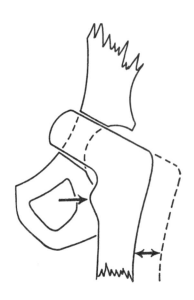

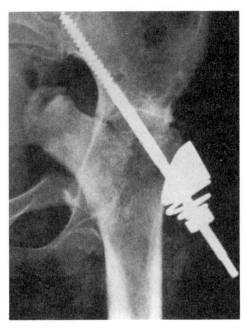

*Diagram illustrating the principle of central dislocation arthrodesis of the hip as carried out by Charnley. (From* Compression Arthrodesis *by courtesy of Churchill Livingstone.)*

*Radiograph showing the appearance one month after operation with fixation by a compression screw. (From* Compression Arthrodesis *by courtesy of Churchill Livingstone.)*

consistent, and not a single patient has been disappointed as have been some of our arthroplasties' (it should be recalled that he was writing in 1952). However, he was determined to obtain bony fusion, and his next step was to use external compression. He devised a rather cumbersome apparatus which projected through the wound, but infection became such a problem that the method was abandoned after he had performed the operation on six patients. None the less, osseous union occurred in five out of the six hips. Charnley went on to design an internal spring-compressor mounted on a strong coarse-threaded screw which passed through the upper end of the femur into the bone of the pelvis so that the two were held together and compressed.

The book had an interesting appendix which made points about the design of Steinmann nails and the compression clamps. Charnley also recorded here his second failure of compression arthrodesis of the knee in Charcot's disease and his final paragraph recalled another case:

> Lest it be thought that we are trying to force our memory and imagination into line with our thesis, our friend, Mr T. J. Fairbank, who operated on this patient while in Manchester in 1946, in the interests of science has very generously given us permission to report that he did not use the arthrodesis clamps, and that he merely tied the outer ends of the nails together with string.

Fairbank, now living in Cambridge where he was the senior orthopaedic surgeon, still remembers the incident clearly. It occurred at a time when Charnley was making the clamps in his workshop in the medical school the night before an operation was planned, and bringing them to the operating theatre immediately before they were needed. But on this occasion, he failed to provide his friend with the clamps. Fairbank writes:

> One day he let me do a compression arthrodesis (a Charcot joint!)but I had no clamps, of course. I think he was a bit disappointed that my do-it-yourself method led to fusion, though it was less efficient than his own.

Although tibial osteotomy and later replacement of the knee joint have largely superseded arthrodesis for osteoarthritis, Charnley's compression technique remains the standard method of arthrodesis and has stood the test of time.

A point about Charnley's operative techniques may be made here. If he thought out a new, and daring, surgical approach, he had no hesitation in carrying it out after due consideration of the anatomy involved. For example, few surgeons would have had the courage to make a hole through the wall of the pelvis at the base of the acetabulum, and then displace the femoral head through it. Further, when he found that the standard approaches to the ankle did not give him sufficient access to the joint, he made a transverse skin incision and divided all the extensor tendons and the anterior tibial artery and nerve. He had satisfied himself that this would not produce any permanent damage which would be detrimental to the patient, but such a radical step must have required courage to take for the first time – particularly as he must have been aware that his colleagues would have considerable reservations about this manoeuvre, if not downright disapproval of it. This courage was one of the qualities which singled Charnley out as an inspired orthopaedic surgeon who was able to rise above the conservative conventions of his day.

*Compression Arthrodesis* was reviewed by Philip Newman in the British volume of the *Journal of Bone and Joint Surgery*; he commented:

> Only one joint has seemed to make the author hesitate – the hip. Here there has been a searching for perfection, as no less than four different operations are described, and one wonders a little how high must be his ideals when the results of the first method seem to have been so satisfactory.[9]

Certainly, Charnley had devoted a great deal of time and effort in perfecting methods of central dislocation arthrodesis and many surgeons became interested in his work. We have, however, already seen, when reviewing his papers on the subject in the previous chapter, that he acknowledged that bony union did not always occur, so that he began describing the operation as 'stabilisation' of the hip rather than arthrodesis.

Over 800 copies of the book were sold in the first two years, which seems reasonable in view of its appeal to a relatively limited audience. After this, it continued to sell steadily, although in decreasing numbers each year, until it went out of print in 1969.

A final word on the effect of compression was written in a letter by Sir Louis Matheson:

> I recall, I hope correctly, Charnley telling me years later, when he was visiting Melbourne, that the significant requirement had turned out to be

that the bones had to be rigidly held so that there was no relative movement until they had fused. He had earlier thought that the clamping force was critical . . .

But this was no longer a burning issue to Charnley, as it had been in the days when he was arguing with Watson-Jones.

In recent years, arthrodesis has been needed less and less often and a stiff joint is no longer acceptable to most patients with osteoarthritis. Nevertheless, even after he had perfected his arthroplasty of the hip, Charnley still taught that arthrodesis was the operation of choice in young patients for a limited period. When they became older, and found a stiff hip more burdensome, the arthrodesis could be converted into an arthroplasty.

Although his contributions to surgical technique were important, it is the original observations which Charnley made about the effects of compression on bony union which have proved to be of lasting significance.

Charnley also contributed to several textbooks during this period. In a chapter on 'Fracture Treatment' in *Modern Trends in Orthopaedic Surgery*, which, in 1950, was edited by Sir Harry Platt, two passages indicate his views on this subject:

> There is little doubt that we are now at the start of an era in which the treatment of fractures will be based on principles evolved from the basic sciences . . .
>
> The fracture surgeon has often thought his mechanical methods to be above reproach but, seen through the eyes of the professional engineer, his methods are sometimes childish, being often unsuited to the nature of the material and the magnitude of the forces involved. From the histological laboratory and the engineering department . . . principles may eventually emerge which will enable us to secure osseous union with the certainty we expect from soft tissues.[3]

Writing chapters in textbooks for students can be a chore, and one which was often passed by a senior to one of his juniors. We do not know how Charnley came to write in the *Encyclopaedia of British Medical Practice*, but the invitation may have been passed on to him in this way, perhaps by Platt or Osmond-Clarke. His contribution in the 1951 edition was on 'Epiphyses, Diseases and Injuries'[4] – a subject which does not seem to have been of special interest to him before or since. His review, which filled 14 pages, was a well-balanced account of various epiphyseal disorders with a full list of references.

Charnley also wrote the chapters on 'Orthopaedics' in the 10th, 11th, 12th and 13th editions of *A Short Practice of Surgery* by Hamilton Bailey and Love which were published from 1956 to 1965. This book became, after its first edition in 1932, a popular text for many generations of medical students. In the earliest editions, the orthopaedic section was written by the authors, who were both general surgeons and felt able to encompass the whole field of surgery themselves. In 1952, they acknowledged that Sir Reginald Watson-Jones had 'contributed a considerable amount of material' to the chapter on fractures. It was after this that Charnley was invited to write the orthopaedic section; this included six chapters on injuries and diseases of bones and joints, and on muscles, tendons and bursae, and deformities. The volume is large and these chapters made up 177 pages in the 10th edition. Charnley used the previous format, but introduced much new material and many new figures. Osteoarthritis of the hip was illustrated by a radiograph of a patient with a Smith-Petersen cup arthroplasty on one side and a Judet acrylic femoral head on the other – which represented two forms of surgical treatment being used at the time (Chapter 9). It is perhaps significant that in 1962 the orthopaedic section was promoted from the very back of the book to near the front. Charnley continued contributing his chapters with very few changes, but in 1965 he allowed himself a revealing sentence:

> Research is in progress in methods of replacing the acetabulum and the femoral head, and the early results of this technique are spectacular.[5]

This was unchanged in 1968, and the whole section was subsequently taken over by M. A. R. Freeman of the London Hospital.

In the last two chapters all Charnley's written work up to 1960 has been reviewed, giving an overall impression of his contribution to general orthopaedics before he concentrated exclusively on the hip joint. His literary style was fluent and he had the knack of expressing himself vividly when the occasion arose. He was also an entertaining speaker who would enliven any meeting, whether he was making a formal presentation or speaking impromptu from the floor. Orthopaedics was the richer for his contributions, many of which remain enjoyable to read and relevant to today's problems.

*Chapter 7*

# TURNING POINTS
### 1957 and 1958

*Looking back over these last ten years I am quite certain that if I had not made myself financially and geographically independent from the teaching hospital, this project could never have succeeded.*

Charnley 1970

IN SPITE OF his outward successes, Charnley became progressively disillusioned with the work which he was able to do in Manchester. There were several reasons why this was so and why the conditions which he had hoped for when he returned from the Army were not fulfilled. Money was short in hospitals and universities in the 1950s and this made it difficult for him to obtain the facilities which he needed for his research.

Lloyd Griffiths had been in charge of the orthopaedic department at the Manchester Royal Infirmary since 1952 and John Charnley was not the sort of man to sit comfortably in second place. It is true that he never sought position for its own sake, but he preferred to be his own master and in charge of his own unit. He was allotted 18 out of the 36 orthopaedic beds at the Manchester Royal Infirmary, but most of them were filled with patients suffering from the results of road traffic accidents and old ladies with fractures of the femoral neck. The amount of operating that he could do was restricted; as in so many general hospitals the nursing staff in the theatre changed frequently, and he did not like being assisted by junior nurses who were not familiar with his technique. He had 25 beds under his care at Park Hospital, Davyhulme, where he had more control over what went on and where he preferred operating.

There is no doubt also that he gradually became less enthusiastic about teaching medical students and delegated it whenever possible. When he first returned to Manchester he was actively involved in teaching and the success of his demonstration at the meeting in 1947 shows that he was taking it seriously.

81

Furthermore, he was prepared to contribute to the students' magazine and to write chapters on orthopaedics in standard student textbooks. As time went by, however, his involvement lessened and he came to prefer philosophising with the residents over orthopaedic problems and he continued to be a popular postgraduate teacher. Lloyd Griffiths, on the other hand, was always a stimulating teacher of undergraduates.

Radical changes had taken place in the pattern of orthopaedic surgery. The scourges of tuberculosis and poliomyelitis were gradually being eliminated. All orthopaedic surgeons were pleased to see the end of these dreadful diseases, but as a result a great deal of fascinating reconstructive surgery was lost to them. There were, of course, congenital deformities and other disorders of childhood, but these conditions formed only a relatively small proportion of an average orthopaedic surgeon's work. A large part of familiar orthopaedic practice had disappeared, although the management of fractures and other injuries, which had previously been treated by general surgeons, occupied an increasing amount of time. This had nothing to do with the National Health Service, except that it was now easier for patients to come to hospital and demand treatment for relatively minor conditions. Orthopaedic surgeons took on the care of patients with all sorts of musculo-skeletal aches and pains, particularly backache and pain in the neck. Much of this work Charnley found unattractive as it usually did not provide the intellectual challenge which he liked, or demand his surgical skill.

His contract with the National Health Service allowed him to do a limited amount of private practice and he had a consulting room in St John Street (Manchester's Harley Street), but this was only a minor diversion for him. His dissatisfaction in Manchester never had a personal financial basis. Writing in 1956, his views on private practice were both realistic and amusing:

I know that in five years of private practice (even on two half-days a week) I have learned more about Surgery than in the other twenty years of daily hospital routine. In orthopaedics more than any other branch of surgery it is imperative that an experimental, mechanically-minded, operator should have something to restrain his imagination. One might suggest that mere humanitarian considerations ought to offer the same restraint to any decent-minded surgeon irrespective of the type of patient; in practice this is not so, because British patients are loyal, and disciplined, and whatever the surgeon may say tends automatically to be correct, and the resident rarely tells the surgeon absolutely all the truth. The ultimate test of a newly-evolved mechanical operation is for the inventor to try it on a neurotic private patient and himself be the house surgeon throughout.

Charnley's attitude to administration can be dismissed in a few words. He took his turn as chairman of the committee of surgeons at the Manchester Royal Infirmary and was a member of the committee of management, but when his stint was over he did no more work of this sort regarding it as a waste of time. He also never, or very rarely ever, attended meetings of the Manchester Medical Society, and so did not really take an active part in the city's medical life.

On the other hand, he went to many orthopaedic meetings, as the list of his recorded contributions shows (Chapter 5). He had become a fellow of the British Orthopaedic Association in 1948, and he regularly attended meetings of the association, which are held twice a year, and, in the ten years from 1951 to 1960, he either read papers, or is recorded as taking part in discussions, on twelve occasions. He also contributed to the triennial meetings of the International Society of Orthopaedics and Traumatology in Stockholm, Bern and Barcelona in 1951, 1954 and 1957, respectively. He was a guest at a meeting of the South African Orthopaedic Association in 1955, and visited the country several times subsequently. It is clear that he was well in the mainstream of national and international orthopaedics, and there is no doubt that he was a successful and popular speaker. His original, and sometimes outspoken, ideas did not conform to received wisdom and meant that he remained outside the orthopaedic establishment of London, some of whom regarded this young man from Manchester as rather beyond the pale.

At home, he came to feel that the Manchester Royal Infirmary could not offer him the facilities he needed for his work, and in 1956 he made his first move to free himself from the constraints which he considered were limiting the developments he wanted to achieve. He decided that, in order to carry out research, he would give up three or four of his clinical sessions at the hospital, and he approached both the Nuffield Foundation and the Medical Research Council for support. The risk was clear to him: he might not be able to regain his 'lost' sessions in the National Health Service if his research was not 'self-sustaining' after five years. He wrote:

> . . . this is a risk I must take because: (1) I am sure that I can make a success of the plan finding as I do . . . that the older and more experienced I become the more fruitful my ideas seem to be, and (2) I am a bachelor with private practice (which I conscientiously restrain to two sessions a week, doing no domiciliary consultations) and if the worst came to the worst I would perforce have to develop this source of income.

His basic plan included two interrelated aspects of research: clinical, in relation to the treatment of patients with osteoarthritis of the hip; and biomechanical experiments, to determine the fundamentals of bony union and the conditions governing the spontaneous regeneration of articular cartilage. Although he was convinced that pressure stimulated bone formation in arthrodesis operations, he wanted to apply this principle to animals in order to elucidate the reasons for its success. He was well aware of the difficulties of mimicking his compression techniques in small animals, but he was confident the problem could be overcome. Friction and the lubrication of joints, and the forces acting on the head of the femur, were other matters he intended to study. He wanted also to make and test 'arthroplastic devices', and to test and grade the results of operations using them according to 'engineering principles allied to the mechanical efficiency of machines'.

An essential element in his design was to set up a 'pilot centre for hip surgery', probably at Park Hospital, Davyhulme, provided it was possible to 'obtain official recognition, and official liaison with the University and the Manchester Royal Infirmary':

> The unit I visualise is not conceived on a grandiose scale. The running costs would be low because the project depends on paying for man-hours rather than material. Apparatus would be made in the Department of Engineering and other expenses would be no more than would be needed for . . . rabbits, etc.

Laboratory accommodation would probably be available in the clinical sciences building of the university. Charnley was fortunate because J. H. Kellgren, professor of rheumatology since 1948 and director of rheumatological research, had 'offered to help me in numerous ways, not least in the training of a laboratory technician . . . in bone histology'.

In addition to his own salary for four sessions a week, he was looking for the salaries of a full-time technician and a half-time secretary in his laboratory, and a physiotherapist at the hospital to be attached to his unit. Rather than attempt to establish a post for an engineer, he decided (after discussion with the professors of engineering) that it would be better 'to have the advice and help of various lecturers . . . for individual problems as they arose'.

His proposals were viewed favourably by the clinical research board of the Medical Research Council who offered Charnley a part-time appointment to the Council's external scientific staff for a period of five years in the first instance, on the basis of four research sessions a week. This was minuted in March 1957 and was a notable achievement on Charnley's part. The Nuffield Foundation had also agreed to contribute to the cost of the project.

After all this effort, it is surprising to read the minute of May 1957:

> Mr Charnley had decided, owing to a change in his personal circumstances, not to take up the part-time appointment, which had been offered to him . . .

There is no record of the cause of this volte-face on Charnley's part, but a possible reason is not far to seek. He had met his future wife early in 1957 and was married in June of that year (Chapter 8). Moreover, he may have come to believe it would be possible to set up his centre for hip surgery at Wrightington Hospital; indeed he may have been considering this and his original scheme in tandem. It seems likely that both Sir Harry Platt and Dr F. N. Marshall, who was senior administrative medical officer at the Manchester Regional Hospital Board (Chapter 10), supported the Wrightington scheme and persuaded him that this was the better course for him to take. It also had the advantage of relative safety as he would not have to give up any of his sessions in the Health Service. The two men had considerable influence, both with him personally and in the Manchester region, and they may have been able to assure him that he would get the facilities he needed, which included a biomechanical laboratory. These may well have been the deciding factors. Undoubtedly, he would have thought the whole matter over carefully and at length. Whatever prompted his course of action led to progress which was favourable to him personally and professionally. And it was not long before he made his next move.

In 1958, he wrote to the committee of surgeons at the Manchester Royal Infirmary and requested that he should relinquish three of his four sessions at the United Manchester Hospitals to allow him to set up a centre for hip surgery at Wrightington Hospital (where he had continued doing a certain amount of orthopaedic work). He pointed out that he needed more beds and operating time than were available at the Manchester Royal Infirmary. The committee's minutes of November 10, 1958, show that his colleagues were sympathetic and appreciated the problem as he presented it. They supported his desire to advance his work 'for which he already has an international reputation'. In view of the urgency to set the plan for a regional centre in motion, and in order to defer what would be an irrevocable decision in which Mr Charnley would all but sever his connection with the hospital, two recommendations were made:

(1) that Mr Charnley be granted leave of absence for three of his four sessions for a period of three years, after which the decision would be reviewed.

(2) Mr Charnley would retain one session with the United Manchester Hospitals for an out-patient clinic which would probably be devoted to cases of hip disease.

This generous and far-sighted scheme was supported by the medical board and finally by the Board of Governors medical advisory committee. The fact that his colleagues were not prepared to see him go completely, unless his unit at Wrightington proved to be a success, shows the regard they had for him and his work.

His remaining session at the Royal Infirmary was used for an out-patient clinic for hip disorders, and again he was helped by Professor Kellgren who referred many suitable patients to him for operative treatment. He finally resigned from the Manchester Royal Infirmary and Park Hospital, Davyhulme in 1962. He was, however, able to maintain his many informal contacts in various departments of Manchester University.

The critical events of 1957 and 1958 were an undoubted turning point in Charnley's life. He was now in a position to move forward with his research into disorders of the hip joint. Before coming to Wrightington, we shall look at some aspects of his life at home, and then go on to trace his thinking in the 1950s which led directly to the development of the low friction arthroplasty.

*Chapter 8*

# PERSONAL INTERLUDE

## 1957–1977

*It has been said that the shortcomings of great men are the consolation of ordinary folk. That would explain why people like reading about the eccentricities, bad behaviour, and misfortunes of geniuses.*

Dr Edward Hare 1988

THIS CHAPTER is not intended to represent an interlude in Charnley's life; rather it is an interlude between the chapters which describe his orthopaedic accomplishments, and it will deal with rather more personal matters. The period chosen is also somewhat arbitrary, although 1957 marks an important point in his life; we shall, however, go forward beyond the stage we have reached in his surgical career; and return in subsequent chapters to earlier years when he began his work on the low friction arthroplasty. Personal and professional life are inevitably interwoven, but here it seems convenient to consider them, at least to some extent, separately; although aspects of his orthopaedic career and some of the honours he received will be included at the end of this chapter.

Charnley by 1957 had been settled for ten years in his apartment at Rusholme Gardens and appeared to be living the comfortable life of a bachelor; working long hours in the hospital or his workshop in the medical school. He had contemplated marriage in previous years; it is said that he almost had been persuaded to the church door on one or two occasions, but he always managed to find some reason for avoiding matrimony – perhaps because he valued independence in his single-minded attachment to orthopaedic surgery. None the less, he came to realise that he did not want to 'end up' like some of the elderly bachelors who were living in the same apartment block, or so he told more than one of his friends.

Early in 1957, during his annual skiing holiday in Zürs, an event occurred which changed and enhanced his life. He met Jill Heaver on the slopes and within three months they were married. She was twenty-six and he was forty-six years old. The plan was for a wedding in September, followed by a trip to

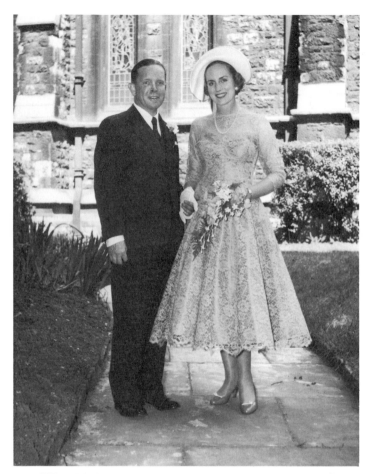

*Jill and John Charnley on their wedding day, June 15, 1957.*

the United States, but there was some hesitation on Charnley's part. Jill, who was working as personal assistant to Sir Norman Joseph, a director of Lyons' catering empire, had no such hesitation. She went to Manchester for the weekend of June 8, and they agreed that if the step was going to be taken, it should be taken straight away. Jill was both determined and a good organiser; she returned to London on Tuesday and, having obtained a special licence, she arranged the wedding for Saturday, June 15, at St Mary Abbott Church in Kensington, followed by a reception at the Cumberland Hotel, Marble Arch. The wedding was a small affair, with twenty-five family and close friends; Brian Thomas was Charnley's best man and Edgar Somerville an usher. The honeymoon was a weekend spent in a riverside hotel at Hurley-on-Thames.

For some months the newly married couple lived in Rusholme Gardens, and Jill Charnley remembers being conscious of the 'old men' looking at her 'over the top of their newspapers' during meals in the restaurant. The kitchen in their flat, which had served at one time as a laboratory, was minute with only a very small Baby Belling electric stove, so life was not altogether easy. It was a relief when they were able to move into a house in Hale in Cheshire about ten miles south-west of Manchester.

Charnley had been invited to lecture at a meeting in Sao Paolo, Brazil, in 1958, and afterwards he and his wife were lent an apartment in Rio de Janeiro for a short holiday; indeed this was really a delayed honeymoon. Most of their time was spent on the Copacabana beach where an episode occurred reminiscent of the title of a poem by Stevie Smith – *Not Waving But Drowning*. Charnley was not a particularly strong swimmer and one day swam off a part of the beach where bathing was not allowed – or so they discovered too late. Jill thought that he was waving affectionately to her, but he was waving for help as he was being sucked under by a fierce undertow. He had to be rescued, somewhat ignominiously for him, by a very large, very dark local lifeguard. He recovered, but developed acute bronchitis and had to spend the rest of his stay in bed. Their first child was born nine months later.

The house which they had found in Hale was called Naemoor, and the previous owners must have been somewhat sentimental Scots; because, in spite of the spelling of moor, the anglicised version was presumably 'nevermore'. One of the first things Charnley did was to convert the attic into an office for his secretary and, more important, a workshop for himself. Helped by Mr Harry Crossley, he moved his tools there from the room which he had been using in the medical school; his lathe created a problem as there was some anxiety as to whether the ceiling would stand its weight. His method of assessing this risk was to lie on his back and draw on paper all the cracks in the plaster – repeating the process every three months until he was sure the cracks were not spreading.

Charnley had come across Crossley when he was looking for a plastic material for the socket of his artificial hip joint (Chapter 9). Crossley was an outspoken Lancastrian with a practical engineering ability which appealed to him. They enjoyed each other's company and met regularly over work and at home.

Some years later, a disastrous fire broke out in the attic, as a result of an electrical fault, while the Charnleys were in Sweden. The workshop was then moved into a prefabricated hut in the garden.

Charnley was interested in his house and accepted Le Corbusier's dictum that it should be 'a machine for living in'. One of his major aims was to achieve efficient and economical heating. He wanted to burn the cheapest British coal, and he went to see the house of a radiological colleague in Knutsford who had an elaborate, but old-fashioned, system of central heating. Naemoor already had a large cast-iron Robin Hood boiler which he set out to adapt. A hopper, which had to be filled once a week with industrial washed shingles, automatically fed the furnace by a large worm. A specially designed mechanism pressed down the clinker as it accumulated in the furnace. At times, when the fire was going full blast, the room was like a blacksmith's forge. If the hopper was not fed regularly, and this chore was often forgotten, the house became filled with smoke. Coal was delivered in loads of three tons and Charnley built a new wall for the coal bunker. He approached this task with his usual careful preparation and attention to detail. He began by reading the appropriate section in the *Encyclopaedia Britannica* on brick-laying to learn how the Romans did it. This activity may not have been unconnected with his admiration for Winston Churchill, who had been an ardent wall-builder in moments of relaxation.

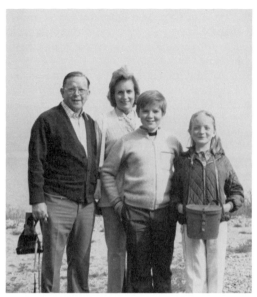

*A family holiday on the Isle of Mull 1970: John, Jill, Tristram and Henrietta.*

The problem of efficient combustion obsessed him for a time and, as with everything he undertook, he pursued it with enormous enthusiasm. On one occasion when he came to lecture in Nottingham, he kept his host up till the early hours of the morning, drinking brandy while expounding on the virtues of his method of fuel combustion. At times, he seemed to feel that his use of solid fuel would be the salvation of Britain's coal-mining industry – if only others would do likewise. This, of course, was a time when oil central-heating was increasingly popular in this country, and when cheap fuel began to become available after the war; cold rooms were no longer considered a virtuous mortification of the flesh.

The house heating episode has been described at some length because it illustrates many of Charnley's characteristics. Any problem he tackled at home, or at work, absorbed him totally; he would read and ask advice, his solutions were sometimes unorthodox, but he carried them out with practical skill.

Ambitious 'do-it-yourself' was certainly well within his grasp. Some years later, an interior designer was asked to produce a scheme for changes in Naemoor. The proposed plans were in the Charles Rennie Mackintosh style and did not appeal to Charnley who wanted something modern and Swedish – his idea was to convert two living-rooms into one, leaving a central fireplace and chimney. He embarked on this himself quite suddenly and unexpectedly one day when Jill was ill in bed. The first she knew about it was when she heard the noise of crashing masonry and came downstairs to find the operation well under way with her husband demolishing the walls with a sledge-hammer. Fortunately, at the time they had a very large strong Dutch girl who was staying with them au pair to look after their small children. She removed seven tons of rubble from the room to the garden in a wheelbarrow. Only a little imagination is needed to conjure up this remarkable scene. Charnley clearly was as intrepid in a new domestic venture as he was when carrying out a new surgical procedure, also he had the ability to persuade someone else to do a great deal of the heavy work. Later Crossley came to help, as he had done before, and they inserted a reinforced joist to support the ceiling. Charnley's friends said that the outcome was a very effective new room.

This kind of domestic activity was meat and drink to Charnley, since he could apply the direct approach, together with the mechanical principles, which was the basis of his orthopaedic surgery. Becoming a family man was a different matter. His son Tristram was born in May 1959, and was a constant surprise to him, as if he never really had expected to become a father. He doted on the new baby, which Jill Charnley says 'was the image of him – apart from the collar and tie'. He would rush home from hospital and go straight to the cot to make sure that everything was all right. He was constantly worried that Tristram might be bored and devised amusements for him. Henrietta, Hetta for short, was born in 1960.

Charnley was an enthusiastic father to his small children, and was good at inventing ingenious games for them. One called 'What'll you do' was usually played in bed on Sunday mornings when he made up complicated stories about grotesque monsters. Another involved Major MacQuerry, a mythical Scotsman, whose elaborately constructed adventures provided hours of amusement. If school homework was difficult, he would apply himself to it; Hetta remembers that, after an evening trying to solve equations, her father presented her the next morning with a poem he had written after she had gone to bed, which explained the method in a way she could easily understand and remember.

Holidays were something of a problem and had to be purposeful as Charnley never could accept the 'bucket-and-spade' type of family holiday at the seaside. A motor launch on the river Nene in Northamptonshire was successful and was followed by similar excursions: one on Lough Erne in the north of Ireland provided some adventure. They sank their boat, a Penguin made of seacrete, in the middle of the lough on a submerged rock. While the family were busy bailing out, their father stood in the stern filming them with his 8 millimetre cine-camera. In other years, they went to Devon, Scotland, once to Finland and their last family holiday together was on the canals of France.

Parents are often a liability to their children as each grow older. Tristram and Hetta were particularly embarrassed by their father's eccentricities when he was away from home. He did not like exposing himself to the sun and always wore both sun glasses and a visor; in France, he even made himself a hat of aluminium foil to prevent the sun from 'boiling his brains'. The family were convinced that this would have precisely the opposite effect. He also shamed them by loudly reciting Chaucer while walking through the streets of Canterbury.

Hetta feels now that she was very much 'Daddy's girl' when she was about ten or twelve years old, but both children went away to boarding school and were swept up by the pressures of adolescence in the 1970s. Shoulder length hair for boys, for example, was an anathema to Charnley. Hetta would lie in a bath to shrink her jeans which he thought extraordinary. The children thought the same when he wore his ski-boots in the bath to soften the leather. There were aspects of his children's life which Charnley simply was not able to comprehend or accept, and he gradually grew apart from them as they approached adulthood; acknowledging with regret that there was a two-generation gap between him and his children. Happily, towards the end of his life, mutual understanding and respect developed.

In the late 1960s, the Charnleys decided they needed a bigger house; Charnley told his wife that if she could find a piece of land within ten minutes' drive from the M6 motorway, she could buy it. Wrightington is only two or three miles from the motorway, going north from Manchester, and he was wanting a rapid drive to work. By chance, Jill Charnley discovered a plot of land at Mere, near Knutsford, which fulfilled his criterion, and so they bought it. An architect was consulted and produced plans which they did not like. At some expense they disengaged themselves from him, and decided to start again. A lecture tour to Finland seemed a good opportunity to see what they thought would be the best of modern architecture, but their hosts all lived in apartments, and they did not get any ideas. On the way back, while waiting in Copenhagen airport, they sketched out their own plan. Expense was not spared, although this resulted in a considerable financial burden for a time, to make the house easy to run and economical to maintain. They found a second architect who agreed to put their scheme into practice. An unusual feature was that the main living-room was upstairs so that they had a view over the top of the trees which gave the house its name – Birchwood. The floors of all the downstairs rooms were tiled with travertine, and the walls were of natural wood and exposed brick; only the bedrooms were plastered. A special system of blown-air central heating was installed to avoid the dirt from conventional radiators. The prefabricated workshop from Naemoor was transferred to the garden.

Charnley had rather scorned the idea of a swimming-pool, but Frau Müller (the wife of Professor Maurice Müller from Bern, Switzerland) was staying with them and told him firmly 'you must swim' – so a pool was built. Birchwood was Charnley's pride and joy; designing it as an efficient house and living in it gave him great pleasure. The garden was entirely Jill Charnley's creation, and he took no part in looking after it.

In the early years of their married life, Charnley usually arrived home from hospital at about six o'clock in the evening, and expected to eat straightaway. After relaxing for an hour or so, he retired to his study to write, or to his workshop. This pattern changed over time, he slept less well and would get up before dawn. He had a small room next to the main bedroom, which his family called the 'monk's cell', where he could read when he was unable to sleep; and a small kitchenette for making tea which he would drink in great quantities.

As he grew older and worked even harder, a gin and tonic was called for to revive him when he arrived home tired. Although not a wine drinker, he had installed a temperature controlled wine cupboard which was lined with polystyrene – and the excess heat from the unit was used to warm the lavatory next to it. He smoked only intermittently, but took it up out of sheer perversity when the statistics about the link with lung cancer were first put forward. He considered that the connection had not been proved and smoked out of defiance for a time.

Christmas was not a day he enjoyed. He did not go to church and the secular festivities held little appeal for him. He might go to Wrightington in the morning, return home for lunch, and then work again at the hospital in the evening. He resented the increasing length of the Christmas–New Year holiday and might show his boredom by retiring to bed on Boxing Day. He did, however, at one time take an interest in the technical aspects of cooking the turkey without making it dry. He suggested cooking it upside down and also injected liquid butter under the skin. He was prepared to do his duty and carve, with some reluctance, but his family say that he did so rather badly.

Charnley disliked cocktail and dinner parties and avoided them whenever possible, although the residents from the hospital were entertained regularly to Sunday lunch. There were also parties for incoming and outgoing groups of doctors from the hospital. He did not enjoy small talk, but he was always ready to discuss any aspect of orthopaedics. As more surgeons came to see his new operation, one or two were invited to stay at Birchwood on most weeks. Dr Lou Brady from Winter Park, Florida, visited Wrightington with Dr Bill Enneking in 1970 and they and their wives were invited to dinner:

> That evening we discovered that the formidable figure at conference and in surgery was truly a warm and charming host who was complemented by his even more charming hostess wife, Jill. The roots of a lasting and cherished friendship were put down that evening.

Later Brady wrote:

> I rather suspect that the majority of those who came in contact with John looked on him as cold and aloof . . . I was privileged to know [him] as a warm, kind and almost shy man. His love for his family . . . and concern for the welfare of his children . . . was touching and very real.

It would be unfair to say that orthopaedics was Charnley's only raison d'être, although perhaps his tongue was in his cheek when he completed his entry in *Who's Who*. Under 'recreations', he first gave 'skiing two weeks a year, otherwise none', and later changed this to 'other than surgery, none'; but this was never wholly true.

He certainly continued skiing; and for a time he had what he described as a 'nest-egg' in St Moritz where he went for a number of years. He joined the British Orthopaedic Ski Group at its second meeting in 1970 and went with them to Zürs for the next two years. He gave up in 1973 writing to say that 'he could not take the risk of breaking a leg with so many people relying on him' – presumably to do their hip replacements. He had only ever skied with orthopaedic colleagues; neither Jill nor the children ever joined him, although he taught Hetta to ice-skate.

Fly-fishing occupied him for a time in the 1970s; he practised casting on the lawn at Birchwood, and occasionally fished in Scotland. He was never particularly successful, but enjoyed the names of the flies and the knot-tying. After an orthopaedic meeting in the United States, he and Jill were taken deep-sea fishing off the Florida Keys by their hosts, Dr and Mrs Lou Brady. The weather was appalling, but Charnley insisted on going out. He ignored the high seas and caught a dolphin which he hung on the wall of his study at Birchwood. In order to repay their hospitality, the Charnleys invited the Bradys to a holiday in Corfu in 1973, with his old friend Brian Thomas and his wife. This is one of the very few times that Charnley ever took a holiday that was not preceded or followed by an orthopaedic visit or meeting, or which had some other active purpose.

He remained an enthusiastic motorist, but he no longer did his own repairs and maintenance. The Aston Martin DB4, which he had bought in 1954, was irreparably damaged in an accident when he was returning from a meeting in Liverpool in 1959 – fortunately he was not hurt. Perhaps it was in recognition of his family responsibilities that he now bought a Humber Supersnipe, a large staid car. He wished to buy British, but after a second Supersnipe, he decided that the only reliable car for him was a Mercedes Benz, whose workmanship he appreciated in spite of his feelings of guilt at buying a German car. An Australian registrar remembers that the car did not always start readily on icy winter evenings, having been parked at the hospital all day. He is quite certain that Charnley's method of drying the distributor was to pour methylated spirits over it and apply a match which was followed by an alarming whoosh of flame. This seems somewhat unlikely (do Mercedes ever fail to start?), but there is more than a spark of truth in the story. The method was characteristic as Charnley was an impatient man and would not want to waste time drying the distributor and points in the conventional way – also, although what he did was risky, it was effective.

Reading when he had time for it, remained a pleasure and he returned to his childhood favourites, re-reading, for example, *Tristram Shandy* on several occasions. But the classics take time to read, and it cannot be denied that he was primarily absorbed by orthopaedic literature. He was, however, able to become remarkably well informed on subjects which caught his interest – Darwin's theory of evolution, for instance. He read *The Origin of Species*, *The Descent of Man* and *The Journal of a Voyage in HMS Beagle* critically and was convinced that Darwin was wrong. He would expound his own ideas for hours on end with family and friends. *The New Scientist*, a weekly magazine, provided him with a wide view of scientific matters, and he read it regularly for some years. He argued passionately with his residents at Wrightington about the rights and wrongs of various scientific theories.

Charnley had always enjoyed listening to classical music, but a curious idiosyncrasy made it impossible for him to go to concerts or, for that matter, the theatre. He was quite unable to tolerate extraneous noise, in the same way as he could not bear hearing people snore. Coughing or the crackling of sweet-papers were unbearable distractions, and he could not stand those near him crunching toast or an apple – indeed, his wife learnt to avoid eating such food in his presence.

Rather surprisingly, he was untidy and not at all well organised. His office has been described as a 'nightmare' and his workshop a 'shambles', and he did not have a simple method of dealing with the ordinary affairs of life. He relied very much on other people to tidy up after him, and to make sure that he fulfilled his social obligations.

Bad temper could be sparked off easily, and often he was not able to control his irritation. This was the case at home and at work. The stimulus to such outbursts was, more often than not, his feeling that the recipient of his wrath had been either lazy or stupid, or both. He always demanded the highest standards of work and behaviour in himself, and in others. When he had been unfair or unjust, a willingly given apology often restored the situation. Relatively small things seemed to produce a disproportionate disturbance, and on more serious matters he could become emotional and easily moved to tears when he was deeply upset.

But the overwhelming impression which Charnley gave to those who met him was his bubbling enthusiasm, although those who failed to come up to his expectations saw a different side. He could be highly critical of others when they did not meet his approval. Friends and those who supported him received the utmost loyalty. Manchester contemporaries continue to hold him in the highest regard, not only for his contribution to orthopaedic surgery, but as a good friend over many years.

Charnley's political views were basically right wing. He did, however, loyally read the *Manchester Guardian*, but when it became *The Guardian* he changed to the conservative *Daily Telegraph*. He became progressively disturbed by his belief that the British people were becoming dilatory and lazy. He felt that the Conservative government had let things slide in the 1960s and, he believed, when Harold Wilson became prime minister of a socialist government, the new theme of 'white-hot technology' might bring about a revival; but his conversion was short-lived. Strong patriotic instincts led him to write vehement letters to the newspapers – which he usually committed to the waste-paper basket in the cold light of the following morning.

One letter to the *Manchester Guardian* on January 28, 1960 was published under the heading 'Weakening the NHS'. Many British doctors were emigrating to North America and Charnley did not think that the fact should be allowed to pass unnoticed:

> While this emigration is going on the resident posts in our hospitals are frequently being filled by coloured doctors on a temporary basis. Does this indicate a healthy, self-sustaining medical service? Does the fabric of my old teaching hospital, the Manchester Royal Infirmary, indicate buoyant economy in nationalised medicine?
>
> We would all like to see our Health Service prosper but it seems to me that it is still functioning largely through the backbone of men whom it inherited during the first five years of its existence . . . if British medicine is permanently to hold its world-wide prestige, the public and the Government will have to consider a formidable increase in the annual budget.

Underlying this letter is a hint of Charnley's chauvinism and his colour prejudice. The latter issue is much more sensitive now than it was then, and he did not hesitate to let his opinion be known. It was a side to his character which cannot be ignored, but it is important to understand that his opinions were not the product of superficial prejudice, but were based on careful thought. He expressed his views in a letter written to a friend in 1970:

> I hold strong racialist views . . . which I consider to be noble and intellectual . . . I hold that sloppy thinking in Britain will destroy the character of this country for our children . . . Only will respect for the coloured people be acquired (and in particular I mean the most dangerous of the lot – the Asians) until they stay in, or return to, their own countries and build them up into proud nations by getting rid of the corruption, nepotism and avarice which has reduced them to their present state – which national characteristics they are bringing into the British scene with I know not what consequences for our children. I was one of the first to see the dangers of emigration of British doctors to Canada and to write to the Manchester Guardian about it ten years ago [this is the letter just quoted] when it was pooh-poohed as sensationalism . . .

Although Charnley's dramatic predictions have not come about, the problem has not gone away.

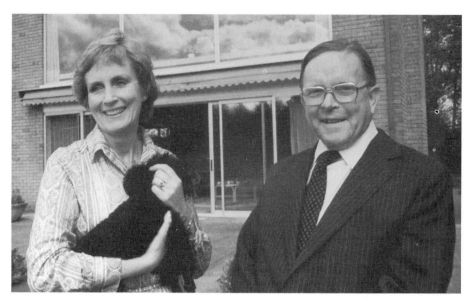

*John and Jill Charnley at Birchwood in the late 1970s.*

At one time he was considered for senior office in the British Orthopaedic Association, and after a long discussion with his wife, he thought that he might accept the proposal which had been put to him. But, waking at five o'clock the following morning, he replied:

> I saw everything with the extraordinary clarity which this time of day brings and I was absolutely sure that I was right to decline . . . The older I get the more urgent seems to become the tempo of life. I live as tho' I might have only a year or two left to me and I must get everything into it while there is time. Anything which takes me off my main purpose is frustrating and tedious.
>
> I feel rather like someone running a race or exploring an area where time is against me; I deliberately shed things which could be of value later in life merely to make sure I gain the nearest objective safely.

He goes on to say that he has recently 'shed the University', and that he had not gone to orthopaedic meetings in Australia and Mexico, and declined an invitation to be the president's guest lecturer at the American Academy of Orthopaedic Surgeons meeting.

> . . . I am now more absorbed when than I was as a young man – I think because I have retained something of my enthusiasm and creative urge and this has now become grafted on to a rather amazing fund of experience accumulated in one field – the result is a very effective 'think-tank' and I feel that if I don't make full use of it I am sinning in the New Testament parable sense!
>
> . . . but I am so engrossed in the hip-joint that I fear I shall let it spoil in the latest stages . . . now that the main challenge is over. And this is

not from lack of interest – it is merely that I cannot permit myself to spend the number of hours needed to think and think and plan when there are other matters I find more urgent and unexplored.

It is clear that this letter was written under some emotional stress. None the less, it does reveal several aspects of his character. He was prepared to sacrifice professional advance, which many of his colleagues would have considered important, in order to avoid the distractions of administration.

A year later his work was publicly recognised when he was made a Companion of the Order of the British Empire. Moreover, although he said he had 'shed the University', he accepted a special chair in the University of Manchester in 1972, and thenceforward was Professor Charnley. Later in his career, when he was more certain of the success of his aspirations, he accepted other honours and awards, and he was prepared to travel overseas to attend meetings and to lecture (Chapter 16).

We now need to return to the early 1950s and consider the ideas which led to the development of Charnley's successful low friction arthroplasty.

Chapter 9

# THE GROWTH OF AN IDEA
## 1951–1961

*The cart has been put before the horse; the artificial joint has been made and used, and now we are trying to find out how and why it fails.*

John Charnley 1956

IN THE YEARS after the war, and while he was working in Manchester, Charnley gradually evolved his concept of a low friction arthroplasty. He had become intrigued by the way animal joints were lubricated and he carried out laboratory investigations in collaboration with engineering colleagues to test his ideas. This led to the search for a new material with a low coefficient of friction which could be used in an artificial joint.

The history of arthroplasty of the hip has been recorded by Professor Scales[25] who gave credit for the first such operation to Thomas Gluck in Germany in 1890; followed by the Robert Jones gold foil arthroplasty in 1895 and Hey-Groves' replacement of the femoral head with an ivory prosthesis in 1922 – the last two procedures being carried out in the United Kingdom. The first total hip replacement is credited to P. W. Wiles[28] and was inserted into a patient in 1938 at the Middlesex Hospital in London. This was a stainless steel device, the femoral and acetabular parts being fixed to the bones with screws. None of these procedures were successful enough to be adopted generally. But, as so often is the case, failure resulted in subsequent improvements.

Scales described Dr M. N. Smith-Petersen, of Boston, Massachusets, as 'the doyen of arthroplasty of the hip'. Smith-Petersen introduced the mould or cup arthroplasty, using glass, in 1923. The first metal cup was inserted in 1938[26], and the operation began to be used in the United Kingdom after the war. An advantage was that very little bone was removed, so further procedures might be undertaken, if necessary. Many surgeons found that their results were disappointing, and some welcomed the idea of replacing the patient's femoral

99

head with an acrylic prosthesis. This operation, devised by the Judet brothers[20] who were orthopaedic surgeons in Paris, had been introduced in London by Mr St. J. D. Buxton and Mr K. I. Nissen. It was simple to perform and the immediate results were remarkably good. Unfortunately, the acrylic wore and broke in many of the patients, and invariably became loose in the bone. Moreover, the method of fixation was inadequate and the material itself was not sufficiently durable. Further, a large piece of bone was discarded so any subsequent operations were difficult and unsatisfactory. As a result of this experience, orthopaedic surgeons acknowledged that collaboration with engineers was essential if any kind of satisfactory artificial joint was to be designed to replace an arthritic joint in the human body.

In a grant application written in 1956, Charnley recorded that he had developed an arthroplasty of the hip ten years previously. This was similar to the Judet operation but after a preliminary trial, he abandoned his method as being unsatisfactory. He then embarked on what he acknowledged was regarded as the retrograde step of concentrating on improving methods of arthrodesis. Outwardly, he remained sceptical about the possibility of a successful arthroplasty ever being devised. He said in 1951 that such an operation, if carried out in the first half of life 'would probably not last more than ten years, and that it rarely increased the range of movement'[1]; and it was many years before he changed this opinion. The British Orthopaedic Association held a debate on the motion 'in the opinion of this house all methods of arthroplasty of the hip have failed to achieve their purpose' and Charnley spoke in support.[2] He was still uncertain in 1955 about future developments as his reported comments at a meeting of the South African Orthopaedic Association make clear: replacement arthroplasty of the hip was 'doomed to failure if only because of the coefficients of friction involved between metal or acrylic material on the one hand, and bone or cartilage on the other'.[4] And as late as 1957, he was still advocating his central dislocation type of arthrodesis for osteoarthritis when only one hip was involved.[5]

Notwithstanding the difficulties, Mr G. K. McKee in Norwich was certainly not in any way discouraged in his search for a total joint replacement. By 1940 he had designed and made model prostheses[23], but these were never actually used in patients as World War Two intervened. McKee served in the Royal Army Medical Corps and began working on artificial joints again after he was demobilised. In 1951, he reported to a meeting of the East Anglian Orthopaedic Club[22] that he had inserted artificial hip joints into three patients, and he showed these patients at a clinical session of the British Orthopaedic Association in Cambridge in the same year. The design was a ball and socket joint made of stainless steel, and the components were held in position by screws. Two of these prostheses became loose, but the third had screws made of chrome–cobalt alloy and these remained tight in the bone. He redesigned the joint in 1953 using a femoral component similar to the Thompson femoral head prosthesis[27] which he had seen during a visit to America. The metal used was vinertia, a form of chrome–cobalt alloy. This model was put into 40 patients between 1956 and 1960 with a success rate of 54%, and he recognised that failure was due to loosening of the components.[23] McKee was an exceptionally versatile and inventive orthopaedic surgeon who devised many new operative techniques, including a method of fixation used in arthrodesis of the hip. He deserves great credit for persevering with total hip replacement, at a time when Charnley was still pessimistic about the outcome of this type of operation.

Suffice it to say at this point, that McKee realised that the bone cement which Charnley had introduced in the late 1950s (Chapter 11) was likely to be the answer to the problem of loosening.

We must now leave the pioneering work in Norwich and return to Manchester. While these developments had been taking place, Charnley had begun to think about arthroplasty of the hip; although, in practice, he was still advocating arthrodesis. He continued to carry out this procedure until the early 1960s, but he cannot have been entirely satisfied with it as he acknowledged that research was needed to find a reliable arthroplasty, 'even if its use is confined to bilateral osteoarthritis and rheumatoid arthritis'.[9] This was a measure of his conservatism since arthrodesis or a stabilising operation is not a practical proposition when both hips, or other joints, are badly damaged by chronic arthritis.

It is important to understand that Charnley's response to the challenge of producing a successful arthroplasty was not now to devise an ingenious new implant and start using it in patients as soon as possible. To the contrary, he thought deeply about the problem, and his first approach arose from following up a chance observation; an example, indeed, of the serendipity which he had commended to del Sel (Chapter 4). A patient, who had had his femoral head replaced with a Judet acrylic prosthesis two years previously, was attending the out-patient clinic at the Manchester Royal Infirmary and reported that his artificial hip squeaked when he leaned forward. The noise was so loud that his wife avoided being in the same room as him whenever possible.[17]

Charnley had become aware of a similar phenomenon in other patients who had had this operation. The squeaking was usually short-lived and occurred only in patients who had had osteoarthritis, and never in those in whom the femoral head had been replaced as treatment for a recent fracture of the neck of the femur. He attributed this to the fact that in osteoarthritic hips the articular cartilage of the acetabulum was worn away by the disease, whereas after a fracture the articular cartilage was normal. This was the observation which led him to suspect that loosening of the femoral prosthesis was related to the degree of frictional resistance developing between it and the floor of the acetabulum.[11] When the squeak stopped, he reasoned that it was not because lubrication had improved, but rather because the prosthesis had loosened. He proposed that the problem should first be tackled by investigating friction and lubrication in normal joints, before searching for a suitable material from which to make an artificial joint. His first approach was, therefore, essentially biological rather than mechanical.

Charnley's ideas were developed in discussions with engineering colleagues, particularly Drs F. J. Edwards and R. I. Tanner who were lecturers in Professor Diamond's department of mechanical engineering in the University of Manchester. His close collaboration with these two men taught him a great deal about lubrication and was vitally important to the whole of his future thinking on the subject.

The classic paper on joint lubrication was written in 1932 by M. A. MacConnaill[21], who was professor of anatomy in Cork University. MacConnaill inferred that, since the surfaces of joints are not congruous, there must be wedge-shaped films of synovial fluid at their edges, and therefore hydrodynamic lubrication was present. In this type of lubrication a very thin film of fluid separated the joint surfaces, and the friction present depended on the viscosity of the film. The essential features were the geometry of the surfaces and the viscosity of the fluid.

Charnley realised, even before beginning experimental work, that there were 'serious theoretical criticisms which make the hydrodynamic theory unlikely'. His arguments can be briefly summarised: first, articular cartilage was resilient so the surfaces must be intimately applied to each other when carrying loads; second, hydrodynamic lubrication was known not to be suited to conditions where the motion was reciprocating since the fluid film would be destroyed; and, third, it was not easy to achieve such lubrication with slow-moving surfaces.

Boundary lubrication, on the other hand, had the opposite characteristics since its essential features were the quality of the substances making up the sliding surfaces and the nature of the lubricating fluid. In this situation the lubricant had an affinity for the surface it lubricated, so that when motion took place it was between monomolecular films of lubricant chemically adherent to the underlying surface. This type of lubrication was exactly suited to conditions in which hydrodynamic lubrication was not: slow reciprocating motion under heavy load.

Charnley argued that there were theoretical grounds for believing that the conditions of lubrication of human joints were more akin to boundary than to hydrodynamic lubrication. He was, however, aware that in engineering practice it was unusual to find a pure example of either type on its own; both mechanisms usually occurred together and this was known as 'quasi-hydrodynamic' lubrication. These considerations were undoubtedly informed, not only by reading, but after discussion with his engineering colleagues. They have been described here because they illustrate Charnley's basic approach to the problem.

His next step was to attempt to measure the coefficient of friction ($\mu$) of articular cartilage. This could be done quite simply in an engineering laboratory, but it was not so easy in animal or human joints since the cartilage cannot be fashioned into a plane surface. Charnley was able to find only two papers which were relevant. These were written by a Dr E. S. Jones in 1934 and 1936 and published in *The Lancet*. Jones is rather a mysterious figure and is said to have been a general practitioner in Leeds, or sometimes Newcastle. As a matter of record, his entries in the medical directories of the 1930s show that he had qualified at Birmingham University in 1918, and that he became a general practitioner in Droitwich, near Worcester. No details are given of his research. In his first paper[18], Jones described experiments he had done with horses' stifle (knee) joints using a simple apparatus. He found that the coefficient of friction was remarkably low ($\mu = 0.02$) when the joint was lubricated with either synovial fluid or saline. In his next paper[19], he reported he used an amputated finger joint moving in a modified Stanton pendulum. This device had originally been used by Dr Stanton, who was an engineer working in the National Physical Laboratory, to study friction in heavily loaded bearings, and it consisted of a pendulum swinging through a few degrees with the bearing under test as its pivot.

Charnley believed that Jones' experiments were open to various theoretical objections and decided to make measurements on a freshly amputated human knee joint. An apparatus was built by his engineering colleagues, and set up in part of the physiology laboratory in the medical school. All the ligaments and soft tissues were removed from the knee and the arrangement was such that the femoral condyles were allowed to slide against the corresponding articular surface of the tibia. Seven experiments were carried out and the coefficient of friction in the human knee was found to be quite remarkably low ($\mu = 0.005$–$0.023$,

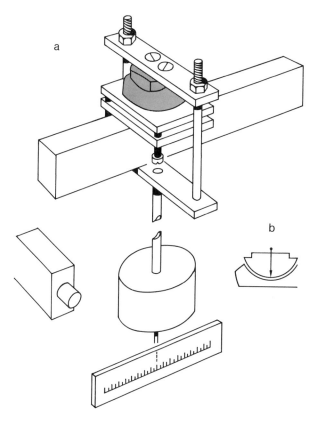

*An illustration showing Charnley's experimental rig to determine the coefficient of friction in a cadaveric human ankle (shaded). The inset b shows the shape of the surfaces which are upside down in relation to their position in the body.*

average 0.013) and there was no difference when the joint was dry or when there was an excess of synovial fluid on the moving surfaces.[6]

The next step was to repeat the Jones finger experiments, but in order to overcome some of its defects, Charnley used the human ankle. A new pendulum rig was built which was also a modification of Stanton's pendulum. Again different results from Jones' were obtained and Charnley concluded that the predominant mechanism in joint lubrication was a boundary phenomenon.

The extraordinarily low coefficient of friction in animal joints was better than that of a skate sliding on ice ($\mu = 0.03$); this intrigued Charnley and led him to wonder whether synovial fluid might possess properties as a lubricant not known in engineering. He deduced from the experimental evidence of other workers that this was not likely. Although synovial fluid had the property of providing strong films, which might have some action in stationary joints under load, there were no grounds for supposing that such films could explain the low friction of a joint in motion. To prove this he and his colleagues constructed an artificial joint which had the basic shape and average dimensions of an adult ankle joint. The engineers insisted that the joint should be lapped to a fit of 1/10 000 of an

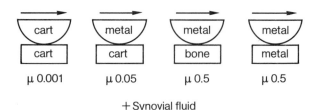

μ 0.001          μ 0.05          μ 0.5          μ 0.5

+ Synovial fluid

*Charnley's diagram drawn to show typical coefficients of friction in a normal joint (cartilage on cartilage) and between different materials used in hip arthroplasty in the 1950s (metal on cartilage, metal on bone, and metal on metal).*

inch, but even then the results showed that synovial fluid was unable to maintain hydrodynamic lubrication. Indeed this could not be maintained even by the thickest lubricating oil at a load less than half that of an adult at a rate corresponding to walking speed. Perhaps it should be said at this point that, in the 1990s, pendulum testing is considered to be insufficiently sensitive to make relevant measurements of friction in human joints, and more sophisticated techniques have been developed.[14]

Charnley had begun his investigations in the early 1950s, and in 1954 he read a paper at the autumn meeting of the British Orthopaedic Association on 'the "slipperiness" of articular cartilage'; and in this he gave a report of his experimental work.[3] He also published papers on 'the lubrication of animal joints' in the *Proceedings of the Institution of Mechanical Engineers*[6] and in *The New Scientist*[7] in 1959. In the same year he gave a similar paper to a joint meeting of the British Society of Physical Medicine and the Heberden Society when he also discussed the relevance of his results to 'surgical reconstruction by arthroplasty'.[8] (The account of his work which has already been given in this chapter, and some of that which follows, has been summarised from these publications.)

Charnley's thinking and collaborative research ultimately led to the concept of what he called a low friction arthroplasty which was one of his most important contributions to the design of a successful total hip replacement. His aim was to find two bearing surfaces of dissimilar materials and with a low coefficient of friction which would not need artificial lubrication. The forces on the two components of the joint would thus be reduced thereby decreasing the risk of loosening.

Further tests were carried out using the pendulum rig to compare the friction found in a normal joint with that encountered between bone and the materials commonly used in arthroplasties at that time; for example, stainless steel, cobalt–chrome alloy and polymethylmethacrylate (acrylic or perspex). Even when lubricated with ox synovial fluid, which was the best experimental substitute for human synovial fluid, the coefficient of friction of bare bone against these artificial substances was always high ($\mu = 0.4$ compared with $\mu = 0.013$ in a normal joint). The kind of squeak which had occurred after an acrylic femoral head replacement (Judet) could be reproduced. Furthermore, normal articular cartilage retained its remarkable low friction property when tested against steel or perspex. This confirmed his clinical observations which have already been described.

In the late 1950s, most orthopaedic surgeons were replacing the femoral head with a metal prosthesis (if they were attempting any form of arthroplasty), and this operation can be properly called a hemi-arthroplasty – replacement of one half of the joint. This type of prosthesis had a metal head and a long stem which was inserted into the medullary canal of the femur. The hope was that the greater strength of metal, as opposed to plastic, would eliminate wear and breakage. Unfortunately, there were other disadvantages: loosening still occurred (in spite of the improved fixation) and the metal head could penetrate the abnormal bone of the acetabulum in patients with arthritis. A more promising approach was to replace the whole joint, rather than only one half of it, and McKee developed this method using metal for the bearing surfaces; a procedure Charnley now followed, but with a very important difference.

Since his experimental work had suggested that an artificial joint could not be adequately lubricated by body fluids (and there was no practical prospect of introducing an external lubricant), Charnley began looking for a 'slippery substance' which would be suitable for the socket of a total hip replacement. As was his habit, he sought help from experts in the field; it is known that he went to the plastics division of the Imperial Chemical Industries Limited (ICI). He also acknowledged valuable advice from Dr Philip Love who was scientific director of the Glacier Metal Company, at Wembley in London. ICI, who were developing new types of fluorocarbon polymers, put Charnley in touch with Henry Crossley (Packings) Limited of Bolton, Lancashire, a firm using these materials in engineering applications such as in making valve seatings and non-lubricated bearings. Charnley thus was introduced to polytetrafluorethylene (PTFE) which was known in industry as Teflon or Fluon. The coefficient of friction was very low, but its characteristics in the human body were not known, although biological assay indicated that it was exceptionally inert. Charnley worked closely with Harry Crossley and eventually he decided that it would be justifiable to use PTFE in patients because it seemed to have the ideal properties for the socket of an artificial hip joint.

It is not clear from Charnley's writings exactly when this surgical experiment was begun. In one paper, given at a meeting in July 1959[8], he said: 'this material has been used in arthroplasty of the hip . . . for nearly three years' which suggests late in 1956. Later, he wrote that he 'decided in 1958 that the only chance of success in lubricating an artificial joint would be by using surfaces which were intrinsically slippery on each other . . . This led to trials of PTFE . . .'.[12] Although it would be satisfying historically to be able to record the exact date on which the first low friction arthroplasty was carried out, it will become apparent in due course why this date is not especially significant. Furthermore, since most surgical techniques evolve by small steps, exact dates do not necessarily have great significance.

PTFE is white, semi-translucent, looking rather like articular cartilage and it can be cut with a knife. Charnley wrote in 1961 that it 'is chemically the most inert plastic so far discovered'.[11] In the first instance he used it as a 'synthetic articular cartilage', lining the acetabulum with a thin shell of the plastic and covering the femoral head, which he re-shaped, with a hollow cup of the same material. The use of PTFE was original to Charnley, and this type of 'double cup' arthroplasty was re-introduced many years later by other surgeons using different materials; long after he had decided that the principle was incorrect.

The absolute relief of pain in Charnley's earliest cases, and the range of hip movement under muscular control, were impressive within the first three months

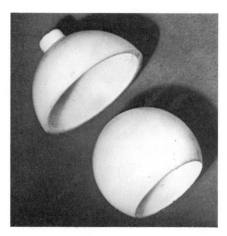

*Charnley's original 'double cup' made of PTFE (Teflon).*

after operation. One of the merits of this technique was the conservation of as much as possible of the bones of the hip joint, only a very small amount being removed and discarded. But Charnley soon appreciated that, in pressing the plastic sphere over the re-shaped femoral head, the blood supply to the bone was likely to be damaged so that a limited area of the bone might not survive. This complication had also occurred after Smith-Petersen's original cup arthroplasty, and in the double cups (now called surface replacement) introduced in more recent years by other surgeons.

Charnley moved on to a more radical solution. He excised (and discarded) the head of the femur and replaced it with a metallic implant which was already in use. He chose the Moore prosthesis[24] and combined it with a low friction PTFE socket inserted into the acetabulum.

An entirely new factor was now introduced. Charnley began using dental acrylic cement to fix the prosthesis in the femur (but not to fix the socket at this stage). This step revolutionised the development of total hip replacement and is so important that Chapter 11 will be devoted to describing the origins of the method and its consequences. At this point, the reader is asked to accept without question that bone cement is a satisfactory method of fixation.

The results of the PTFE socket with a cemented Moore's prosthesis were 'gratifying' (Charnley's word[11]), but he was not satisfied. His engineering colleagues had pointed out to him that the best engineering practice would be to use the smallest diameter of ball on the femoral prosthesis which would withstand the expected load. The main advantages of this would be: firstly, to reduce frictional torque; and secondly, to allow a thicker PTFE socket to be used. With a thick socket and a small femoral head, the difference in radii between the two favours the socket remaining stationary in the acetabular bone; this is not the case when the difference in radii is only small. Furthermore, there was more material if wear occurred in the future. The diameter of Moore's prosthesis was 42 mm ($1\frac{5}{8}$ inch) and Charnley began by reducing this to 28 mm ($1\frac{1}{8}$ inch); then to 25 mm (1 inch), and finally to 22.25 mm ($\frac{7}{8}$ inch). At the same time, he redesigned the configuration of the stem. The minimum size of head

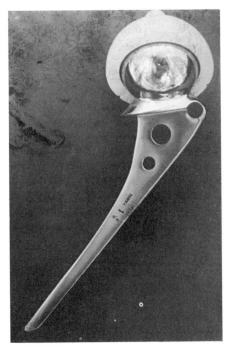

*Hip replacement using a PTFE (Teflon) socket and a Moore prosthesis. (This illustration has been taken from an old lecture slide.)*

was determined by the need to avoid the risk of dislocation, although Charnley later came to believe that the stability of the artificial joint depended entirely on the fibrous sleeve which develops to form the new capsule. He was totally convinced of the correctness of the theory behind the small head and, although many orthopaedic surgeons thought he was wrong (and were worried about dislocation), he never wavered in his opinion. Other reasons for his preference will be discussed in subsequent chapters.

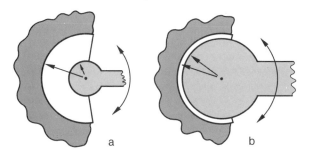

*Diagram showing the low friction principle and the advantage of a small femoral head. Charnley's legend read: "Original illustration of the low friction torque principle applied to hip arthroplasty.* **a** *Thick socket – small femoral head: difference in radii favours socket remaining stationary;* **b** *not so with only slight difference in radii". (From* Low Friction Arthroplasty of the Hip [LFA] *by courtesy of the publisher).*

So now we have seen that the operation evolved through two stages and Charnley described them, together with his third (and, for the moment, final) modification in an article in *The Lancet* published in May 1961.[11] The third design consisted of a PTFE socket with a central spigot on its outer surface, which was hammered into a hole drilled in the floor of the acetabulum; and a stainless steel femoral component with a small head and a long stem that was fixed inside the femur with bone cement. The hip was approached by raising the greater trochanter with its attached muscles; the trochanter was re-attached with wire at the end of the operation. Initially, the patient was put into a plaster cast, which included the trunk and the leg on the side of the operation, for three weeks after the operation. It was soon found that this immobilisation in plaster was not essential – which was fortunate for the patients.

Two important features had been established: the first was the low friction principle; and the second was the use of bone cement. These formed the basis of all his subsequent designs.

The report in *The Lancet* was based on 97 arthroplasties carried out between January 1960 and the time of writing the paper, so the follow up period was relatively short. There were no deaths, except for one due to a heart attack occurring six weeks after operation. The patients were kept in hospital for an average of eight weeks, and then were able to walk without sticks and with a slight limp. The results were claimed to be satisfactory, especially with regard to the relief of pain. The only disappointing cases were those who had had a previous operation; and salvage operations are never easy.

PTFE is radiolucent and so invisible in radiographs; its rate of wear in the body would be suggested if serial films showed that the metal appeared to get nearer to the bony floor of the acetabulum. Charnley wrote that 'while long-term results are awaited . . . close scrutiny of the radiographs of the patients who had been transmitting the full weight of the body through this implant for ten months has shown negligible wear'. He was, however, cautious because he emphasised that the stresses imposed on hip joints of patients with arthritis were only a fraction of those borne by normal people. The operation was only performed in 'subjects with the poor muscles and relatively feeble morale which so often accompany long-continued ill-health and old age'. His attitude was nevertheless optimistic as he published these early results, and he must have felt confident that he was close to finding a satisfactory total hip replacement.

The stainless steel femoral components were manufactured to his design by Chas. F. Thackray Ltd, but Charnley made the PTFE sockets himself, turning them on his lathe in the medical school, and later at home when he had moved his workshop to Naemoor.

The next chapter will describe the disastrous consequences of using PTFE and will recount the way he coped with the major problems which this failure produced.

Before completing this part of the story, it is convenient to look at two other aspects of his work: first, his collaboration with engineers; and, second, his general approach to the clinical problems of the surgery of the hip joint.

It has already been made clear that, although Charnley had no formal engineering training, he was a good workshop craftsman and he had an innate mechanical sense. Certainly, he learnt from his engineering colleagues and collaborated with them, both in experimental work and in writing scientific papers, always acknowledging their help and frequently naming them as co-authors. He was associated mainly with the department of mechanical engineering at Manchester University and later at the University of Manchester Institute of Science and Technology (UMIST). He also sought advice from departments of engineering in other universities, notably Leeds, and from many sources in industry. In short, he went wherever he thought he could best get the information and help he needed.

His published views on the realities of collaboration between surgeons and engineers are, therefore, somewhat surprising. An annotation in *The Lancet* on the matter in 1961[13] stimulated this response in a letter from Charnley:

> In my view the failure of British surgeons and engineers to cooperate lies with the engineers. The British Orthopaedic Association has a remarkably large number of fellows and members with natural mechanical talents who are doing their utmost to teach themselves mechanical theory.
>
> Almost daily the orthopaedic surgeon is endeavouring to bring his technical problems before engineers; but only if he happens to have unusual creative mechanical talents, and persistence and tenacity, and if he is not put off by a cool reception given to his ideas, will he get anywhere.

Here he might have been speaking of his own experiences, but surely he had overcome these difficulties himself? He next apportioned blame for what he clearly regarded a poor situation:

> The failure of engineers to cooperate positively with surgeons is easily explained. While they frequently show goodwill at the start of a project, this field simply does not offer a career for a first-class engineer. The best a British university department of engineering can offer is occasional help from a junior lecturer whose work is overshadowed by the preparation of his own thesis. The tendency is for the engineer to feel himself a "stooge" for the surgeon. In Sweden they are more realistic: for example, the University of Uppsala pays a salary which makes it worthwhile for a senior engineer . . . to supervise the work done in the biomechanical laboratory for one whole day a week.

Although he seemed to be unkind to engineers, he was recognising an important issue, the resolution of which would have helped the lot of an aspiring bio-engineer. He ended:

> To sum up, it is purely a matter of paying adequately for these services.[10]

Money was not the only problem, and some academic engineers may have resisted the development of what they regarded a minor speciality. But the right man in the right place has sometimes solved the problem. A number of universities have now set up excellent departments of bio-engineering; for example, Glasgow, London, Salford and Guildford.

To return to Charnley's clinical approach to the hip joint. In March 1959, he gave a lecture to the East Denbigh and Flint Division (these were two small counties in North Wales which became part of Clwyd in 1974) of the British Medical Association entitled 'Surgery of the hip joint – present and future developments'. This was published in the *British Medical Journal* a year later.[9] He reviewed the whole subject comprehensively, and his general observations are interesting because they indicate his thinking when he was just beginning to devote all his time to the production of a successful joint replacement.

He began by recognising in the 'modern world' patients wanted operations for 'degrees of discomfort which less than twenty years ago were regarded as inevitable'. This led him to state:

> A surgeon accepts great responsibility if he recommends surgery before a patient needs a stick, and it takes much soul-searching to decide whether the results obtained in early cases are commensurate with the time and money involved in treatment.

He reminded his audience of general practitioners that there were four basic procedures (arthroplasty, arthrodesis, osteotomy, and excision of the head and neck of the femur) available to treat the seven main groups of disorders of the hip. He listed these as: osteoarthritis, rheumatoid arthritis, ankylosing spondylitis, old congenital dislocation and subluxation, complications of fractures of the neck of the femur, miscellaneous infections of the hip (excluding tuberculosis), and the salvage of unsuccessful operations. The permutations and combinations of four operations and seven conditions were increased by four additional considerations: (1) what was suitable in middle age might be unsuitable in later life; (2) what was suitable for disorders of one hip might be unsuitable when both hips are affected; (3) what was suitable for a mobile hip might be unsuitable for one which is stiff; and (4) what was best for a labourer might be unsuitable for a clerk. Consequently, the surgeon was faced with a range of possibilities to choose from.

> A successful arthroplasty would eliminate the intellectual task of choosing the best operation for the individual problem, but until this happy day arrives it is obvious that the surgery of the hip, far from being a small sub-speciality, is the beginning of a large subject. This type of surgery demands a training in mechanical techniques which, though elementary in practical engineering, are as yet unknown in the training of a surgeon. Nowhere in the locomotor system would a liaison with university departments of engineering and colleges of technology be more rewarding than in the biomechanics of the hip joint. For this reason, one of my aims is to indicate the need for establishing surgical centres to concentrate on the study of the reconstructive surgery of the hip joint; in these centres men could be trained to master a repertory of different techniques and abandon the tendency, so common in the past to be a "one-operation man". In such a centre it would be possible to acquire concentrated experience of numerous techniques and to decide the spheres of usefulness of different operations, both old and new.

These remarks would seem to rehearse the arguments he must have already put forward for the establishment of the Hip Centre at Wrightington Hospital, and they certainly suggest that he was not expecting to find an immediate solution to the problem of joint replacement. When he had eventually achieved this, perhaps by 1967, he himself found that there was little need for the 'older' types of operation and, indeed, he became very much a 'one-operation man' himself. However, he was in a pessimistic mood in 1959 for he went on to say:

> It is important to realise that factors exist which will for ever limit the scope of arthroplasty of the hip, no matter how we may study and improve

the biomechanical design. It is all too easy to consider the reconstructive surgery of the hip as an exercise in engineering based on the mechanical distortion of the bones as revealed in the radiograph; but the bony changes are only part of the process which affects the soft parts and which produces the thick capsule and weakened muscles . . . If the head of the femur is replaced by a polished sphere of steel or plastic, surely it is a vain hope to expect an elderly patient to balance securely on the summit of this slippery "universal joint" if strong muscles do not exist to pull the body into balance. It is an axiom in hip joint surgery that mobility and stability are incompatible . . .

How wrong he eventually proved this to be. He continued:

Though these are the factors which limit the quality of an arthroplasty, this must not be taken as an absolute condemnation of arthroplasty, because there exist many patients in whom valuable amelioration has been obtained even though the results fall far short of perfection . . . no matter how well the patient co-operates, the quality of the final result depends on the quality of the tissues and on the sound mechanical design of the procedure.

This attitude was shared by many of his colleagues and reflected the despondency which followed from the unsatisfactory results of the arthroplasty operations then available. It also indicated that his mind was open to any future developments which he, or anyone else, might produce. Not only did he stress that the solution would never be entirely mechanical, he emphasised that in selecting patients for any operation it was necessary to consider their 'temperament and personality'.

The rest of his talk evaluated the place of osteotomy and arthrodesis. He said that osteotomy is 'still a reliable method of abolishing pain in an osteoarthritic hip'. The operation was a logical procedure when there was a fixed deformity to correct, but he could not accept that there was any rationale for it when the hip was mobile. He did, however, hint that if it was agreed that the mechanical problem was subsidiary, then a new approach to the 'treatment of pain as a vascular problem' might follow. This rather cryptic remark acknowledged the possibility that osteotomy might have a mysterious biological effect, but he never became an advocate of this procedure and it was never an operation he liked carrying out.

He still preferred his 'central dislocation stabilisation', or arthrodesis, when the osteoarthritis was confined to one hip joint. He concluded by suggesting that the place for arthroplasty might be suitable for patients with rheumatoid arthritis:

. . . it now seems possible that the restricted demands required of an arthroplasty by patients whose activity is limited by disease in other joints may make it possible for them to benefit greatly by techniques which would not stand the wear and tear inflicted on them by less disabled sufferers.

Some weeks later, the journal published an anonymous editorial[16] on the subject which expressed the view that central dislocation arthrodesis had found a place in many clinics, but arthroplasty was not acceptable as a routine procedure. Correspondence followed; and amongst the ten letters there are two by Dr J. L. Brailsford.[15] Brailsford was a distinguished radiologist and the tone of what he wrote suggests that he may have had an osteoarthritic hip. He quoted Sir James Walton's words to an audience during a lecture on gastric surgery:

maybe in the lifetime of many of you, these marvellously skilled operations will cease to be performed and will be regarded as curiosities of the past.[29]

Brailsford commented somewhat cynically:

How true this is of osteoarthritis of the hip.

The need for gastric surgery has been greatly reduced by new drugs, whereas in osteoarthritis medical treatment is at present ineffective and, thanks to Charnley, there now is a 'marvellous' operation for it.

His conservative attitude, when talking to general practitioners in 1959, may seem overcautious when viewed in retrospect. He was after all in the process of developing his low friction arthroplasty which he described the following year, and which was considered earlier in this chapter. There is, however, no doubt he believed that the whole range of disorders of the hip would be investigated at the Centre for Hip Surgery which he was planning to set up at Wrightington; and perhaps this would allow him to devise new operations for them. There is no hint that he anticipated inventing an arthroplasty which would solve most of the problems of replacing arthritic hips (except those in young people) – but there were exciting years ahead before this was to come about.

# Chapter 10

# THE PLAN FULFILLED: WRIGHTINGTON
## 1959–1969

*Yesterday at Wrightington was a triumph. The next steps are urgent.*

Platt to Charnley 1966

CHARNLEY SAID that he first began to consider the possibility of setting up a unit at Wrightington for the treatment of what he then called 'non-tuberculous' hip conditions as early as 1956.[11] There were obvious difficulties because of his commitments in Manchester; but in November, 1958, his surgical colleagues at the Royal Infirmary suggested he should take 'leave of absence' for three years (Chapter 7) which allowed him to concentrate on Wrightington. He was then aged 49 years and he had married eighteen months previously. The pattern of his life had changed and he now moved forward with increasing momentum towards the goal he had set himself. He had a clear sense of purpose and undoubtedly believed that he had a special contribution to make in orthopaedic surgery.

The reasons why he chose Wrightington for his Centre for Hip Surgery need to be explained, but first it is helpful to understand the background of the hospital.

In 1913, Dr Lissant Cox was appointed as the first central tuberculosis officer to the Lancashire County Council and one of his major responsibilities was the provision of proper sanatorium facilities in the area. World War One delayed progress, but in 1920 the council bought Wrightington Hall (and part of the estate) for £16,473, with a view to converting it into a tuberculosis hospital with 480 beds. The hall had belonged to the Dicconson family for centuries, but the estate passed to a 'spendthrift with a fanatical attachment to blood sports' who had died in 1918 and money was needed to settle death duties. The house was an early 18th century mansion standing above a lake in attractive country between Standish and Parbold, six miles north-west of Wigan. There were, however, delays and it was not till 1926 that the Ministry of Health agreed to a modified

113

scheme in which the beds were reduced to 226. In spite of much pressure from Dr Cox, building had not begun until the same year. The hall itself was adapted as a nurses' home and five single-storey pavilions with open verandahs were built. By 1932, it was possible to accommodate 218 patients, most of them suffering from bone and joint tuberculosis (and a number with pulmonary tuberculosis). Cox persuaded Mr H. Platt, of Manchester, and Mr T. P. McMurray, of Liverpool – who both became professors of orthopaedic surgery in their respective universities – to become the first consultant orthopaedic surgeons. Wrightington was, of course, not one of the country orthopaedic hospitals which were set up under Sir Robert Jones' and Girdlestone's national scheme (Chapter 4) and which were largely founded by charitable organisations. It was a Lancashire County Council hospital for patients with surgical tuberculosis, and not for the generality of cripples.

Seven 'temporary' wards were added for the Emergency Medical Service during World War Two. After the war, four of these wards were used for chest diseases (and thoracic surgery) and one for a genito-urinary unit; the remaining two were converted to accommodate male nurses. The introduction of the National Health Service in 1948 meant that the hospital was transferred from the authority of the County Council to the Ministry of Health. This was followed by a general refurbishment of the buildings, and consultants from Wigan in all the major specialities were appointed to the staff. Charnley had become a consultant orthopaedic surgeon to the hospital in 1947 at the time of Sir Harry Platt's 'first' retirement (Chapter 4); his colleague, in the first instance, was C. H. Cullen from Manchester; later they were joined by E. W. Knowles (Wigan) and R. S. Garden (Preston).

The tradition in tuberculosis sanatoria was to have a medical or surgical superintendent in charge of medical administration. Dr J. Dobson had been appointed in 1943 and he had published papers on tuberculosis of the hip and spine in *The Journal of Bone and Joint Surgery*. Dobson was succeeded by K. L. Barnes, who had been a senior orthopaedic registrar in Manchester, in 1959. This was a fortunate appointment as Barnes took all the responsibilities of administration from Charnley. The two men, who had completely diverse characters and abilities, formed an effective partnership each recognising what the other could contribute to the efficient working of the hospital.

During the late 1940s, there had been about 250 beds available for the treatment of bone and joint tuberculosis. Basic treatment was prolonged bed rest and the tempo of the hospital was slow. Charnley visited once a month from Manchester when he saw the patients in the wards and carried out any necessary operations. The incidence of tuberculosis began to decline as a result of improved living conditions throughout the country and the pasteurisation of milk. Then, at the beginning of the next decade, effective anti-tuberculous drugs were introduced (at first, streptomycin and para-amino-salicylic acid). The disease could now be controlled in a way which had not been possible before, and more radical surgery could be safely undertaken. As a consequence, there were not only fewer patients to be treated, but those who had to be in-patients stayed in hospital for a much shorter time. Sanatoria and orthopaedic hospitals all over the country were faced with the same predicament – how to use effectively that large number of beds which had been available for tubercular patients, and which were now no longer needed. Some of these institutions failed to find a proper solution and were closed, or their function was totally altered. Others found new aspects of orthopaedic surgery in which to specialise and went from strength to strength. Wrightington was saved by the creation of the Centre for Hip Surgery. But why did Charnley choose Wrightington? The most obvious reason would seem to be that both he and the hospital 'were there', but there were a number of special factors which were important.

Wrightington celebrated the 50th anniversary of its official opening in 1983 and an excellent small book was produced, edited by Dr W. R. Swinburn, to mark the event.[17] Various members of the staff contributed and Charnley wrote an account of the development of the Centre for Hip Surgery. He listed what he called the 'bits of luck' which made this possible and there is no better way of understanding his reasons for choosing Wrightington than by going through the 'bits of luck' one by one (paraphrasing his words where necessary).

The first was that there was only one other orthopaedic surgeon (Cullen) on the staff initially. It is not easy to see why he rated this as being of prime importance, but presumably he felt that it was easier for him to make changes when he did not have to battle with half a dozen awkward colleagues (and he and Cullen were old friends).

Secondly, there was a rumour that a North–South motorway was going to be built somewhere in the region. Charnley showed foresight in realising that if patients and visiting surgeons were to come to what some would think the back of beyond in Lancashire, they would only do so if there was quick and easy access from, say, London by car. He therefore wrote to Mr Drake, the county surveyor, explaining the problem and enquiring about the planned motorway. Drake was helpful, and it was fortunate that there was to be an access point on the M6 motorway within half a mile of the hospital gate. Thus there was a direct motorway link from London to the hospital. Charnley was delighted; had the junction at Wrightington been twenty miles further north or south, 'it would', in his words, 'have been useless for my plans'.

Thirdly, Wrightington did not belong to a hospital group and so had its own management committee with direct access to the Manchester Hospital Regional Board. This was an advantage because it meant that there was less competition for money, and direct access to the board without going through an intermediate administrative committee.

Fourthly, the senior administrative medical officer (SAMO) at the regional board, Frederick Marshall, was an old friend. Marshall had been a demonstrator in the anatomy department at Manchester in the 1930s (and not a senior lecturer as Charnley recorded); he had taught Charnley as a student and had continued to take an interest in his career. He was quick to see the merit of the plans for a centre for hip surgery and gave Charnley every support. This was critical because an unhelpful SAMO could have made any development very difficult. Another favourable point was that the hospital secretary, Mr H. Bibby, had worked at Wrightington since 1948 and his career had been dedicated to building up the hospital. He did a great deal to help Charnley and acted as a valuable intermediary between him and the regional board.

Another 'bit of luck' which Charnley recognised was the generosity of his colleagues in Manchester who had recommended that he should be granted leave of absence. He particularly was grateful to Mr R. T. Johnson, a neurosurgeon, who was chairman of the surgeon's committee. Johnson had been a colleague of Charnley's in Manchester since the war.

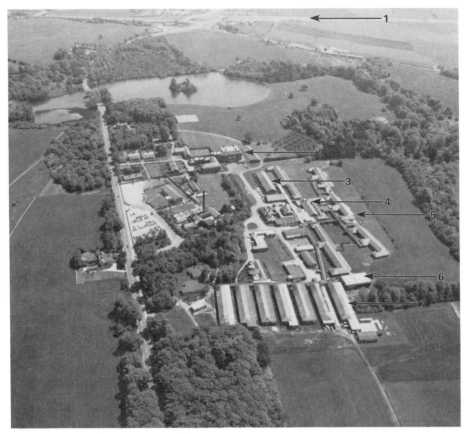

Key: 1 – M6 motorway with exit to Wrightington; 2 – The 18th-century mansion; 3 – Hip Centre; 4 – Operating theatres; 5 – Wards; 6 – Biochemical Research Laboratory and workshops; 7 – Wards.

*Aerial photograph of Wrightington Hospital after the development of the Centre for Hip Surgery. (From Mr J. H. Nuttall.)*

Charnley was now coming to Wrightington every Tuesday and Thursday. He had about fifty beds under his care (later this increased to 100); he held an out-patient clinic, and he operated all day on Thursday. He continued to do general orthopaedics while the number of patients with hip disorders gradually built up. He had gained a reputation for dealing with complications after fractures, bone tumours and children's orthopaedics, and his colleagues in Manchester referred 'difficult' cases to him. During the remainder of the week he worked at Park Hospital, Davyhulme, where he did routine elective orthopaedics and was responsible for the fractures; he had a clinic at the Manchester Royal Infirmary for patients with hip disorders, and he also saw private patients in Manchester.

Charnley's first aim at Wrightington was to find the money to build a biomechanical laboratory, and then a clinical research centre. But before any of this came about he obtained the salary for a workshop technician from the regional hospital board. The post was advertised by the hospital authorities and in June 1958 Harry Craven attended for an interview. He was aged twenty-eight years and had worked in industry as a turner–fitter, becoming a foreman at Metal Box Company Ltd. He had also taken a full apprenticeship in the ventilation of mines at the Wigan College of Mining Technology. Craven was interested in the job, but it was not until September he was told that he was appointed. This was a new type of post for the National Health Service and there was no appropriate grade for him. He was paid as an orthopaedic appliance fitter, and Charnley supplemented the salary from his own pocket.

To begin with Craven was allowed to use the hospital engineer's workshop, but he went to Naemoor on three days a week where he worked on the lathe in Charnley's attic. His main jobs were to make prototype instruments and the PTFE sockets which Charnley was using at the time. Craven would often go to the operating theatre to see what was needed. After he had produced an instrument, Charnley would modify it more often than not; when it was finally correct, it would be manufactured by Chas. F. Thackray Ltd in Leeds. Charnley would also make prototypes himself at home. The sockets were made as they were needed on the night before the Thursday operating list – so Wednesday night became 'socket night' at Naemoor.

Times were difficult with little money and not much in the way of materials, so undoubtedly there were frustrations. One Friday, Craven had worked very hard all day, but had little to show for it. On the following Monday morning, Charnley telephoned and cursed Craven roundly for 'not getting anything done'. But this outburst was followed by apologies and the two men subsequently got on well together.

The Manchester Regional Hospital Board's research committee granted Charnley £6,500 to build a biomechanical workshop and laboratory. This was a single-storey hut situated on the west side of the main hospital buildings. It was open in time for a meeting of the British Orthopaedic Association, which was held in Manchester in April 1961, when about 200 orthopaedic surgeons came to a clinical demonstration at the hospital. Charnley wrote in a report:

> The singular absence of professional jealousy at or after this meeting encouraged ideas for the future, and the title "Centre for Hip Surgery – Wrightington Hospital" was officially adopted.

It was at this Manchester meeting that Charnley spoke to orthopaedic surgeons for the first time about his new low friction arthroplasty using PTFE (and before his article was published in *The Lancet* – Chapter 9). He had by then operated on 51 patients. The subsequent discussion was reported and Charnley made two points which he probably regretted[1]: the first was that 'engineers were quite happy about the durability of Fluon [PTFE], which did not cause any soft tissue reaction' – how wrong this was to be proved; secondly, he said that chrome–cobalt alloy 'would be better than steel and he would use it in the future' – in fact, he never did. Nobody has ever been right about everything, and Charnley was prepared to change his views in the face of strong evidence to the contrary.

The formal opening ceremony of the biomechanical workshop was performed by Sir Harry Platt on June 23, 1961, one month after the British Orthopaedic Association meeting. Work could now go ahead on a larger scale and a wear-

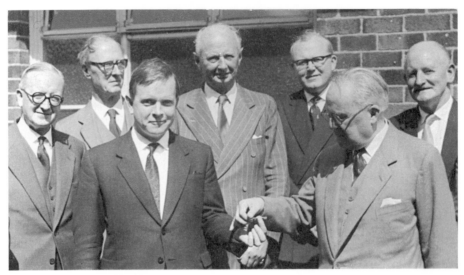

*Sir Harry Platt handing the keys of the biomechanical laboratory and workshop to John Charnley after the official opening. Mr H. Bibby, the hospital secretary, is on the extreme right. (By courtesy of Mr H. Farrimond.)*

testing machine was installed in 1962 which was used to examine the wear of PTFE, and other plastics against stainless steel.

There still was not enough money for equipment; Charnley worked hard to collect more, and there was a 'thrift box' in the workshop for small contributions. He had persuaded the management committee to provide two beds for private patients; this may seem a modest allocation, but there had been none previously. It was not until 1964 that the number was increased to ten. Charnley had a part-time contract with the National Health Service and so was allowed to have private patients in the hospital; this was a side-line for him, but he found it a useful source of money for research (and, of course, he was able to charge a fee for himself). At the time there was a regulation that the charge for a major operation in a private National Health Service bed could not be more than £75. Charnley would then persuade his private patients to contribute a similar sum to his research fund which was administered by the hospital management committee.

Commercial firms were approached by letter and money obtained from them; for example, two organisations each made covenants for £3,000. When he started work on the sterile enclosure in 1960 (Chapter 12) a grant was made by the Medical Research Council. Pilkington, the country's leading glass manufacturer, provided the large sheets of glass for the enclosure as well as technical information. Grants to pay for staff were also received from Smith, Kline & French and the Wade Trust.

In 1966, he came to an arrangement with Chas. F. Thackray Ltd that, in consideration of 'waiving his right to royalties on the sale of prostheses bearing his name', the firm would pay to the research fund a 'sum of £1 per complete prosthesis' sold by them. This is going ahead in time, but it is a good indication of the way in which Charnley managed to acquire money for his research.

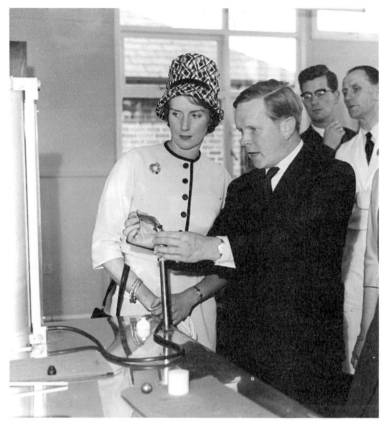

*Charnley showing visitors around the biomechanical laboratory and workshop. Jill Charnley is on his right.*

He was successful in obtaining a grant of £20,000 from the National Fund for Poliomyelitis and Crippling Diseases (this charitable organisation later became Action Research – the National Fund for Research into Crippling Diseases) which enabled the clinical research department to be built. This had space for offices for consultants and secretaries, a large conference room where patients could be seen before and after operation, a pathological laboratory and other rooms which had a variety of uses. The centre was officially opened on May 30, 1962 by Field Marshal Lord Harding, Chairman of the Fund.

In 1965, the National Fund made a grant of a further £1,500 for building and installing an apparatus for recording the gait of patients with disorders of the hip before and after operation. The basic idea had already been used in a prototype designed by Charnley and used in the workshop. Dr J. Skorecki, a lecturer in mechanical engineering at UMIST, produced a new design which eliminated errors in the original apparatus (Chapter 14), and made it possible to record the gait of out-patients in a form which could be used immediately as part of their clinical assessment. Cine-films were also taken of the patients walking; at one stage this was a job the residents were expected to undertake and the studio was the hospital corridor.

Charnley had from the outset always insisted that standardised records must be kept so that the long-term results could be evaluated. New data processing facilities were introduced into the centre in 1965 with the help of a further grant of £6,476 from the National Fund. An expert, who was invited to advise, agreed that an information retrieval computer would be no more effective than a new type of punch-card system (a so-called poor man's computer), and this is what was installed.

We have seen in the last chapter that Charnley was carrying out the third modification of the PTFE low friction arthroplasty at Wrightington in 1960. His aim then was to do an operating list of six major hip operations a week which would deal with the waiting list for admission. The rise in number of operations done for 'degenerative' arthritis was striking: from 109 in 1959 to 452 in 1962. The last increase coincided with the time that Charnley stopped going to Park Hospital so that he was able to work for eight 'sessions' (4 days) at Wrightington. It should be emphasised that these operations were not all arthroplasties, but included the central dislocation stabilisation, arthrodesis and various types of osteotomy. Charnley now had two registrars to assist him: Mr J. Read, from University College Hospital, London, who stayed at Wrightington for almost five years, and Dr J. K. Houston from Canada. These two were the first of many assistants who worked at the hip centre; over the succeeding years young men came from all over the world to learn from Charnley.

But before this came about, Charnley had a setback which might have crushed a lesser man. Sometime in 1962, it became clear that PTFE was not a suitable material for hip replacement. Charnley's own description was:

> Then came the dreadful weeks . . . PTFE proved unsuitable not so much because of its low resistance to wear as by the adverse tissue reactions caused by the wear debris.

Particles of PTFE in the tissues produced a severe granulomatous reaction with masses of amorphous caseous (cheesy) material forming around the implanted joint; the prosthesis came loose in the bone and the hip became painful. In nearly all cases a further operation was necessary. Charnley continued:

> It may seem strange that it took us some 300 operations and between three and four years to arrive at this conclusion [that PTFE was unsuitable], but there were a number of different reasons. First, the results up to three years were so spectacular, and the patients so pitifully grateful, that we could not bring ourselves to face the suspicion that, in such highly successful results, the x-rays were showing incipient harmful evidence. Second, by its chemical nature PTFE was so extremely inert we felt that even if wear debris was present it would be harmless. Third, though we could see wear of the order of 1 mm after about a year in the x-rays, I thought that this was not unexpected and could be explained by the "bedding-in" of the head in a socket which was deliberately machined to have an internal diameter larger than the head. It was only when the first year's wear was more than doubled in the second year and more than tripled in three years that the seriousness of the problem became evident.

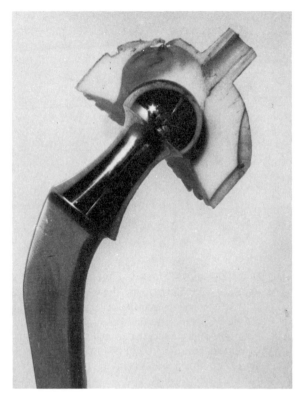

*Wear of a PTFE socket after three years in the body. The abraded particles produced a severe granulomatous response.* (LFA)

Other surgeons had to be warned about the adverse tissue reaction to PTFE. Charnley had hoped to do this when he found that a report was to be made about using PTFE in the knee joint at a meeting of the British Orthopaedic Association in the autumn of 1963. He intended to speak, but the chairman vetoed discussion for lack of time. He therefore wrote a letter to *The Lancet* which was published on December 28, 1963.[2] He described the masses of white amorphous material (sometimes as much as 100–200 ml) that formed around the new joint and how this material destroyed nearby bone. Fortunately, surgical removal of the material resulted in complete healing. He went on to report an experiment he had done on himself:

> I have introduced subcutaneously into my thigh, by means of a wide-bore needle . . . two specimens of PTFE prepared in finely divided form. After nine months . . . the two specimens are clearly palpable as nodules, and have been stationary in size for the last six months. They are almost twice the volume of the original implant.

He concluded with a strong warning against the use of PTFE in the body where abrasion with liberation of particles was likely.

Certainly, his self-experiment showed an element of courage, and indeed rashness, which can but be admired, although it was not quite so dramatic as the bone graft which he had taken from his leg in 1946. The material might have led to the formation of a cancerous tumour, but fortunately there were no long-term ill effects.

The consequences of the PTFE disaster gradually unfolded before this letter was written, and Charnley came to terms with it in a remarkable way. He accepted the responsibility and, as he felt he had a debt to the patients, he performed all the revision operations himself. This should not be underestimated – these operations were all difficult, time-consuming and there must have been a worrying uncertainty about the eventual outcome. Hardinge[12] has quoted one of the assistants at Wrightington as saying that every time Charnley did a PTFE revision it was 'like observing a monk pouring ashes over his own head'. This may be an exaggeration, but it does convey Charnley's distress at that trying time, and he wrote:

> In surviving this worrying period I must pay tribute to the loyalty of my team and nursing staff . . .

At home, Charnley was in a state of despair and the failure was the main topic of conversation. He would arrive back from the hospital without a smile, even for his young children. He fell asleep from sheer mental exhaustion, and would wake in the early hours. Jill Charnley remembers him sitting up in bed with his head in his hands. She felt that 'everything was grey and there was an all-pervading gloom'. He was determined to find a solution, and once he began to see his way ahead, the gloom lifted quickly. The period of total despair lasted for weeks rather than months.

It was characteristic of Charnley that he would analyse any failure in great depth in order to learn from it, and he obtained a good deal of valuable material from his PTFE cases which he published in due course. He also came to appreciate how much pain patients with osteoarthritis had to put up with:

> We all thought that once the news got round that second operations [revisions] were having to be advised, there would be a total disappearance of new patients in a matter of weeks. But nothing of the kind happened; new patients still came for consultation in undiminished numbers and they often said "I hear the operation only lasts two years"; they were evidently quite prepared to have it even for only two years of relief. Others, when told they would have to have the operation repeated with a new socket of a different plastic material, often made such remarks as "Well, it was worth it, it was the best three years of my life".

He continued to look for a new type of artificial joint and he had two unsuccessful attempts. His first idea was to produce a 'sealed' ball and socket consisting of a conventional metal-on-metal joint with a silicone rubber bellows to keep grease in and tissue fluids out. There were insuperable difficulties; for example, 'the impossibility of achieving an adequate range of motion without the silicone being destroyed and crushed at the extremes of the range'. Laboratory testing convinced him that this system would not work in practice and these prototype joints were never used in patients. Second, he tried to improve the wear of properties of PTFE by 'filling' it with glass fibre, or by using a synthetic proprietary substance (Fluorosint-Polypenco). The wear tests of Fluorosint in the laboratory were

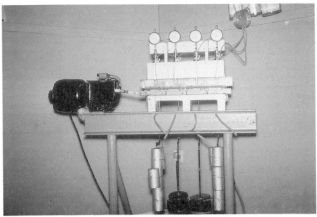

*The four-station wear testing machine in use in the early 1960s. (From Mr J. Read.)*

twenty times better than PTFE. The plastic became highly polished, but Craven remembers the material was so hard that it wore the stainless steel against which it was being tested. Charnley decided that it would be justifiable to try Polypenco in the human body and used it in about twenty patients. Unfortunately 'it behaved very badly' as he reported later[10], wearing as much as PTFE had done, and worse still the filler acted as an abrasive and lapped the metal as Craven had predicted.

The other burden which Charnley had to carry during this early period was that he was working in what he later described as 'the crudest of operating theatres', which was responsible for an unacceptable incidence of serious wound infection. The way he coped with this is a story in itself and will be described in Chapter 12.

These were bad times, but he regarded it as another 'bit of luck that we were only about nine months in the doldrums – not daring to do any more PTFE hips and having no good operation to offer the flood of patients still coming to our clinics'. But when the solution appeared, it was another instance of serendipity.

Some time in May 1962, Craven was telephoned by the hospital supplies officer and told that he had a young man (Mr V. C. Binns) with him who was trying to sell plastic gears. It is remarkable that the supplies officer should have thought of telling Craven, and it is one of the advantages of being in a small specialised hospital where everyone is aware of what is going on. Craven found that Binns had a plastic material which was made in Germany and which was being used for gears in the weaving trade in Lancashire. Binns did not know much about its qualities, but he gave Craven a piece three or four inches in diameter. This was high molecular weight polyethylene (HMWP). Craven decided, on his own initiative, to try this new material on the four-station testing machine which he had built in the biomechanical laboratory. When shown the material, Charnley dug his thumb-nail into it and walked out, telling Craven that he was wasting his time. But Craven too had a stubborn streak and persisted with the test: after the first day there were no signs of wear, and only 1/2000 of an inch at the end of two days, which was incomparably better than PTFE. Meanwhile Charnley went to a meeting of the British Orthopaedic Travelling Club which was held in Copenhagen from May 29 to June 3. He described what happened when he returned:

> My office door opened to reveal Craven who asked me to come down to the lab . . . Down I went to see the HMWP. After running day and night for three weeks this new material, which very few people even in engineering circles had heard about at that time, had not worn as much as PTFE would have worn in 24 hours under the same conditions. There was no doubt about it: "we were on".

In spite of his initial scepticism, which was perhaps not surprising in view of his previous experience with plastics, Charnley at once accepted Craven's results. He immediately grasped the potential of HMWP, and despair was overcome by enthusiasm. He wrote to the manufacturers, Ruhr Chemie, for information and his account continued:

> By its chemistry, polyethylene had a very good chance of resisting attack by body fluids. With 200 to 300 hips where PTFE had been used, and which eventually would need some sort of salvage, there were real problems ahead and this new substance fitted the bill.

His relief was evident. But what he did not mention was that he had implanted HMWP into his own thigh before using it in patients. An account of this was included in the letter which he wrote to *The Lancet* about PTFE in 1963.[2] The specimen of HMWP 'could not with certainty be detected by palpation' after six months, and he took this to indicate that 'there were grounds for believing that high density polyethylene (not necessarily ordinary polythene) did not produce any tissue reaction when implanted in a finely divided state'. The letter is noteworthy because it was the first time the medical profession were informed about his use of HMWP.

After this self-experiment and further wear tests, he was prepared to use the new plastic in a patient, and the first HMWP socket was inserted in November 1962.

About this time a revealing incident occurred which has been described by Mr P. H. Newman:

> John invited three of us [all were friends and orthopaedic colleagues who had been with him in America in 1948] to spend a weekend at Naemoor to discuss the problem [of PTFE] . . . We spent a whole day at Wrightington seeing and talking about many of the patients. . . On the Sunday we had a full discussion. All three of us had come to the same conclusion, that the operation should be abandoned and we told him so.
>
>      This was John's big moment. He said "No – I've got the answer now, I have found a much harder plastic . . ."

The plastic, of course, was HMWP. Newman's story makes clear Charnley was confident that he had found the solution. And, indeed, he was right – as HMWP has now stood the test of more than twenty years' use in patients.

There was a great deal of work to be done and now Charnley operated on two days (Tuesdays and Thursdays) a week, and occasionally on Mondays and Fridays. Wednesday became the day for the teaching conference, followed by a ward round in the morning, with an out-patient clinic in the afternoon (Chapter 14).

Although he had been through a devastating experience, Charnley had developed a sound operative technique for arthroplasty of the hip before the failures occurred; in particular he had designed the instruments, learnt more about the use of bone cement (Chapter 11), improved the theatre conditions (Chapter 12) and he had improved the basic design of the prosthesis. Consequently, when the HMWP became available, he was well prepared to use it. He at once began a prospective study of all the patients who were operated on, and by 1965 he had collected the group who were thereafter always called 'the first five hundred'. This continuous review and assessment of all his cases was one of the most important features of his organisation at Wrightington. It depended on keeping accurate records of clinical and operative details, which was done by using standardised pro formas, and by expressing the result for each patient numerically.

A technical point arose at once because the new plastic was found to have a relatively high coefficient of friction in the laboratory, at least compared with PTFE. But the coefficient of friction of HMWP decreased when it was subjected to high stress, and it was also capable of a modest degree of boundary lubrication by synovial fluid. The latter statement meant that it was an exception to his earlier belief (Chapter 9) that 'no substances were available for joint replacement which could avail themselves of synovial fluid as a lubricant'. Charnley could hardly have minded having to change his previous opinion.

The newly designed HMWP sockets were fixed in position with bone cement, as was the small head femoral prosthesis. Six months after the operation, radiographs often showed a line of demarcation between the cement and the floor of the acetabulum, and Charnley thought that this might foreshadow loosening and failure – particularly since such lines were almost non-existent around the femoral prosthesis after five years. He therefore designed a 'press-fit socket' to use without cement. This was made of HMWP encased in a stainless steel shell with a spigot of the plastic protruding through a hole at its summit. The bony acetabulum was precisely shaped with an expanding reamer and a hole drilled

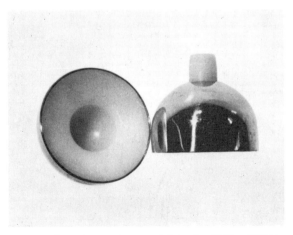

*A press-fit socket used as a trial in the 1960s.* (LFA)

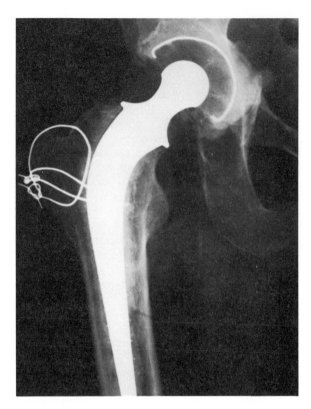

*Radiograph showing a low friction arthroplasty 11 years after its insertion in 1965. The plastic socket and the femoral prosthesis have both been cemented in position (the wire in the socket is purely a marker for assessing the position of the socket and wear).* (LFA)

through the floor of the acetabulum into the pelvis. The artificial socket was hammered in so that fixation was obtained by an 'interference' fit. These press-fit sockets and the standard plastic socket were used in alternate patients between 1963 and 1965. Almost 300 press-fit sockets were inserted, but they were then given up for a number of reasons: the clinical results were not as good as they were with the cemented sockets, and the demarcation around the cemented sockets, which had caused anxiety at six months, did not get worse after the first year.[10]

The operation now settled into a routine. Charnley introduced a standard technique and imposed a strict surgical discipline on himself and his assistants. On the other hand, he was always prepared to make modifications and to take any steps which he thought would be an improvement, frequently inventing new instruments. Such large numbers of operations were carried out that it was possible to make a valid comparison of the results.

The HMWP sockets were made in the biomechanical workshop at Wrightington and each took about 45 minutes to complete. As the number of operations increased, there was clearly a need to speed up production and in 1963 Charnley

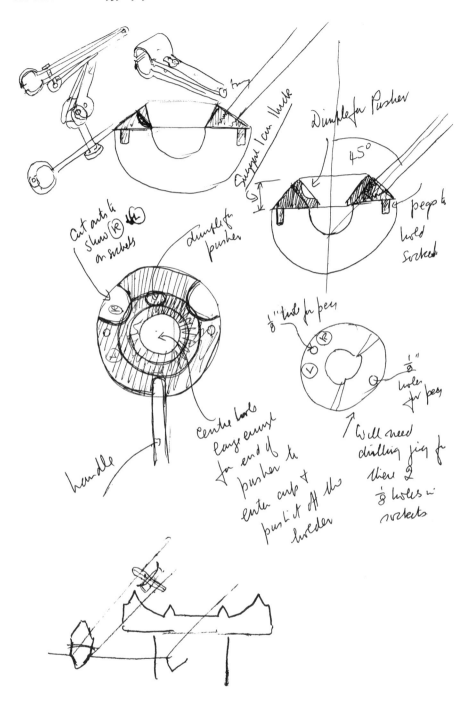

*An example of a sketch by Charnley illustrating an instrument (in this case, a socket holder) which he wanted made in the workshop. The technician would work from this drawing. (From Mr Geoffrey Middleton.)*

asked Craven to build a machine to automate the manufacturing process. Charnley was sceptical about Craven's efforts, but Craven persisted and was successful – the new machine could turn out a socket in four or five minutes. The machine was sold to Thackrays who continued to use it for a time. The stainless steel for the femoral prostheses was produced in Sheffield where it was forged into a rough shape; it was then machined and worked at Thackrays in Leeds. The final lapping and polishing was done in the workshop at Wrightington until 1968, after which Thackrays took over the whole manufacturing process.

Craven, who had made a continuing contribution to the development of Charnley's ideas, left in 1966 and Mr G. Middleton, who had joined him as an assistant in the previous year, was then in charge of the workshop. Thackrays took over the payment of the technicians' salaries from the National Health Service in 1970 and this proved a much more satisfactory arrangement. In 1971/72 the workshop was doubled in size to meet the increasing amount of work which was required. Middleton had been joined by Mr K. S. Marsh in 1970 who took over in 1973 (when Middleton left), and continued in post until 1982. Mr F. Brown started in the workshop in 1973 and was still working there in 1989. These four men, whose work with Charnley spanned twenty-five years, made a very considerable contribution to the development of the low friction arthroplasty; especially by helping him with the mechanical testing of materials and by making the prototypes of the instruments he designed. Each regarded Charnley as 'a good friend' or 'a good man to work for', in spite of the occasional row; they all felt very much part of a team and enjoyed their work. Middleton recalls 'these were very exciting times, with lots of original ideas being developed'.

Charnley's confidence had been shaken by his experience with PTFE and, although he had taken all steps open to him to evaluate HMWP before implanting it in patients, he was extremely cautious. He would only do the operation on patients who were old (over 68 years in the early days) and who were very disabled. This was a wise precaution and he kept to this rule stringently – refusing those patients who did not fit his criteria. He was sometimes criticised for selecting those patients who would not be very active after the operation, or who might not be expected to live for a great many years. As time went by and the results were seen to be good, he widened his selection and he began to operate on patients in their early sixties. While the operation was considered still to be 'under development' (at least up to 1969), he continued to take the line that patients must be reassured that their pain would not inevitably get worse and that nothing was lost by delaying the operation as this would not prejudice the final result. He wrote:

> Using this type of approach, it is usually possible for the surgeon to avoid having his arm twisted, and at the same time to afford [by reassurance] genuine relief to the patient.

Charnley also did something very unusual for a surgeon – he delayed publishing his results for as long as he reasonably could. This remarkable attitude can at least partly be explained by his experience with PTFE and his fear of having to be responsible for a further cataclysm of failures in the future. He wanted to avoid other surgeons taking up the operation before it was proven; this would not only be bad in itself, but it would reflect on his reputation if problems were to arise subsequently. Money was certainly not a factor which caused him to place an embargo on the sale of the prosthesis. At this stage there were no patents; and money from Thackrays was paid into his research fund. Some surgeons criticised what they regarded his 'dog in the manger' attitude, but this was quite unreasonable and the same critics would have complained even more vociferously if he had encouraged the widespread use of his method prematurely.

Even after he had had five years' experience, he gave Thackrays permission to sell the prostheses only to those surgeons to whom he had given his personal approval. The restriction was on the purchase of the prostheses; the special instruments were readily available and could be used for other hip operations. Any surgeon who wished to perform the low friction arthroplasty was required to spend two and a half days at Wrightington to learn the theoretical basis and the surgical technique (Chapter 14). When an individual surgeon had fulfilled these conditions, Thackrays were told and that surgeon was then permitted to purchase the implant. There were some who thought they should be exempt from this ruling, but Charnley remained firm and this did not endear him to some of his senior colleagues.

Charnley wrote to Thackrays on April 22, 1968:

> I realise that the snowballing effect of the operation is getting out of hand, and with the passage of time and the accumulation of experience, my views are now being forced into a different line from the extremely cautious and rather obstructive attitude which I have taken heretofore. The essence of this letter is: (1) that my extended experience clinically and in my theoretical laboratory indicates that the low friction arthroplasty is mechanically better than the rival McKee operation; and (2) the time has now come for me to declare that this procedure has been tested for five years in the human body and can now be fully developed.

He made it clear that by using the word developed, he meant that it was not yet time for a 'general release'. Thackrays must have been disappointed because commercially it was difficult for them to continue with restricted sales. The complex relationship between surgeon and manufacturer continued over many years to the mutual benefit of both parties; and this will be explored further in Chapter 13. In due course, Charnley stopped making a personal selection of surgeons, and agreed that any surgeon who spent two days at Wrightington could purchase the prosthesis without specific approval. Of course, his assistants were privileged and obtained the equipment at a reduced price from Thackray. It was not until the early 1970s that the operation was generally released and available to anyone who wished to do it. The publications[6,8] in which Charnley revealed his early results are considered in Chapter 14.

Notwithstanding his restrictive policy, Charnley 'characteristically freely exchanged information' with visiting surgeons.[16] If they were innovators and if they had the facilities, there was no reason why they should not incorporate his ideas into a prosthesis of their own design, and this happened in several instances. Professor M. E. Müller of Bern produced a new prosthesis in 1963[14] which he named the Charnley–Müller prosthesis for a number of years (Chapter 13). Another example was Professor W. Bucholz, a general surgeon from Hamburg, who visited Wrightington in 1961 and 1963, and then developed his 'Modell St Georg' replacement. HMWP and cement were used, but he and Müller preferred chrome–cobalt to stainless steel, and a larger femoral head (33 mm or 38 mm diameter in Bucholz's case). At a third visit to Wrightington in 1969, Charnley did not approve of the large head, neither did he then accept Bucholz's use of

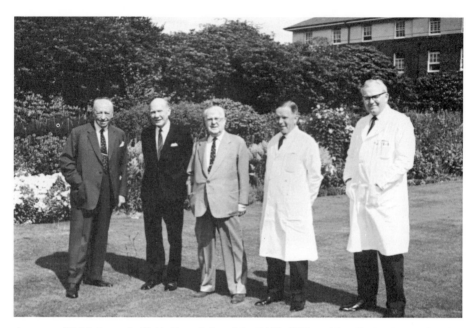

*A group at Wrightington in 1966. From left to right: Philip Wilson (New York), Scottie Garden, Harry Platt, John Charnley and Keith Barnes. (From Mr R. A. Elson.)*

antibiotics in cement. After this there was very little contact between the two men, but in 1982 Bucholz invited Charnley to inspect the Endo-Klinik which he had set up in Hamburg. This hospital was one of the only centres in the world concentrating almost exclusively on joint replacement. Mr. R. A. Elson, who is now an orthopaedic surgeon in Sheffield and had worked with both Charnley and Bucholz, accompanied Charnley on a very successful visit. Charnley was favourably impressed; indeed this was the sort of organisation which he believed was necessary for teaching and research on joint replacement.

Alternative forms of arthroplasty had also been introduced in England in the 1960s. We have already seen that McKee conceived and inserted into patients a total hip replacement with a metal-on-metal bearing before Charnley produced his low friction arthroplasty. McKee published his results in 1966.[13] There was undoubtedly professional rivalry between the two men, but they remained on friendly terms and skied together with the British Orthopaedic Ski Group. As far as their operations were concerned, Charnley was reported as saying at a meeting of the British Orthopaedic Association in 1965 that 'metal on metal is not a good friction surface, but it seemed to work in the human'.[4] Charnley certainly thought the McKee prosthesis good enough to justify comparing it with his own in patients who were having both hips operated on – he would do a low friction arthroplasty on one hip, and insert a McKee prosthesis in the other. He was nevertheless worried about the high friction and believed that the metal-on-metal 'stuck' when it was bearing weight. He was also satisfied that the McKee prosthesis had a higher incidence of mechanical failure within the first 18 months after operation. When giving the founder's lecture to the Chartered Society of

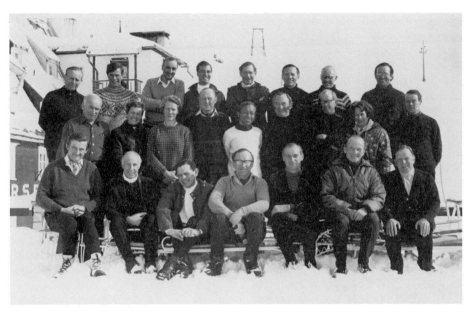

*The British Orthopaedic Ski Group in 1971. Charnley is sitting on the extreme right. Ken McKee is next to him. Other members in the front row from left to right are: Robin Denham, Denys Wainwright, Alan Apley, David Evans. (From Mr Roy Maudsley.)*

Physiotherapists in 1968[5], he referred to the two 'archetypes of hip replacement', commenting 'and it is very nice to know that they are both British!'. He described the differences between the two operations and said:

> It is a mysterious fact that in the human body both these prostheses work extremely well, and it is the future alone which will decide which pattern will be the one to be universally taken up.

In the late 1960s Mr P. A. Ring, an orthopaedic surgeon at Redhill, Surrey, also developed a metal-on-metal hip replacement which was designed to be used without cement.[15] Ring, like McKee, later converted his prosthesis to a metal-on-plastic bearing and made other modifications to it, but he never found it necessary to use cement with the type of mechanical fixation which he had devised. Neither McKee nor Ring placed any restriction on the sale or use of their prostheses as Charnley had done.

In a booklet produced by the Wrightington Hospital Management Committee, there is a record of Charnley's appearances on national television:

> Many who read this will have seen and heard Mr Charnley explaining his techniques on his two BBC television appearances. The first in the *Your Life in Their Hands* programme and the second on December 30, 1965 in *Challenge* when important scientific developments of 1965 were reviewed.

Charnley had gradually built up an organisation within the hospital which he ran with firm discipline. He was an authoritarian and laid down exactly the way everything should be done. Consequently, the very highest standards were maintained in the wards, in the out-patient clinic and, above all, in the operating theatre. Although he was always prepared to listen to intelligent suggestions, he was absolutely unable to tolerate stupidity or idleness. Doctors, nurses and technicians, who worked with him, respected his dedication and were extremely loyal. A momentary outburst of temper was invariably followed by an apology. He had been known to run down the corridor after a junior doctor to make amends. Even if he did not apologise, the episode would be quickly forgotten and normal relationships resumed, provided the offence was not heinous. An anonymous American visitor made the apt comment that Charnley was 'like electricity, he flows and flows, but every so often there is a short circuit and he blows a fuse – it is always repaired'. Many of the men who worked with him remained his friends for life, returning to Wrightington or writing to him when they needed advice.

Dr B. T. Hammond, an Australian who was at Wrightington in 1965 and 1966, was 'impressed by the loyalty that Charnley showed to his "men" – the ones who had shown devotion to him'. Hammond 'found him easily approachable – but one soon found one could not take liberties. . . he couldn't stand waffling. . .'. He particularly admired Charnley's ability to

> grasp the essentials of any idea – and discard the non-essentials. He could go right to the core of the matter, extremely lucidly and quickly . . . he was quite prepared to abandon an idea or a method . . . if he thought there was something better . . . It was a tremendously exciting time to be at Wrightington, we felt we were on the frontier of something new . . .*

A measure of the respect held for Charnley by the surgeons who worked with him was the formation of the Low Friction Society. Charnley himself initially rejected the idea when it was first raised, but in due course he was persuaded. When the inaugural meeting was held in 1974, 45 members attended (membership was limited to those who had worked at Wrightington). Meetings have been held every three years in the United Kingdom since then and there are now about 100 members. The society has chapters in Europe, North America, Australia and the Far East, South Africa and Latin America.

Many of Charnley's registrars came from overseas, but he was concerned about the difficulties which United Kingdom graduates were having in their orthopaedic training. This seemed to him to revolve around the Fellowship examination of the Royal College of Surgeons of England (FRCS) which was, and still is, a necessary qualification for any surgeon. He was stimulated to write a long and critical letter in the correspondence columns of the British Medical Journal which was published in 1964.[3] He put forward a plea for a Fellowship in orthopaedic surgery (rather than only in general surgery) as a specialist examination:

> This letter is prompted by experience that I have in my own unit with registrars in orthopaedics. During the last three years my registrars have produced five quite valuable papers on orthopaedic subjects, but not one of these registrars . . . [was] born or educated in the British Isles. While

---

*These remarks are paraphrased from a tape-recording made by Lady Charnley when she visited Hammond in Australia in 1988.

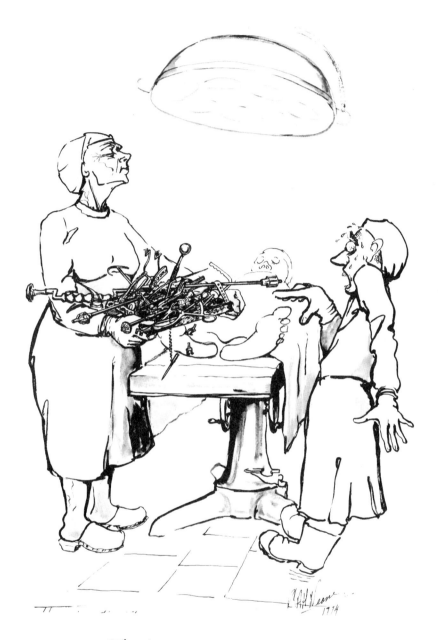

*The house surgeon who asked
for a "Charnley's"*

A cartoon presented to Charnley at the inaugural meeting of the Low Friction Society in 1974.
(By courtesy of Wrightington Hospital.)

these overseas residents were working on research projects, my British registrars have had to bury themselves in general reading in a desperate attempt to get the Final Fellowship, and they had not been able to afford time away from parrot work to experience the beneficial exercise of attempting original work under guidance and encouragement . . .

Charnley elaborated his theme at some length, and he was expressing an opinion which was shared by many of his provincial orthopaedic colleagues; although no one had had the courage to express them so forcibly in a medical journal. This was an outspoken attack on the surgical establishment in London and he did not endear himself to it by a remark in his penultimate paragraph:

I would like to add to this a criticism of the fact that the FRCS examination is competitive. Competitions should be reserved for games and beauty queens . . . Merely to pass the top 10% is a dodge to make life easy for busy examiners and keep the College coffers full.

Not surprisingly, numerous letters followed; some were critical, some in support of his opinion. He himself wrote again to emphasise his views, and to retract the sentences which have just been quoted.

. . . but the point is not important to my argument and it is evident that at that stage in my letter I was carried away by my own rhetoric.

Charnley made no headway on this particular issue; he was up against an immovable object in the Royal College of Surgeons. The controversy has continued until the present time and many orthopaedic surgeons continue to press for a specialist fellowship in orthopaedic surgery.

Sir Harry Platt had taken a continued interest in Charnley's orthopaedic career and had strongly supported him in many ways, particularly in regard to the development of the Centre for Hip Surgery. Even after his retirement, Platt remained an influential figure in Manchester. The two men liked each other and shared a mutual respect. They corresponded regularly over the years and a number of their letters from 1963 to 1969 have survived. Platt usually wrote by hand, often almost in note form, and his letters are sometimes difficult to decipher. On February 7, 1964, he wrote after a visit to Wrightington:

My reactions to yesterday's delightful and stimulating experience are – the hospital rests on one man, yourself, a hazardous situation. The pupil you need now is a young man on the eve of consultancy . . .

Platt went on to suggest that other facets of orthopaedics could be expanded into beds remaining after 'the elimination of urology and chest diseases'. He also said that 'operating theatre extensions are urgent' and no doubt his support helped Charnley to achieve this. The letter ends:

The times are critical; we are on the wave of the scientific and technological revolution . . . obviously your links with both the University teaching and Colleges of Advanced Technology research should now be strengthened.

Again on March 31, 1966:

Yesterday at Wrightington was a triumph. The next steps are urgent. (1) The *blueprint* of the hospital in the *near* future – and its staffing requirements. We still need to get more free monies as well as Regional Hospital Board support. (2) An additional consultant . . . to be bracketed with the faithful . . . Keith Barnes, you need the best young man available – good enough to succeed you . . . (3) The university "recognition", in whatever form, should come quickly – the International Centre exists now, but it needs the material trappings.

For a number of reasons, Charnley was unable to appoint a consultant colleague until 1971. He replied to Platt on April 4: 'your letter . . . was the biggest compliment I ever had'. He went on to discuss 'the possibilities of setting up a private clinic within the hospital funded with private monies'. This was a revolutionary idea, but Charnley was prepared to consider any approach which might benefit the hip centre. His next comments throw light on his attitude:

The point about getting a private clinic to which we could attract foreign patients, and in which the professional fees would be ploughed back, and the surgeon paid a salary, is a very important part of my future planning . . .

At the moment we have only enough private beds [for] . . . one consultant in the field, and I am exploring methods of getting private monies to extend our private clinic. I think this would not be difficult, but the main objection might be [from] the Ministry [of Health] and administrative problems of having a clinic built with private money inside the compound of a National Health Service hospital.

I think you know me well enough to accept my statement as being absolutely true that I have no great interest in private practice from the financial point of view. I am very interested in private practice from the point of view of prestige and international relations as they bear on the development of this clinic. I think you might well be exactly in the right position to put this point of view to important people in the Ministry . . .

Disappointingly, Platt's reply is not in the file. But Charnley must have known that his proposal was impossible within the framework of the National Health Service, particularly with a Labour government in power, as was the case from 1964 to 1970.

The next letter from Platt dated August 25, 1966, is brief and is typed:

This is just to thank you for putting on such a splendid show at Wrightington for Philip Wilson [a distinguished orthopaedic surgeon from New York]. His three days of "brain washing" showed him that we now have a Manchester School of Orthopaedics. It is not for me to say that it is now Number One in Great Britain.

Although Platt was moving in international surgical circles (he was president of the International Federation of Surgical Colleges from 1958 to 1966) and was travelling widely, he remained loyal to Manchester and proud of the success of his protégé.

On April 10, 1968, Charnley wrote to Sir Harry:

I really do think that I have now hit the "jackpot" and that money for an Institute or a Research Department at Wrightington is available if I can get together a plan of action . . . The active and creative goodwill comes from Lord Netherthorpe, who is Chairman of Fisons and Costains [two large industrial companies]. . .

Lord Netherthorpe had been a patient at Wrightington, his operation had been successful and he had been very impressed with the work going on in the hospital. He made contact with 'a number of influential personal friends' and returned to discuss Charnley's ideas for research. Charnley wrote that the 'sum mentioned is certainly in excess of £100,000 and I imagine could safely be put at £150,000'. He invited Platt to take part in preliminary discussions in London and went on to outline some of his proposals. He was convinced that the research institute should stay within the very specialised field of hip surgery, and the effort should not be diluted by taking in general orthopaedic surgery. He outlined his plans for gathering together a group of scientists who would investigate all aspects of hip replacement.

Lord Netherthorpe had made it clear that no Trust would give money merely to subsidise the National Health Service. He was, however, prepared to support a private clinic for the benefit of the international reputation of the unit. Charnley added a postscript to his letter:

I want to make the best use of any money by spreading it in salaries rather than in bricks and mortar. I plan, at the moment, for a ten year programme rather than for posterity – posterity will get the results of the research, not the empty shell of a building.

Charnley was clearly excited by the prospects which the future seemed to hold for him. There is no record of how negotiations proceeded. The next letter in the file is dated September 3, 1968, and it is frustrating not to know what went before. Charnley's words were a sudden let-down:

I am no further forward with the £150,000 target, purely because I am so engrossed in my work. I have two important papers on the stocks which for me are more urgent than the getting of money which may take me away from my research bench.

This can hardly have been the real, or at least the only, reason for him being unable to grasp this wonderful opportunity. The rest of the letter hints at what must have been an important consideration:

The National Health Service has been a very important part of my expansion at Wrightington . . . but its narrowness now completely cramps the ability to move in original ways . . .

It is impossible for me to claim the money from Netherthorpe etc with the dogma of the Ministry of Health vis-a-vis private practice in its present state. I am therefore completely blocked and cannot move forward.

Although Charnley had fully supported the concept of the National Health Service, he became disillusioned with the way it was manipulated by politicians. He wrote elsewhere some years later that 'the NHS was destroyed by politicians of such quite different kidney as Mrs Barbara Castle and Sir Keith Joseph'.[11]

In spite of these frustrations, and the failure to set up a research institute at Wrightington, Charnley had already achieved a great deal by 1968.

The Centre for Hip Surgery, as Sir Harry Platt had written, now had an international reputation, and surgeons were coming from all over the world to learn about the operation (Chapter 14). Charnley summarised his main aims at Wrightington: (1) to carry out research and development; (2) to deal with large numbers of patients; (3) to use a standardised system of documentation; (4) to train all echelons of staff; (5) to be cost-effective, and (6) to maintain a high general level of excellence.

The number of operations carried out is impressive: Charnley wrote that in 1967 700 or 800 were being done each year; after the second clean air operating enclosure was opened in 1970 (Chapter 12) the numbers increased to about 28 operations a week. The organisation required to undertake this volume of work, and to follow up the patients subsequently, cannot be underestimated.

His dedicated hard work resulted in success and he had no doubt that it would not have been possible for him to achieve so much had he stayed in Manchester. He believed that his relative isolation at Wrightington had positive advantages and he addressed this matter in two papers in 1970 and 1972. The first, with the title *Subspecialisation or superspecialisation in surgery?*, was published in the *British Medical Journal*[7] and described the benefits of concentrated experience in dealing with one problem. He visualised the establishment of a 'limited' number of centres like Wrightington which would train postgraduates in the surgical technique; deal with problem cases, and cope with secondary operations which he regarded as inevitable, once the operation was being carried out on a large scale. As far as isolation was concerned:

> Many of the criticisms . . . are not as sound as they appear at first sight. In a great teaching hospital the isolation of different "firms" can be quite astonishing, even though they are separated by only fifty yards of corridor . . . Furthermore, my experience is that it takes no longer to get the opinion of a consultant in another speciality from the Wigan Infirmary . . . than from just up the corridor in a teaching hospital.

The title of the second article, published in the *British Journal of Hospital Medicine*[9], was *The organisation of a special centre for hip surgery*. He concluded:

> Looking back over these ten years I am quite certain that if I had not made myself financially and geographically isolated from the teaching hospital this project could not have succeeded.

But he was very concerned about postgraduate training of orthopaedic surgeons and the difficulty of devising rotational schemes which would allow a trainee to work at different centres in order to gain a wide experience. To this end he was convinced that Wrightington would have to forge links with a number of different teaching hospitals.

It is not surprising that Charnley, who prided himself on his colloquial French, was unable to resist quoting two comments from a visiting surgeon, Dr Chandeclerc:

> Chaque prosthésé est mise en place selon une rhythme immuable, avec une facilité déconcertanté et une régularité presque monotone car on aimerait de temps en temps assister à une autre intervention.

This seemed to confirm the picture of a man reduced to a machine. But later in his report, and apparently without the intention of relating it to the former image, the same surgeon said:

> Les trés bon résultats sont ici suprenant par leur fréquence et leur régularité. Il est exceptionnel, parmi les malades revus, de recontrer un mécontent et l'enthousiasme quasi général des opéré contraste avec la satisfaction toujours nuancé des nos consultations hospitalières.

Charnley had pointed out that a 'new surgical industry' was emerging and he estimated that 'some 20 000 hip operations' would be needed a year in the United Kingdom. At the time, this seemed almost unbelievable, but it was in fact an underestimate, as by 1988 over 30 000 hip replacements, of various kinds, were being carried out. Charnley, more than any other single person, had made this possible. He was undoubtedly responsible for a revolution in the science and art of arthroplasty, especially of the hip, which influenced the whole of orthopaedic surgery.

Further very important aspects of the work at Wrightington will be described in the following two chapters which deal with the use of bone cement and the prevention of wound infection.

*Chapter 11*

# BONE CEMENT: GROUT NOT GLUE

## 1958–1982

*A very important piece of original work in my unit has been the development of cold-curing acrylic cement . . . This fundamental technique has completely revolutionised hip joint surgery.*

Charnley to Hawtin 1964

THUS FAR the reader has been asked to accept that the use of bone cement was an integral part of Charnley's low friction arthroplasty, but now it is time to consider how and why he came to introduce this material into the operation. At the outset, it should be made clear that he was not the first person to use acrylic cement in orthopaedic surgery, but his meticulous studies of its application were of great importance in demonstrating the manner in which fixation was obtained and in the interpretation of the long-term changes in the neighbouring tissues.

Kiaer and Jansen of Copenhagen had attached plastic cups to the femoral head with acrylic cement, and reported this to an international orthopaedic meeting in 1951[22] which Charnley is known to have attended. He was there giving a paper on lumbar disc protrusions (Chapter 5), but it is not known whether he heard the Danish contribution on cement, although he may well have done so. Two years later, Dr Haboush of New York published an article in the *Bulletin of the Hospital for Joint Diseases*[20] which indicated that he had used acrylic cement as a seating compound to distribute load from a femoral prosthesis over the bone of the femoral neck.

In the early 1950s, Charnley met D. C. Smith, who had trained as a chemist (and was not a dentist), and who was then a lecturer in the department of material sciences at the Turner Dental Hospital in Manchester. Charnley had first gone to the laboratory to ask advice about measuring the temperature in the flue of his chimney at Rusholme Gardens – this was a reflection of his interest in combustion (Chapter 8). He became a regular visitor to the department to discuss this and other subjects, and Smith remembers that in 1956 or 1957 Charnley asked him whether he knew of a suitable material to fix a femoral

139

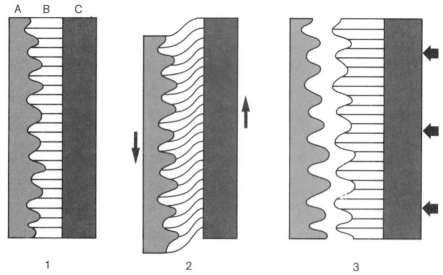

**Fig. 9.5.** *1* *A*. cement; *B*, cancellous endosteal lining of femur; *C*, cortical bone of femur. *2* In shear we visualize elastic deformity taking place within the thickness of the layer of cancellous bone without relative motion occurring at the cement-bone interface. *3* (Surfaces distracted to illustrate absence of adhesion.) When under compressive loads there will be no relative motion between the surfaces

*The bone–cement interface.* (LFA)

prosthesis inside the femur. First they tried dental plaster which was very hard, but the presence of blood retarded its setting to an undesirable degree. Smith was working for a PhD and his subject was acrylic materials in dentistry, so he next suggested Nu-Life, a self-curing acrylic cement which was used as a dental repair material. Smith remembers that they then were working very much in isolation, and were not aware that neurosurgeons had already used acrylic cement in some of their operations.[17,18,25]

Self-curing acrylic cement, properly called polymethylmethacrylate cement, is made by mixing a powder (polymethylmethacrylate plus an activator) with a fluid (methylmethacrylate plus an inhibitor). The process is done in a bowl with a spoon or spatula. The mixture becomes creamy and then doughy. After three or four minutes, it begins to set, and as it does it becomes hot; the monomer evaporates from its surface producing a characteristic smell. The material having become viscous, is plastic, then elastic before becoming solid. The setting time when it was used initially was about fifteen minutes and depended on a number of factors, such as the ambient temperature and humidity. The monomer is self-sterilising, but Charnley sterilised the powder with formaldehyde vapour from formagene tablets.

He experimented with mixing the powder and liquid in the laboratory, and made a plastic femur which he mounted in a box – this became his 'stuffing

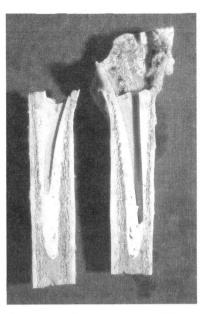

*An early case in which a femoral prosthesis was cemented in position in the treatment of a fracture of the neck of the femur. The patient died four years later. The shaft of the femur has been split open to demonstrate the naked eye appearance of the bone and cement. (From Mr J. Read.)*

box', and was used to practise the insertion of cement and observing how it flowed into the hollow core of the plastic bone (which represented the medullary canal of the femur).

After all the investigation and rehearsal that was possible outside the body, Charnley decided it would be justifiable to use cement in elderly patients who had sustained a fracture of the neck of the femur for which the insertion of a femoral prosthesis was an accepted orthopaedic procedure. If the prosthesis became loose, it was believed to cause pain, so an experiment to achieve a better fixation seemed justified – and in those days there were no ethical committees. The first operation with cement was done in Manchester in 1958 and Charnley reported his first six cases in the British *Journal of Bone and Joint Surgery* in 1960.[1] He made the point that the dough should be 'rammed' deeply into the femur by thumb pressure. The cement acted as a 'grout' and not as glue, so that fixation was by interlocking and not by adhesion. The dough was forced into every crevice in the interior of the femur so that the weight of the body was dispersed over a large area of bone. Heat created during setting was absorbed by the metal prosthesis acting as a 'heat-sink' and did not damage the tissues. None of the six patients had suffered any ill-effects, and Charnley stated that the quality of the results was better than when cement was not used.

The way was now clear for the introduction of cement into the hip replacement operations which Charnley was developing; first to fix the femoral prosthesis, and later the socket. But he continued to observe and study the effects of cement in his original group of patients. Since they were mostly in their seventies and eighties, he was able to obtain some post-mortem specimens, and in 1964 he reported his findings in six such specimens[2] (these were not from the six cases that had been reported originally). No sign of deterioration was seen in histological preparations up to three years after operation, and he concluded cautiously that 'the technique is considered justifiable in elderly patients. . .'. Other publications followed and are listed at the end of the chapter.

In 1964, Mrs Marie Stringfellow was appointed as a part-time histology technician to work in a laboratory in the hip centre with a salary paid from Charnley's research fund. She had very little experience of the techniques which were needed, and Charnley arranged for her to go to Manchester to learn. There were difficulties initially, but she improved and remained in the post until 1978. Her job was mainly to prepare sections to show the microscopic appearance of the interface between cement and bone. She found Charnley not always easy to work for; she remembers that he was a 'perfectionist, and was always prepared to have a go himself'. Charnley showed his appreciation of her efforts when, at the end of a paper[6], he acknowledged her 'careful and patient work in overcoming the technical difficulties in making these histological preparations'. The fact that she stayed for fourteen years is a testimony to their collaboration.

Charnley realised that it was essential to obtain the artificial joints from patients who died some years after their operation in order to study the tissue changes which occurred in relation to the cement. This was a delicate and difficult matter which had to be approached with care.

Charnley undertook the task with his usual attention to detail. He wrote to 'some of my patients [presumably those who lived not too far away] who have had the new operation . . . performed on their hip, at least three years ago'. The following two paragraphs illustrate some of the problems involved:

> I am selecting patients whose ages are such that they are likely to predecease me by more than ten years, in the hope that they will bequeath their hip to medical research.
>
> If the idea . . . should be repugnant to you, there is no need to reply to this letter and I shall take precautions to make sure that you are never bothered again on this score.

Those who agreed were asked to return a signed copy of the letter and give the address of their eldest son or daughter. The letters were all personally addressed and signed by Charnley himself. Sometime later he would write to the son or daughter:

> It is possible that you may have heard from your father about his wish to co-operate in our research.
>
> It is now-a-days a very common practice for the deceased's remains to be taken to the undertaker's premises to await the day of the funeral. If I were to be notified by telegram or telephone at this hospital, giving the name and address of the undertaker, I would come by car with the necessary equipment and remove the specimen at the undertaker's premises. This whole procedure would not take more than half an hour and certainly would not delay the funeral arrangements for more than one day at the most.

His approach was effective and it is said that he never had a refusal. Over the years, more than seventy specimens were collected providing invaluable material for research.

An important phase in Charnley's work on cement began with a letter to Mr F. Hawtin on August 5, 1964. Hawtin had been a patient at Wrightington and was a director of the Dental Manufacturing Company. He wrote: 'I have not seen you since your famous ox-roasting, but our professional ways seem to be coming in contact again'. He explained that he had been getting Nu-Life self-curing acrylic cement from a firm in London. When he had asked them about the possibility of their supplying cement 'in a form suited for orthopaedic surgery rather than dentistry', they had replied that they did not manufacture the cement themselves, but were getting it from the Dental Manufacturing Company, which was Hawtin's company. This coincidence led Hawtin to express an interest in Charnley's problems with cement. He wrote:

> I don't mind how much trouble I go to to help you and am quite prepared to bear the expense myself because it is not a commercial proposition to the Company; but don't let that be an obstacle.

This was a very generous gesture, although Charnley had made it clear he was convinced that 'in the next few years very large demands will be made for this material'.

Nothing happened for four months so Charnley wrote again and arranged to meet Hawtin. The upshot was that Charnley was put in touch with Mr G. S. Thurman who was then works manager for CMW Laboratories Limited (the initials stand for Calculated Molecular Weight). The firm was a subsidiary of the Dental Manufacturing Company based in Blackpool, which was conveniently near Wrightington. During the next two years Thurman went regularly to the hospital to discuss the most appropriate way of making cement with the properties that Charnley needed. Their correspondence from 1965 to 1981 is available and provides a good account of the practical problems which they had to deal with.

First, the sterilisation of the powder, and the addition of barium sulphate to make the cement radio-opaque, were discussed in detail. Sterilisation by γ-radiation, carried out by the United Kingdom Atomic Energy Authority at Wantage, was tested but Charnley felt that it altered the setting time and quality of the mixture. A decision was made in April, 1965, to continue with formaldehyde vapour.

Thurman provided various powders with slightly different constituents for Charnley to test, and these were packaged at the hospital in a way which was suitable for use at operation. The aim was to develop a cement which 'would be deprived of all unnecessary additives which creep into it when making it suitable for dental purposes' – one of which was presumably 'pinkness'. By August, powder B10 was found to be best, and the question of commercial manufacture and presentation then arose. Various names were considered: orthocrete, orthocem, osteocrete, osteocem. Perhaps wisely they were all discarded and the product was called CMW Bone Cement. Charnley emphasised the special features which he felt were essential:

(1) The cement has been prepared without any unnecessary additives . . .
(2) The exact constituents should be published . . . 'too many products are on the market with secret compositions [which] . . . ought to be divulged publicly if they are to be used in the human body.

(3) Formaldehyde sterilisation . . . 'a great deal of experimental work (at Wrightington) has shown that this is the best method . . . Incidentally, it is very much cheaper than anything else'.

(4) The inclusion in the package of two measured doses of barium sulphate to allow the surgeon the choice of different degrees of radio-opacity.

In November, 1965, Charnley produced detailed instructions about the way the cement should be used which were to be included with the commercial product. The first invoice for 250 packs of the new cement was issued to Wrightington on January 4, 1966. Two other similar cements were available at this time. Surgical Simplex, made by North Hill Plastics Limited of London, was the cement used in the United Kingdom by neurosurgeons since the early 1950s to fill defects in the skull and to contain intracranial aneurysms.[17,18,25] It was also chosen by McKee for his hip replacements after his colleague Watson-Farrar had visited Wrightington. The other cement was Palacos which was produced in Germany. These can fairly be described as 'rival' products, but Charnley always preferred CMW and he remained loyal to it for the rest of his life.

As bone cement was gradually used more widely in orthopaedic surgery, there was more concern about the possibility that its insertion might cause cardiac arrest during operation. Charnley certainly took this seriously, but felt that cement could not be blamed. In 1967, a senior house officer in anaesthesia at the London Hospital wrote to CMW Laboratories enquiring about the fall in blood pressure which had been observed to occur as cement was inserted into the femur. Charnley was given the letter and wrote a long reply in explanation. He stressed that the cement should be held in the hand until the smell of monomer had completely disappeared, and he discussed why a fall of blood pressure was more likely to occur as the cement was put into the femur than when it was put into the acetabulum. The whole matter was discussed by those most interested (mainly orthopaedic surgeons and anaesthetists), and in 1971 the Department of Health and Social Security set up a working party, which was chaired by Professor R. G. Burwell, to enquire into these aspects of the use of acrylic cement. The report published in 1974[16] vindicated Charnley's opinion:

> The use of cement in total hip replacement on patients with arthritis appears to be associated with no greater risk than that which might be expected in any group of patients in the same age range, subjected to other major operative and general anaesthetic procedures.

They did, however, find there was a greater risk in elderly patients when cement was used with a prosthesis inserted for the treatment of a fracture of the neck of the femur, and in some types of knee replacement.

The risks of hip replacement were raised again in an editorial in the British Medical Journal in 1975[19] which stimulated a response from Charnley[10]:

> During the past four years the use of acrylic cement in hip surgery has multiplied many times, but we no longer seem to hear of these complications in scientific meetings of surgeons who are using this substance almost daily . . .
>
> I think I am right in saying that all experimental investigations have exonerated methylmethacrylate monomer in concentrations likely to be encountered in the blood stream during a surgical operation. . .

He asked 'are these complications occurring in any numbers or even at all?' and invited readers of the journal to write to him. He wrote again five months later pointing out that the experience in his unit 'would give the impression that no problem exists at all'. In 10 356 hip operations performed at Wrightington between January 1963 and June 1975 there were two fatal cardiac arrests, but in one of these there were features which suggested that the monomer was not responsible. He was, however, worried because he had received three replies to his first letter reporting four instances of cardiac arrest which were attributed to the use of cement. He suggested that these cases might have occurred in 'patients whose hearts are already poised for arrest from unrelated causes and that the final stimulus for arrest is not specific for the monomer'. Nowadays, while cement is treated with respect, its safe use is taken for granted, so much so that it is difficult to recall the anxieties of the early days. Charnley's conviction, based on his vast experience, was responsible for overcoming the initial doubts and his opinions have been justified with the passage of time.

As early as 1966 Charnley, after a visit to Chicago, had written to Thurman that 'the Americans have almost no knowledge of cement . . . ' and that he should expect 'a lot of enquiries'. Dr M. Lazansky was the first American to have worked at Wrightington where he was a registrar from July to October, 1965. On returning to New York he began to carry out the low friction arthroplasty at the Albert Einstein College Hospital and at the Hospital for Joint Diseases. At first, he had been able to obtain CMW, and indeed there is evidence in a letter from a director of Thackrays, dated May 13, 1969 that CMW Laboratories 'were still supplying their cement to the United States as they had not yet been informed of any imports being stopped'. Earlier, in April 1960, Lazansky had written to Thackrays to tell them that he 'had the largest individual series in the States, now amounting to some 60 cases'. But acrylic cement had been classified as an 'investigational new drug' by the Food and Drug Administration, and it could only be used under licence. This meant that the operation could no longer be done without such a licence, as the cement was an integral part of the procedure. Professor Jack Stevens, an English orthopaedic surgeon who was then at the University of Chicago, visited Charnley in 1969 and wanted to carry out the low friction arthroplasty when he returned to the United States. He had difficulty in obtaining a licence to use cement, but whenever an orthopaedic surgeon visited the United Kingdom his colleagues would ask him to bring back a few packets so that there was a considerable 'trade' in cement around Chicago for a time.

The first official licence was issued to the Mayo Clinic in Rochester, Minnesota. The first prosthesis was inserted there in March, 1969 by Dr M. Coventry, who had know Charnley since 1954 and had visited him more recently at Wrightington. In due course, licences were granted to other major centres.

However, these surgeons, and those who followed them, were using Simplex cement, not CMW. Charnley had anticipated that there would be problems introducing CMW into the United States. He knew, for example, that the Food and Drug Administration would not readily accept sterilisation with formaldehyde vapour; although he had pointed out that if cement containing barium sulphate (to make it radio-opaque) was irradiated, the setting time was lengthened and some change in colour occurred, both of which he considered undesirable. At this stage (in 1970), he insisted that 'CMW was the only cement on which there has been an extensive series of publication regarding the reaction of human tissues'. There were also difficulties because CMW Laboratories were then reluctant to release their formula in case it was copied, whereas Simplex did not impose the same restrictions on their product. The original CMW application in 1970 was said 'to have become totally "bogged down" in the bureaucracy'.

A number of changes occurred in the ownership of CMW Laboratories, and their parent company was purchased by Dentsply International Inc in 1976. Nothing further was done about the application to the Food and Drug Administration until February, 1980, when responsibility was transferred to the Bureau of Medical Devices. Further data was requested and was filed on fifteen occasions between 1980 and February, 1984, when approval for CMW was finally received. By this time low viscosity cements, which are fluid enough to be used with a cement gun, were being used by 80 to 85 per cent of American surgeons; and the original doughy CMW cement could not be applied in this manner. CMW Laboratories now also manufactured a low viscosity cement and a radio-opaque cement which were licensed without difficulty.

Between 1960 and 1970, Charnley published eight papers dealing with such problems as the way in which prostheses were bonded to bone by cement[2], and the biomechanical factors involved.[3] He also described how fractures of the femur, occurring after hip replacement, healed in the presence of cement.[4] Two important contributions in 1968 and 1970 concerned the long-term reaction of bone to cement. The first was a radiological study of the changes in the femur after an average of four years following operation in 174 patients.[5] This was carried out meticulously and made it possible for surgeons to understand the significance of the appearances they observed in their own patients, and which were not recognised at the time. The second paper was based on the histological findings in 23 specimens collected from patients who had died from one month to seven years after operation.[8] The appearance of the critical bone-cement interface was studied in order to show how the body weight was transferred from the cement to the shaft of the femur. This was found to occur at isolated points through fibro-cartilaginous tissue which had formed in response to load.

The culmination of this stage of his research was the publication of his book, *Acrylic Cement in Orthopaedic Surgery*, in 1970.[7] All aspects of the subject were covered in 130 pages which were packed with relevant information. He concluded with a list of the 'attractive features' of self-curing acrylic cement and which he regarded 'as highly satisfactory and not to be lost in any new modification':

(1) Insolubility of the cured resin

(2) Setting time adapted to surgical practice, i.e. six to eight minutes

(3) Sharp end point to mark setting

(4) Setting not impaired by admixture with blood

(5) Tendency to expansion while setting; certainly not a contraction

(6) Consistency of the acrylic dough excellent

(7) Strength of cured cement adequate

(8) Easily sterilised without changing chemical structure. . .etc

As far as (5) is concerned, it is now considered that Charnley's conclusion was incorrect[21]: all cements contract to a varying degree on setting, but CMW substantially less than most. These are rather technical matters, but they indicate (in his own words) the range of properties which he considered to be of practical importance.

Although CMW Laboratories had used γ-radiation to sterilise the powder since 1967, it was 1972 before Charnley accepted the method. Presumably his change of view was a concession to demands from the United States. But the CMW which Charnley used continued to be sterilised by formaldehyde.

The importance of pressurising cement during its introduction into the joint was recognised in the early 1970s; the aim being to force the dough into every crevice in the bone so that extensive interlocking was achieved. Charnley had always relied on forcing the cement into a narrow opening in the femur with this thumb, but the acetabulum presented a problem as the cement tended to flow out around the edges of the socket as it was pushed into place.

Mr R. S. M. Ling of Exeter had designed a new type of hip replacement, in conjunction with his engineering colleague Dr A. J. C. Lee, which was first used in 1970.[23] They were concerned about the cement technique and after laboratory research devised a new method of pressurising the cement in the acetabulum while it was setting using a rubber, water-filled tampon; the socket was then pushed into the cement at precisely the correct moment. They chose Simplex because it was more fluid than CMW. Charnley was interested in this technique and went to Exeter to see it used. He had already (in 1969) altered the direction of reaming the acetabulum from oblique to horizontal in order to keep the socket at a lower level. Tension in the soft tissues was maintained, so reducing the risk of dislocation, and the length of the leg was restored. But the cement tended to flow out of the acetabulum above the rim of the socket, so pressurisation was poor. Instead of applying pressure by the Exeter method, Charnley changed the

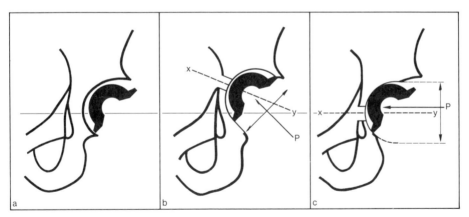

**Fig. 7.3. a** Socket in acetabulum which will fit socket better when deepened. **b** Deepening at 45° keeps rim of socket concentric with rim of acetabulum; good for pressurisation of cement; but centre of rotation raised above anatomical level. **c** Socket deepened transversely to keep centre of socket at anatomical level; but renders rim of socket eccentric to rim of acetabulum; bad for pressurisation of cement in roof of acetabulum

*Diagrams showing the effect of changing the direction in which the acetabulum is reamed, with Charnley's comments.* (LFA)

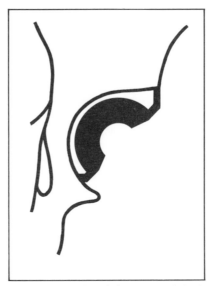

*Diagram showing the way in which the rim of the pressure injection socket retains the cement within the acetabulum.* (LFA)

design of his socket by adding an oval rim so that the cement was retained while it was setting. The rim, which was inclined 45° away from the face of the socket, was 1 mm thick and could be trimmed with stout scissors to fit the acetabulum. The effect of this new design was implied by its name: the pressure injection socket. A further modification to the socket to improve cement pressurisation is discussed in Chapter 13.

In preparing the bone to receive cement, Charnley made three 12.5 mm holes in the floor of the acetabulum to anchor the cement, and he now added a number of shallow holes (6 mm) for additional fixation. Blood and debris were washed away by irrigation with saline from a syringe, and fibrous tissue was removed with a rotary nylon brush. These improvements in cement technique could be expected to produce better long-term results. Charnley was able to report in 1978 that mechanical failure at the bone-cement interface in the socket occurred in only 2.2% of cases which had been followed up for an average of 8.3 years.[14] He concluded:

> because the cement technology used at that time is now considered unsophisticated, mechanical failure is a preventable condition.

Although fixation of the femoral component had never presented as much of a problem as fixation of the socket, improvements were also made here. They came about largely as a result of changes which Charnley had made for other reasons. First, the opening in the upper end of the femur had been enlarged to allow a more valgus (vertical) position of the prosthesis. It was then possible to insert the cement with 'two-thumb' pressure and also to place an adequate amount between the medial part of the prosthesis and the neck of the femur. Second, and probably more important, he had designed a stronger femoral prosthesis (Chapter 13); flanges were added to the shoulders of the new design which

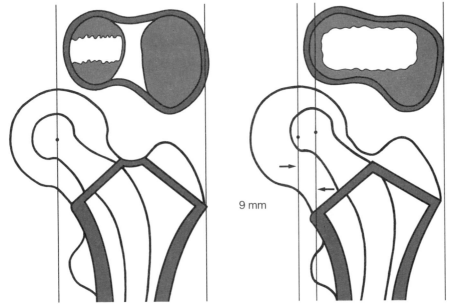

9 mm

**Fig. 6.7.** Change in technique of reaming femoral cavity: before 1969 working through cut femoral neck; later invading the area of the detached trochanter and enlarging medullary cavity for 'two-thumb' technique of inserting cement and more valgus position of prosthesis

*The technique of reaming the femur to receive the prosthesis.* (LFA)

retained the cement and applied compression to it. Since he continued to use the original CMW cement, he was never able to fill the femur with a syringe, as had become popular in many centres where a more fluid (low viscosity) cement was preferred. When one of his colleagues, Mr B. M. Wroblewski suggested blocking the medullary canal of the femur beyond the tip of the prosthesis in order to increase pressurisation. Charnley said it would not work. Four years later, he decided it was a brilliant idea and he adopted it, saying to Wroblewski that he could not understand why he had not thought of it himself.

In making these technical improvements, one thought was dominant in Charnley's mind – he emphasised again and again that it was essential, when doing the operation, to build for twenty years, and not just for the next year or two. Meticulous attention to these details was mandatory if the desired result was to be obtained.

As we saw in the previous chapter, Charnley began publishing the five year results of the low friction arthroplasty in the early 1970s. In passing it is right to mention that this is what he always called the operation – the LFA. Occasionally in papers published in North America, he referred to 'total hip replacement'; but it was other people, not he, who spoke about the Charnley operation.

Five papers, which were specially concerned with bony changes associated with the presence of cement in the acetabulum and in the femur, were published by

Charnley between 1975 and 1980, with various assistants as co-authors.[9,11,12,13,14] His last paper concerning cement was written in collaboration with J. R. Loudon, and described an accurate radiological method of measuring the subsidence of the femoral prosthesis in relation to the femur.[15] It was shown that there was less subsidence with the flanged prosthesis compared with the older design and far fewer fractures of the tip of the cement occured in the former group. Charnley had discussed the significance of these fractures in a previous publication[9] and demonstrated that they were usually related to subsidence of the prosthesis.

Correspondence with Thurman, who had been a director of CMW Laboratories since 1972, continued, and the final letter was written by Charnley on December 2, 1981. He said that he had been using Palacos cement containing gentamycin (an antibiotic). This was surprising since up to this time, as we shall see in the next chapter, he had never used antibiotics because he had devised other methods of preventing wound infection. When asked, one year before his death, why he had made this change, his answer was simple, and understandable: 'I never want to see another infected hip'. He never liked using any cement other than CMW, and the German Palacos was the only cement then available which contained an antibiotic; so Thurman approached a major pharmaceutical company with the idea of producing CMW which would include one of the cephalosporins, which are a group of broad spectrum antibiotics. CMW Laboratories now have introduced two new cements which contain gentamycin.

Charnley continued to collect specimens of hip prostheses removed from patients after their death. Jill Charnley recalls that she drove him from Knutsford to Mansfield, in Nottinghamshire, across the Derbyshire Peaks on a cold wet Sunday afternoon in February 1982 – a distance of more than 60 miles. Charnley wrote in the journal which he kept that year:

> the specimen was waiting for me in formalin in a plastic bucket [the patient had died in hospital and a post-mortem carried out]. This is truly a marvellous climax to my series of more than 70 cases. This one was operated on in 1963 – thus perhaps only six months after the start of the true LFA (with HMWP).

The journey home was somewhat nerve-racking for the driver; she wondered, if they had an accident, how the police would view the hip in a bucket in the boot of their Mercedes car. Charnley dissected the 17-year-old specimen the next day:

> . . . the interior of the joint was perfect and the fixity of the cemented joint in the pelvis, and of the cemented femoral prosthesis, also was perfect.

His delight and enthusiasm are evident. The effort of collecting the specimens cannot be overestimated, nor can their value in a study of the long-term consequences of using cement in the body. A critical factor was that he had detailed clinical records of every case, so that the outcome could be correlated with the pathological findings.

He had intended to review the whole collection of hips himself and he tried to have a small laboratory built at Wrightington in the early 1980s, where he could examine the specimens and make the necessary histological preparations. He became so frustrated by the obstacles created by safety regulations in the National Health Service that Jill Charnley suggested that a small prefabricated laboratory should be put up in the garden of his home instead; it was completed only shortly before he died in August, 1982.

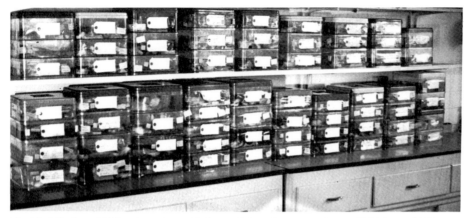

**Fig. 4.1.** Collection of 62 hips donated to medical research by patients operated on at Wrightington 1.5–13 years after surgery

*Autopsy specimens of hips collected by Charnley. The number later rose to 78. (LFA)*

In the end, there were 78 specimens which were bequeathed for further research; they had been in situ for a variable time – from 8 to 23 years. The project has been undertaken by Dr A. J. Malcolm, a pathologist and senior lecturer at the University of Newcastle-upon-Tyne who has a special interest in bone and joint disorders. His work has been supported by a grant from Action Research who provided a salary for a research technician. His investigation has shown that in most cases there is a 'beautiful bone–cement interlock between the viable bone and cement' around the femoral prosthesis, and this confirms Charnley's initial reports that a bone–cement interface could occur and persist for a long period;[24] The situation is different around the socket where there is no such integration and a thick fibrous membrane is formed between the plastic and the bone, but this may not affect the clinical outcome. Another feature is that wear particles, mostly of HMWP, are present in the tissues around the joint and also at the interface in the acetabulum. These particles were only found in the femur in the 18 cases where there was not a bone–cement interface. The significance of these findings is not clear, but it is probable that the tissue response to wear particles might eventually produce a reaction which could lead to loss of bone and therefore loosening. An additional contributory factor is the loss of bone stock which inevitably takes place with age.

Further studies relating these histological results to the clinical condition of the patients before they died are in progress. Whatever the final conclusions, the findings are bound to shed an important light on the natural history of arthroplasty of the hip. It is sad that Charnley was not able to complete the investigation himself as he had planned, but his efforts in collecting and recording this invaluable material have not been in vain.

*Chapter 12*

---

# CLEAN AIR AGAINST INFECTION
## 1960–1982

---

*Postoperative infection is the saddest of all complications . . .*

John Charnley 1982

THE CONSEQUENCES of deep infection around a joint replacement are disastrous and likely to involve the patient in months of treatment; in the past, the outcome was always removal of the components (and cement), although now the prosthesis can be removed and exchanged for a new one. This, however, is not an easy solution because infection will have been associated with loosening and destruction of the neighbouring bone so that the second operation is arduous, and takes very much longer than a routine arthroplasty.

Charnley had faced the problem when he began carrying out arthroplasties at Wrightington in 1960, and he described the situation in the early days:

> Throughout 1960 to 1962 Teflon [PTFE] arthroplasties were performed at Wrightington in the crudest of operating theatres. . . For ventilation it had merely an extraction fan in the roof which pulled air in from the hospital corridor, a corridor which was not even part of the operating suite. Nevertheless this design of ventilation was in use, though in more glamorous surroundings, in what at that time was the most expensive private nursing home in Manchester. . . An extraction fan. . . was merely to keep the operating personnel in reasonable comfort; it was not seen as having any bearing on wound infection.

The infection rate after the PTFE arthroplasties was 7%, which now seems a horrifying figure, but there was an odd feature: the infection might develop three to six months after operation, and often after healing had occurred perfectly in the first instance. The wounds had all the appearances of infection, but if pus was discharged it was frequently reported as sterile – that is, no infecting

153

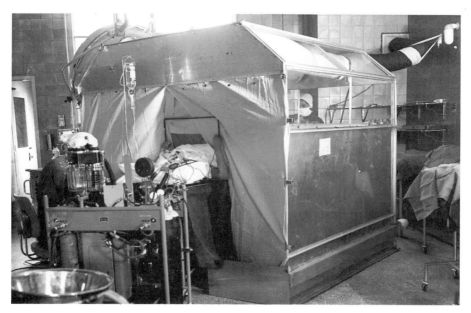

*The first clean air enclosure made by Charnley and Craven which was appropriately named 'the greenhouse'. (By permission of the publishers of the* British Journal of Surgery, *Butterworth & Co (Publishers).)*

organisms were grown in the laboratory by the techniques available at the time. Charnley wrote:

> The explanation itself to my mind was that it must be caused by acrylic cement, because there was no previous surgical experience in the human body of implanting the large volumes needed in this operation.

It was imperative to devise a method of keeping bacteria away from the wound during the operation:

> If I could successfully prevent all bacteria gaining access to the wound . . . then two possible results might ensue: either the infection-like complications would become significantly fewer; or they would continue at the same frequency. In the first case bacteria would be responsible; in the second case the chemical action of the cement would be responsible.

These quotations were written retrospectively by Charnley in *Wrightington – the Story of the First Fifty Years*[9], and they bring the situation to life; we now need to look at the way he tackled and solved the problem.

Orthopaedic surgeons had for many years taken steps to avoid direct contamination of operative wounds, but they had not considered the possibility of eliminating all bacteria from the environment in which they were operating – and this was what Charnley set out to do.

The first step was to establish a base-line which was done by exposing culture plates in the theatre to find out whether they were colonised by bacteria: the

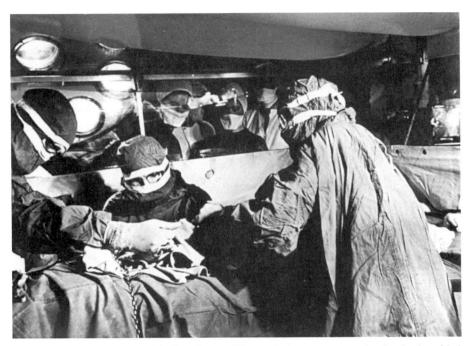

*Charnley operating in the original enclosure. The surgical team are wearing hoods, but this is before the body exhaust system was introduced. Spectators can be seen outside the enclosure. (Photograph from Mr N. W. Nisbet, Orthopaedic Hospital, Oswestry.)*

colony count per hour (cph) in the unmodified theatre was an average of 80 to 90 indicating heavy contamination of the air.

Charnley then sought advice from several air-conditioning firms without making much progress, but he concluded that the answer lay in operating in an enclosure within the main theatre into which filtered air could be passed. The first such enclosure was built at Wrightington by Craven to Charnley's design. Craven had no assistants and had to work at night and on Sunday mornings when the theatres were not being used. The prototype enclosure, which was constructed in 1961, was designed to contain the lower half of the patient's body and the surgeon and two assistants. The walls were made of glass and the aperture around the patient's chest was closed with sterile curtains. Air was ducted in from outside the theatre building and blown in by a small fan with an electrostatic precipitator which removed dust particles on which bacteria are carried. The enclosure took about fifteen minutes to set up in the only operating theatre in the hospital, and it had to be dismantled between Charnley's lists. Its size was seven feet square and seven feet high; to those seeing it for the first time its appearance in the theatre was bizarre, and it was nicknamed the 'greenhouse'. Operating in such a small space was very restricting, but those involved had to learn to cope with the new situation. This prototype was in use between November 1961 and June 1962. Although the air flow was not more than 40 cubic feet a minute (cfm), the colony count was reduced to an average of 25 an hour.

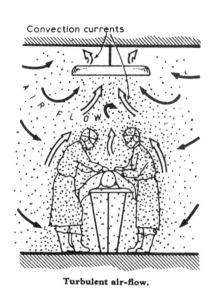
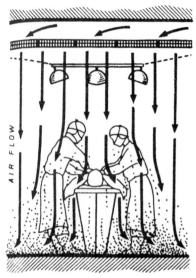

**Turbulent air-flow.**  **Removal of particles by laminar/ linear system of air movement.**

*Diagram showing the pattern of turbulent airflow in a conventional operating theatre compared with the pattern achieved with downward linear flow. (From Scott CC (1970) Laminar/linear flow system of ventilation – its application to medicine and surgery.* Lancet I:989–993. *By permission of the Editor of* The Lancet.*)*

Colleagues in the department of microbiology in the University of Manchester, whom Charnley consulted, put him in touch with Mr F. H. Howorth whose family firm had built air filtration systems since 1854. They were based in Bolton, Lancashire, and Howorth's father had designed filters to remove soiling particles from the air in textile factories which were installed not only in Lancashire and Yorkshire, but as far afield as St Petersburg in Russia and Shanghai in China. In 1919, The Friary Brewery in Guildford, Surrey, had wanted to eliminate bacteria from their fermenting rooms. Howorths did this for them with filters which consisted of bags made with two layers of cotton blanketing and which were 98% efficient against very small particles (up to $2\mu$). The system was later installed in breweries throughout the United Kingdom and used in the pharmaceutical industry where bacteria-free air is needed for some processes. Howorth went to Wrightington on December 10, 1961, for the first of many visits. He was able to provide the operating conditions which Charnley wanted, and indeed to him the problem seemed on a small scale, almost 'like model-making'. Like Hawtin in the cement story, Howorth was convinced by Charnley's enthusiasm and was prepared to contribute his firm's expertise to the project.

The original greenhouse was adapted to take the new air handling and diffusion system which Howorth had designed and donated to the hospital. This was working by June 1962 and continued in use until March 1966. The main improvements were indicated by the flow of filtered air which was increased from 40 to 800 cubic feet per minute, and the number of air changes also increased from 10 to 130 an hour. The fall in the settle plate count was spectacular: from

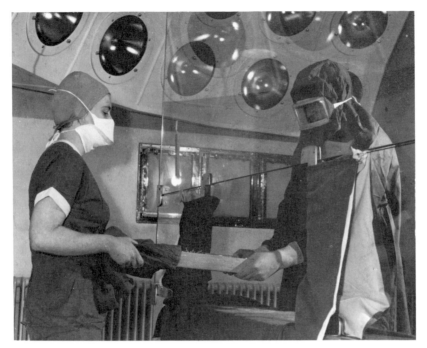

*The circulating nurse is passing a tray of sterile instruments through the service opening to the nurse inside the enclosure.* (LFA)

an average of 25 to 1.8 colonies per hour. At the same time, there was a fall in the infection rate associated with these changes, but for various reasons this was hard to prove.

In any operating room, heat creates up-currents of air and much of this heat is generated by the theatre lamp. Charnley, therefore, designed two quadrants of lights (one for each side) which were placed outside the enclosure and provided excellent diffuse illumination.

Once the surgical team were inside the enclosure with the patient's head and the anaesthetist outside it, a method of getting the instruments inside was needed. A service opening with a shelf was made at the foot-end of the enclosure through which trays of instruments could be passed. Charnley had planned the operation in a number of set stages with every move clearly defined, the instruments for each stage being provided in separate trays (seven in all). This imposed a strict discipline on the way the operation was carried out so that a highly efficient routine was established.

Charnley and Howorth collaborated closely over the many technical details to be overcome. This led to a long association that was usually, but by no means always, friendly; their correspondence from 1963 to 1979 is available and information to be quoted is taken from it.

Howorth now went on to produce the first permanent (mark I) downflow enclosure which was installed in a new, second operating theatre at Wrightington in June, 1966. A grant of £3,199 from the Medical Research Council in 1964

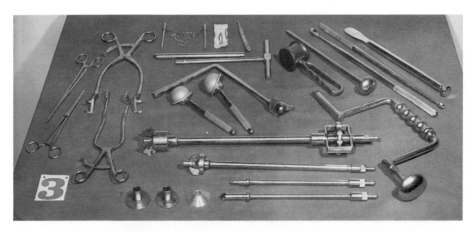

*These instruments would be contained in one tray for a particular stage of the operation. Most were designed for specific purposes by Charnley. Once this stage was finished the tray would be removed and replaced by another. (From Mr Geoffrey Middleton.)*

helped to cover the cost of installation. The air flow was increased from 2000 to 4000 cubic feet per minute, and contamination in the enclosure was extremely low. To test this, Craven had built a slit-sampler which provided a more accurate way of assessing air contamination than settle plates. A great deal of bacteriological investigation was carried out; much of it undertaken by the hospital's pathology technician, Mr F. Dandy, with advice from Dr F. Hillman, who was the consultant pathologist at Wigan.

If problems arose with the new theatre, Charnley never hesitated to write (or telephone) in anger:

> The thermostatic control in our new theatre is really quite a farce. On Monday I spent half an hour in the ventilating plant while operating was going on downstairs. (16.11.66)

He went into great detail about how the valves and water-pump were working and then made suggestions about the humidification of the theatre air. All this was sorted out satisfactorily, although not before some further communication of which this is an example:

> Since my telephone conversation when I expressed my annoyance about the functioning of this installation so very forcibly . . . (22.12.66)

Charnley published two papers in the *British Journal of Surgery* in 1964. The first concerned his experience in developing his method of 'performing a surgical operation in a sterile atmosphere' and described the design of his operating enclosure.[1] In the second, he correlated the occurrence of infection with the amount of bacterial contamination in the air of the operating theatre.[2] He pointed out that the low friction arthroplasty was a very sensitive indicator of deep infection because, in the presence of such a massive implant, infection can never be overcome by the body's normal defence mechanisms. This explained the high incidence (in the region of 7%) when clean air was not used; other major orthopaedic procedures carried out in this environment had not shown such a high incidence of infection. A more detailed paper, written with N. Eftekhar (an assistant from New York) was published in the same journal in 1969.[4] The conclusion was that, even after taking other factors into consideration, the infection rate fell to 3.7%, and then to 1.3%, as the clean air system was improved.

In spite of this considerable reduction in infection, Charnley was concerned about what he called 'the hard core' of 1.3% which was acquired in the operating theatre, and which he had so far not eliminated.

Surgeon's gloves were often punctured during operations, particularly when vigorous manoeuvres were carried out, as was the case during the arthroplasty of the hip. Thus there was the chance that organisms might be transferred from the surgeon's hands to the open wound (in spite of rigorous 'scrubbing up') resulting in infection. To minimise this risk, the surgeon and his first assistant wore two pairs of disposable gloves from 1966 onwards.

From the time when the greenhouse was used in 1961, Charnley had designed methods of diminishing the risk of contamination from the nose, throat, and hair of the surgical team. A cloth hood completely invested the head and neck (but was separate from the gown), and a suction tube near the mouth and nose evacuated expired air. The latter was important because the downflow of air from the filters in the ceiling might otherwise have blown organisms towards the wound.

Everyone sheds scales of skin and bacteria from their body all the time, and in an operating theatre the numbers can rise during activity to as many as 50 000 viable organisms each minute. To some extent this is controlled by the downflow of air in the enclosure, but as movement creates minor turbulence it seemed desirable to try to remove this source of contamination as far as possible.

The type and material of clothing worn by the surgical team was important; and in 1965 Blowers and McCluskey suggested that gowns made of ventile, which is a tightly woven long-staple cotton, were effective in this respect.[10] Their paper was published in *The Lancet* and Charnley replied in the correspondence columns of that journal[3]:

> I doubt whether any of the innovations to surgical clothing will make more than a marginal improvement in the bacterial content of air in conventional theatres.

He described the work at Wrightington with the clean air enclosure and wrote:

> . . . we have had the opportunity under actual operating conditions of making a large number of slit-sampler investigations of the effects of different types of clothing.

The use of suction under the all-enveloping hoods (instead of the conventional surgical cap) made it possible for the surgeons to wear ventile gowns which were otherwise very hot. But Charnley found that there was very little improvement over the cotton gowns with which ventile was being compared. He thought the explanation was that heat from the surgeon's body caused a rising flow of air encouraging particles to escape from the upper part of the gown. This idea brought a solution to the problem:

> Through altering the design of the operating gowns by incorporating the helmet into the gown (like that of the Ku-Klux Klan) and by closing the

back of the gown completely so that it has to be put over the head like a night-shirt), the use of body-suction has now produced a great improvement of the bacterial content of the air inside the enclosure . . .

These precautions sound very elaborate and expensive, but in fact they are neither. Further experience will lead to simplification . . .

To those who are unfamiliar with operating theatres, the ritual which surgeons perform to clothe themselves may appear arcane, but is an important part of surgical procedure. Charnley was now proposing radical changes to accepted practice in his drive to reduce aerial contamination in the environment (and hence wound infection). He did not, however, suggest that these precautions should be used for all operations, but only for those 'demanding conditions of almost perfect air-sterility, necessitating specially designed installations'; and hip replacement was undoubtedly such an operation.

He also realised that another source of direct contamination was through the surgeon's gown. For example, as the acetabulum was reamed, the surgeon pushed his body against a brace-and-bit; his sweat and the patient's blood might, therefore, permeate (from either direction) the material of the gown. Standard theatre gowns were made of 'balloon cloth', a fine cotton material with apertures in it through which bacteria could pass. In a series of tests, Charnley demonstrated the presence of bacteria from the surgeon on the external surface of the gown. He published this work with Eftekhar in *The Lancet* in 1969[5], and they suggested a number of preventive measures: a plastic apron worn under the gown, or a sterile apron of fine woven cloth worn over the gown might help; and disposable plastic or paper gowns might be better than coarsely woven textile.

The attack on the prevention of infection required much painstaking investigation and trial, and it was not until 1970 that the full body exhaust system was introduced at Wrightington. The basic equipment was a headpiece through which suction was applied and an all-enveloping gown of ventile. A lightweight headpiece, which had a window of transparent plastic and internal openings for the suction hose, was fitted first to the wearer's head. Then the ventile gown, having been correctly folded, was put on over the head and allowed to fall down over the body, so that it hung freely from the top of the head, with the opening for the face in the gown coinciding with the window. It was essential that there was no restriction at the neck or waist. The suction was then connected and turned on to give an extraction rate from 15 to 35 cubic feet per minute. Higher rates produced a certain amount of noise to which the wearer quickly became accustomed according to Charnley. He said that at its worst, it was less than that experienced in a private aeroplane. He found this acceptable, but some surgeons did not like it. The pressure under the gown needed to be sub-atmospheric so that when the arms were raised and lowered the 'bellows' action of the gown did not pump skin scales into the theatre air. Maintenance of adequate suction was critical and if it failed the wearer became very hot. This happened once to Charnley when the latest model of enclosure and body exhaust was installed at Wrightington in 1970. He was so upset by the experience that he wrote to *The Lancet* to advise surgeons to test their equipment personally[6]; and to make sure that the pressure within the gown was reduced, in comparison with atmospheric pressure, by one quarter to one half. Further, he described exactly how this could be done quite simply in a 'non-sterile rehearsal'.

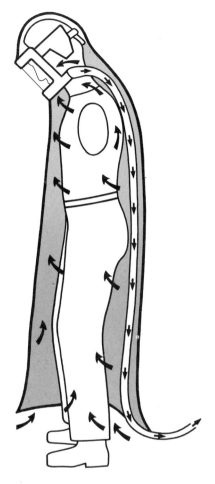

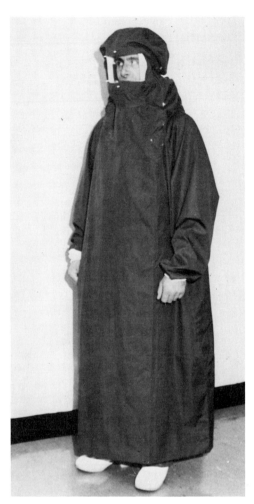

*Diagram showing the body exhaust with arrows indicating the direction of air flow. (LFA)*

*The body exhaust gown as it was worn. (LFA)*

An important point that Charnley stressed about body exhaust was that, even when wearing a heavy ventile gown, the surgeon was cool and comfortable; and felt 'positively invigorated' by the experience – at least he himself did. Indeed, one day when he was in his sixties, he demonstrated that he could do nine low friction arthroplasties in a day, and be fit and fresh at the end of it. This was a remarkable feat of athleticism for a man who took no exercise, apart from operating (and a swim before breakfast in his pool at Birchwood). Others might complain that the gowns were cumbersome and a nuisance to put on, but everyone who worked at Wrightington became accustomed to the routine. An audio system was available, which allowed the surgeon to communicate with his assistants and those outside the enclosure, but Charnley could not 'be bothered' to use it. The operation had become such a well rehearsed routine that he never needed to talk or issue instructions.

The body exhaust equipment was made and marketed by Howorth; patents were taken out and royalties paid into the Wrightington research fund. As always, Charnley was concerned with economy and he wrote in 1973, with regard to the plastic headpieces:

> When one considers that children's space helmets with moving windows and multiple complicated moulded parts are available in plastic for £2.50, it seems to me ridiculous that hospitals should have to be paying £20 for something which is probably a much less complicated moulding. (7.1.73)

No detail was too small for Charnley's attention and this excerpt from a letter is an example:

> The transparent film that we have used for the window of the mask is Melinex Polyester film 100 microns thick, but I think you would do well to order 175 microns thick since the present stuff tends to suck into the window if the suction is high, and I think the thicker material will last longer. (16.4.73)

While the clean air enclosure and body exhaust were being developed, Charnley was making alterations in surgical technique which he believed also helped to reduce the risk of infection: the original T-shaped incision was abandoned and meticulous closure of the fat layer was begun in 1966; antibiotics to put into the wound were used at different times between 1961 and 1966 – and all these factors were evaluated.[4] Charnley's patients were never given systemic antibiotics because he feared the emergence of resistant strains of bacteria. The use of anticoagulant drugs in an attempt to prevent venous thrombosis and pulmonary embolism further complicated the issue. The impression was that more patients developed bleeding into their wounds if they were given anticoagulants, which itself predisposed to infection (Chapter 14).

The whole question of operative wound infection is complicated, and if ever there was a good use for the word multifactorial, it would be to describe the possible causes. Charnley took all the factors into consideration, and became convinced that the clean air enclosure and body exhaust were essential preventive measures which were responsible for lowering the infection rate to 0.61% in 5405 low friction arthroplasties carried out at Wrightington from January 1970 to December 1974 – and that is very low indeed by any standards.

Charnley and Howorth were both enthusiasts who were certain that the clean air theory was correct and worked effectively in practice. Howorth was selling a product, but Charnley wanted to convince his colleagues that he was right. Certainly they had to struggle in this respect, especially in the United Kingdom. Conservatism among surgeons and the proper scepticism of scientists were two factors, but the National Health Service was short of money and needed to be convinced on economic grounds that the Charnley–Howorth·enclosure was really an essential adjunct for hip replacement.

Charnley was comfortable operating in the relatively confined space and as his theatre was only used for hip replacements, the walls of the enclosure did not need to be removed to allow other forms of surgery for which such stringent precautions were not considered necessary. With increasing experience, certain aspects of the design were modified and improved making the enclosure and body exhaust easier to use and so more attractive.

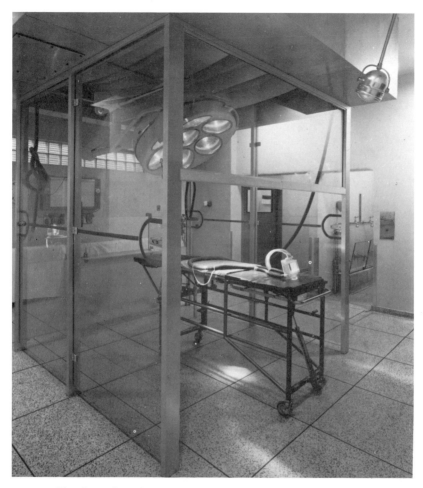

*The clean air enclosure installed at Wrightington in 1970.* (LFA)

A number of changes were made in the theatres at Wrightington. In 1970, a mark II enclosure was installed in the original theatre; the mark I enclosure remaining in the second theatre. A new third theatre was built in 1974 and was fitted with a new DF 10 enclosure with perspex rather than glass walls. Some explanation is needed: the mark II and the DF (downflow) were basically improvements on the mark I (and had perspex side-walls); the number after DF indicates the size, so the DF 10 is ten feet by ten feet with more room for the surgical team. There were now three theatres with clean air enclosures and two additional consultants (J. C. H. Murphy and B. M. Wroblewski) had been appointed and the amount of operating increased.

A mark II enclosure was installed at King Edward VII Hospital, Midhurst in 1969 (Chapter 15) and two at the Nuffield Orthopaedic Centre, Oxford, in 1972. The momentum gradually increased, and subsequent enclosures were either DF 8 or 10 models: there were three elsewhere in the United Kingdom in 1972 and

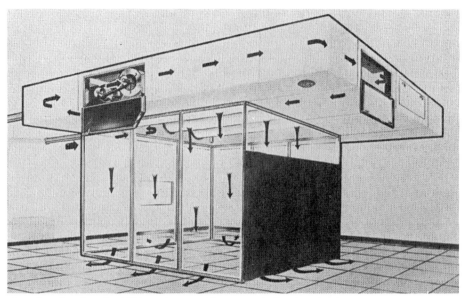

*Drawing showing the 1970 enclosure with arrows indicating the direction of air flow. (By courtesy of F. H. Howorth.)*

four by 1973. Many other countries followed, and by 1976, France had 17 units, Germany 7, United States 6, Ireland 4 and Italy 4. By this time, 27 units had been installed in the United Kingdom, indicating the amount of pressure exerted by orthopaedic surgeons who believed that their patients should have the benefit of this measure.

A feature common to these models was their side-walls, which hung from the ceiling or were supported by corner posts, and so formed an obstruction in the theatre. The walls themselves imposed a useful theatre discipline. Apart from anything else, it was safe for visitors to watch from close quarters as they were 'bacteriologically' isolated from the operation. This was imperative in view of the large numbers who were coming to Wrightington. Some surgeons, however, did not like being enclosed while operating. In a scheme to eliminate the side walls, Dr Allender of the Royal Technical University of Sweden, produced an air-curtain around the operating space with a downward air flow of 120 feet per minute at the periphery. This appeared satisfactory, but Howorth carried out trials which showed that contaminated room air could be entrained into the clean area by induction, and also when personnel or equipment passed through the perimeter of the peripheral flow.[11]

Another solution came to Howorth when he was on holiday in Barbados at Christmas, 1974. Although he took more ambitious vacations than Charnley, neither man ever got far away from their work. Howorth was lying by a hotel swimming pool, when the answer came to him. He realised that a completely opposite concept to Allender's should be used. The highest velocity of air flow should be at the centre, and get less towards the periphery of the sterile area. He immediately applied for a patent, and a model made at Glasgow University worked perfectly. The first prototype of this new exponential flow (EF) system was exhibited at the combined meeting of the English-speaking Orthopaedic Associations at the Festival Hall, London, 1976. At this meeting, Charnley gave the Robert Jones lecture on 'Tissue Response to Implanted Plastic Materials in Orthopaedic Surgery'.

The first EF 12 theatre was set up in the Institut Calot, Berck Plage, France. It proved popular and a further 20 were installed in hospitals throughout France in 1977 and 1978. Over the same period, nine were installed in hospitals in the United Kingdom in these two years, and another nine in 1979. At Wrightington, the original mark I enclosure was replaced by an EF 12 in 1981. Charnley was satisfied with the mark II which he continued to use at Midhurst.

Howorth made changes in the design of the gowns for body exhaust to make them more comfortable to wear, and he credits his wife for these improvements. The weight was taken from the head and redistributed to the shoulders so that it was easier for the wearer to nod or turn his head. A 'mandarin' type of gown was produced with which a conventional cap and mask could be worn, and air removed by a 'necklace' type of exhaust tube. Charnley did not adopt any of these refinements.

A modern system should reduce contamination to less than one colony-forming unit per cubic metre. But is this extreme level of air cleanliness really necessary in surgical operations?

In the early 1970s, many orthopaedic surgeons were convinced by Charnley's results and wanted to install the Charnley–Howorth enclosure and body exhaust in their operating theatres. So far, this has been referred to as producing 'clean' air in the operating theatre, but it is more correct to use the term 'ultraclean' air, since conventional air conditioning was able to produce what could properly be called clean air. Regional hospital boards began to receive many requests for this special equipment, which in 1972 cost about £10,000, and asked the advice of the Department of Health and Social Security; a proper course of action, but one which had the effect of delaying any decision. The department in turn sought guidance from the Medical Research Council about these special ventilation systems and asked whether a controlled trial was necessary to evaluate them. In essence this meant that surgeons, who were able to operate in ultraclean air would be asked to operate on some of their patients (who would be chosen at random) in a theatre with conventional air conditioning. And this created an ethical dilemma.

Charnley knew that his own results were such that it would be morally wrong to expose his patients to anything but the best operating conditions he had available. He went so far as to suggest no doctor would allow himself or a member of his family to be operated on in a 'second class' theatre if there was a 'first class' theatre in the same building; even if that decision was made on emotional and aesthetic grounds, as he admitted it had to be at that time, and without proper scientific evidence. His comments were not entirely fair because the aim of the trial was to compare the good with the better, rather than the worst with the best. No one could deny that his views were personally justified and had to be respected.

Many meetings were held to iron out the difficulties, and in the end the Medical Research Council's committee decided that the trial should be undertaken; but the number of variables presented many problems. It was necessary to compare theatres with conventional and ultraclean operating rooms, in some of which the staff would wear conventional operating clothing, whereas others would use body exhaust suits (or similar protection). It was estimated that about 7500 operations would have to be monitored and, since Charnley was not taking part, this meant that the trial would have to be carried out in several hospitals in order to achieve such numbers. Surgeons were approached in the major orthopaedic centres and, although many shared Charnley's misgivings, enough of them agreed to take part in the belief that it was essential to find the answer. In the end, 19 hospitals were recruited: 11 in England, 4 in Scotland and 4 in Sweden. The first operation in the trial was performed in 1975 and the last in 1979 reaching a grand total of 8316, and of the 8052 that complied with protocol, 6782 were hip and 1270 were knee replacements. Extensive bacteriological testing of the wounds, and of the theatre air was carried out in some special centres, and the state of the wound healing was recorded in all patients. Follow up continued until 1980, with a smaller group continuing until 1984 in order to record the important late infections. Statistical analysis was carried out and papers published from 1983 onwards.[12,13]

It was shown that vertical flow ventilation was the most effective method of reducing bacterial contamination of the air, and that wearing body exhausts produced a further reduction. The question remained: did this affect the incidence of deep infection? Although it is dangerous to oversimplify such a complicated matter, it can be stated that the rate of deep infection was 3.4% in conventional theatres; this was reduced to 1.7% when ultraclean air was used; to 0.75% with body exhaust and ultraclean air, and to 0.2% when antibiotics were given in addition. These remarkable findings substantiated Charnley's ideas about the value of ultraclean air and body exhaust, although he had not expected that antibiotics would be shown to be so effective. Dr Lidwell, who was responsible for coordinating much of the work, wrote: 'there is therefore no conflict remaining between the claims of Charnley and others that operating in ultraclean air reduced the incidence of infection and those who asserted that they could obtain as low an incidence in normally ventilated rooms with the use of prophylactic antibiotics'.[13]

The proof had been a long time in coming; but ultraclean air is now accepted for major joint replacements and units are being installed in many new orthopaedic operating theatres. Most surgeons also take the additional precaution of giving an antibiotic for a short period before and after the operation, or using an antibiotic-loaded cement.

Charnley had written in 1965; 'the sterile enclosure has been, and is, fifty per cent of my life work . . .' and there is no doubt that he made an enormous contribution, not only to the prevention of infection, but to the fundamental understanding of the bacteriological problems involved. Many of his concepts have been vindicated. The Medical Research Council's trial confirmed that contamination of air was related to contamination of operation wounds, which in turn was directly related to wound infection. This was the supposition which Charnley had made in the first place. His early anxiety about cement in relation to wound infection was also correct; recent research has shown that its presence does diminish the body's ability to resist infection.[14]

There is no better way to end this chapter than to quote his published words from a presentation given to the Hip Society in 1982[8]:

Postoperative infection after total hip replacement is the saddest of all complications; it is sad because it seriously limits the success of any subsequent operation undertaken to revise a poor result following a first intervention.

He concluded:

Because of the tragic seriousness of postoperative infection, I am prepared to combine a perfect ultraclean air operating room environment with antibiotic prophylaxis. I hope this demonstrates how very seriously I regard it as our duty to continue in the future to study to eliminate postoperative infection by any means, or combination of means, whatsoever. I say "eliminate" deliberately because I have not yet abandoned hope that we shall achieve this target. In the Medical Research Council report . . . 1500 operations were isolated wherein clean air and the body exhaust system were combined with antibiotics . . . with only one infection in the one to four years following the last operation in the series.

This should remain the last word.

Chapter 13

# THE CHARNLEY–THACKRAY
# RELATIONSHIP
## 1947–1982

*In Britain it is not considered good form to acknowledge commercial*
*undertakings in too glowing terms, even though the work would*
*not have been possible without their collaboration . . .*

John Charnley in *Low Friction Arthroplasty of the Hip* (1979)

IN MANY WAYS the relationship between John Charnley and the commercial firm of Chas. F. Thackray Limited, of Leeds, (referred to as Thackrays hereafter) was the foundation for the development of the prostheses for the low friction arthroplasty. Fortunately, his correspondence with the company from 1968 to his death in 1982 is available and forms a continuing account of considerable interest. It is possible to trace, not only his personal approach to various general problems of manufacture, but the changes in design of the component parts which were made as the operation evolved. But his connection with the company goes back well before 1968, and the history of the firm well beyond that.

Thackrays stems from a pharmacy opened by a Samuel Taylor in Leeds in 1862 which was taken over by Charles Frederick Thackray (1877–1934) and his partner, H. S. Wainwright, in 1902. The business was in Great George Street close to the General Infirmary. In 1905 a steriliser for dressings was purchased, and this led to a diversification from retail pharmacy into manufacturing and a wholesale business. From 1918 the emphasis changed from pharmaceuticals and dressings to surgical equipment. The first instruments were made for Lord Moynihan, a surgeon in Leeds and a national figure, who designed many new instruments for abdominal surgery. Thackray died in 1934 and his two sons, C. Noel and W. P. (Tod) Thackray, became directors of the commercial and manufacturing operations. After the managing director, W. M. Gray, died in 1957, the brothers assumed joint managing directorship.

Their involvement with orthopaedics began in 1947 when various instruments were made for Mr Broomhead in Leeds, and it must have been about this time

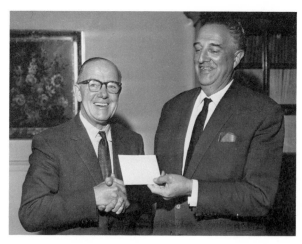

*W. P. Thackray and Arthur Hallam (on the left) on the occasion of the latter's retirement in 1962. (Courtesy of Mr W. P. Thackray.)*

that Charnley approached the company. He had previously had instruments made by Down Brothers Ltd, of London, (Chapter 5), but there were some difficulties, and the instrument curator at the Manchester Royal Infirmary put Charnley in touch with Thackrays. The first instruments they made for him, and which he published in 1950, were used in his method of inserting guide-wires for nailing fractures of the femoral neck. Thus began a close association which was maintained until the end of his life.

One important figure from the first time Charnley went to Thackrays was the foreman in their development workshop. Arthur Hallam was a very talented instrument-maker and a good craftsman whose skills were appreciated by Charnley. He worked closely with Hallam and undoubtedly learnt workshop techniques from him. He remembered him with affection and wrote in 1972: '. . . there is no one with the background of our dear old Mr Hallam'. Charnley undoubtedly also had Hallam in mind in 1970:

> The important thing is always to be suspicious of experts . . . they are of very limited use compared with the unparalleled, and rare, boon of a gifted craftsman at the bench. (24.12.70)

Hallam helped Charnley with the screw he designed for fixing fractures of the femoral neck (Chapter 5) and about this time Thackrays also manufactured his orthopaedic table – described in their catalogue as 'an entirely new design with many novel features'. The price was £308 and it was manufactured from 1957 until 1966; it was then modified for use in hip arthroplasty operations and continued to be produced.

Close collaboration really began with the development of the low friction arthroplasty. Thackrays took over the manufacture of the HMWP acetabular sockets from Charnley in 1963 and made the femoral prosthesis from the outset, the heads being lapped and polished at Wrightington until 1968. The firm contributed £1 for every prosthesis used to the research fund at the hospital.

From the very beginning, Charnley was concerned for the future of the company and appreciated the commercial difficulties created by some of his ideas:

> . . . your firm may have been influenced by my desire to keep the cost of the implant as low as possible . . . I now feel that you have plenty of latitude in the price . . . compared with world prices, to cover a considerable capital investment looking towards a long-term dominance in this field . . . (26.1.68)

The price of the femoral prosthesis in March 1968 was £12 and the socket £3.

Charnley was concerned with minutiae and never hesitated to make criticisms of work done; indeed, he regarded himself as the 'scourge and flail of Thackrays', but it was his intention to be helpful:

> I hope you do not consider my criticisms of the products we have been receiving recently as "complaints". They are of course constructive criticisms for the improvement of the product and I feel sure you welcome these and know they are not just "bellyaches". (4.4.68)

His technicians at Wrightington scrutinised instruments and implants made by Thackrays and, when he felt there had been a decline in standards, he commented: 'I am quite sure that this defective workmanship would not have occurred in the days of Mr Hallam'. When an instrument was satisfactory, he gave credit: 'the femoral punch is an excellent job', for example. And, when necessary, he was prepared to make amends: 'I must apologise . . . as I was operating today I realised that they [the socket-holders] did have R and L marked on them'. There was scarcely a week when Charnley did not write at least one or two letters to various members of the company, and they cannot have found it easy to accept some of the comments. None the less they did; standards were raised and, in spite of what he wrote, Charnley remained loyal to Thackrays and they to him.

The form of words used to go with the purchased implant in 1968, which was carefully amended by Charnley, summarised what was important about its manufacture:

> The Total Hip Prosthesis contained in this package consists of a plastic socket made of High Density Polyethylene for the acetabulum and a stainless steel femoral head. Both components have been developed by Mr J. Charnley DSc, FRCS, at Wrightington Hospital. Chas. F. Thackray Ltd have been granted sole rights of manufacture in return for which they contribute to the Wrightington Hip Centre Research Fund.
>
> All prostheses are manufactured under carefully controlled production techniques which meet rigid requirements as laid down by Mr Charnley. Quality control of the product includes a final inspection of a representative proportion of the products in the Research Laboratory at Wrightington Hospital.
>
> Mr Charnley has authorised the issue of this statement.
>
> Chas. F. Thackray Ltd

There were problems about the prosthesis being copied since it had not been patented; although in the future some inventions were patented, such as the cement restrictor in 1970.

Charnley realised, however, that it was impossible to prohibit imitators from using his name in connection with versions of his prosthesis and suggested their

prostheses would have to be called, for example, 'Vitallium Charnley-type'.
Some years previously, Professor Maurice Müller from Switzerland had visited
Wrightington and had produced a modified version which by agreement was
called the Charnley–Müller prosthesis. This was, to quote Charnley, 'a vitallium
femoral prosthesis with a head approximately 30 mm in diameter, with a rather
slender stem'. He contrasted the essential features of his own prosthesis as '(1) the
22 mm head, (2) the profile of the head and neck, and (3) the shape of the stem
which is considerably more robust than others on the market'. He concluded a
letter to Thackrays:

> I feel if you are permitted to use the words 'Authorised Pattern', and if
> you can beat other manufacturers in price by using stainless steel authorised
> by me, you should have no difficulty in keeping ahead. (19.7.68)

A few days later, he was writing that 'I think I can now see the possibility of
imitators being restrained from using my name in connection with copies . . . it
is for imitators to find a different form of words when using my name . . .'

In December 1968, three orthopaedic surgeons from California, who were
planning to set up a 100 bed centre for hip surgery, visited Wrightington. The
senior surgeon was Dr Charles Bechtol and the Charnley low friction arthroplasty
had been chosen as their 'starting model'. Charnley wrote to Thackray that they
might expect enquiries about the possibility of 'franchise' arrangements being
made.

This was an encouraging development, but the situation with regard to sales
in the United States became complicated. Charnley wrote:

> I am quite certain that there will be large numbers of modifications of my
> instruments made under other people's names . . . but I do not think that
> this in any way infringes Thackray's control . . . my name will only be
> used with devices developed here at Wrightington. (16.9.70)

And again a few days later:

> It is only recently that we decided to attempt to copyright the name
> Charnley itself and, therefore, I would imagine that if letters are in
> possession of other manufacturers in which I give permission to use the
> term 'Charnley-type' this decision can now be rescinded. (21.9.70)

The whole situation was confusing, particularly when Charnley was told that in
the United States surgeons were changing to the Charnley–Müller prosthesis.
Some of the reasons given were: 'you don't have to remove the trochanter'; 'it
has three lengths of femoral necks', and 'I like the size of the femoral head
because it is larger'. This must have been somewhat galling for Charnley:

> Müller attached my name to his prosthesis out of courtesy because we are
> close personal friends and because he was acknowledging my pioneer
> work . . . The situation has now changed in so far as my operation is
> certainly a more extensive mechanical procedure than his . . . those
> manufacturers who in the past have made the Charnley–Müller with the
> 30 mm head should now drop my name . . . (28.10.70)

Although Charnley never changed the size (22 mm) of the head of his femoral
prosthesis, many orthopaedic surgeons felt that it was likely to dislocate

easily, although this was not the case in Charnley's hands. A letter from W. P. (Tod) Thackray throws light on the problem:

> It is certainly not our wish to produce a larger headed model, but all the time we are being pressed by our foreign agents who seem to insist that there is as much demand for the Müller type, as for your small-headed variety, mainly required by the not-so-good surgeon, where he can use an easier operative technique. (19.9.72)

The striking feature of the Charnley/Thackray correspondence is not only the number of letters he wrote, 46 in 1968 for example, but the range of subjects he dealt with. No detail in the design of an instrument was too small to escape his attention, and all the time he was seeking to improve Thackrays manufacturing abilities:

> . . the sales of these instruments and prostheses . . . will be promoted mainly by good design and availability . . . If one can establish a tradition for absolutely first-class design, and not damage this tradition by defective instruments, then a prestige situation develops . . . (5.1.71)

Charnley was always concerned about those working with him. The workshop technicians at Wrightington had been graded in the National Health Service as orthopaedic appliance makers which was not only inappropriate, but provided salaries far below the value of the work they were doing. Early in 1970 the hospital secretary, at Charnley's request, wrote to ask Thackrays if they would consider employing these men and this was very strongly supported by Charnley:

> . . . the existence . . . of the biomechanical laboratory here is a vital part of the welfare of Thackrays in the future, and I think you will agree that our technician is an excellent man in his ability to carry out quite delicate test work in addition to fairly heavy mechanical engineering of an ordinary type. (13.1.70)

Thackrays recognised the importance of the link and the two men were taken on their staff at a proper salary. When there was some difficulty over pensions, Charnley pursued the matter vigorously:

> These two men are of outstanding capacity as regards inventiveness in tackling unusual projects in addition to outstanding technical skills in carrying them out. . . (28.3.72)

By the early 1970s the company was fully committed to the manufacture and marketing of the Charnley instruments and prostheses, and what might almost be called a revolution had taken place in their organisation. After C. N. Thackray died, the family connection remained strong: W. P. (Tod) Thackray became chairman and managing director; his son, John P. Thackray, deputy managing director, and his nephew, C. Paul Thackray, a director. There had been difficulties in achieving the manufacturing volume to meet the demands from surgeons wanting to do the low friction arthroplasty, and an approach was made to Leeds Polytechnic industrial liaison unit for advice. Ron Frank, who was then a principal lecturer there in management studies, was asked (with one of his colleagues) to produce a works organisation report. As a result Jim Boyd, a chartered engineer, was appointed as a new general works manager in March, 1971. Tod Thackray then invited Frank to become group management accountant and corporate planning manager and he joined the company in May, 1971. These two men were the first professionally trained managers from outside industry and their appointments heralded a more modern approach. Charnley had been pressing for the company to move forward, but his appreciation of commercial matters was limited. The way was now open for Boyd to build up Thackray's technical ability, while Frank developed the financial side. Both men became directors in 1973.

Charnley visited Thackrays in Leeds from time to time and, after one occasion, he recognised the improvements which had been made:

> I would just like to thank you for the visit to the works on Friday, September 13, and to let you know how impressed I was with everything that had gone on since I was there last . . .
>
> We all know there is no time for complacency . . . but at any rate I would like you and all your staff to know that I came away with an extremely good impression of the whole show. (17.9.74)

Thackrays were now making about nine to ten thousand hip prostheses a year. Originally, there had been only two types of femoral component and two sockets, but by 1971 there were five prostheses: standard; straight narrow stem; straight thick stem; with an intramedullary extension, and a resection prosthesis (to replace the upper one third of the femur). The sockets had also multiplied: standard; small; small without rim; and long posterior wall. Each variant had been produced to fulfil special needs depending on the shape and size of the bones, and the surgeon's requirements. The development of these, and of Charnley's knee joint, can be followed in the correspondence.

On July 22, 1970, Charnley was advising Thackrays to increase their output to 100 000 a year because he believed that only by this sort of approach would they avoid 'falling by the way as does the British Aircraft Corporation in competition with America (i.e. not enough and too late, but an excellent product)'. The response by Thackrays is not in the file.

The femoral component was made of stainless steel; all Thackrays previous experience in making surgical instruments had been with this material, and their consultant (Mr G. Parkin from whom they sought metallurgical advice) had worked with Harry Brearley who had developed stainless steel in 1913. Air melt En58J, a ductile austenitic steel, was used for the first Charnley prosthesis.

Charnley maintained that the metal femoral head must be absolutely spherical, and that the lapping and polishing was a critical process. He argued that the small-diameter metal femoral heads which he was using could be fabricated cheaply at very high degrees of sphericity. Such a condition, with a high degree of polish, was more expensive to obtain in larger femoral heads. Furthermore perfect sphericity could not be achieved with chrome–cobalt because it had to be cast.

The metallurgical factors involved with implants were extremely complicated and a forum on metallic surgical implants was held under the auspices of the Department of Health and Social Security in May, 1970.[1] Charnley reported the success of stainless steel as a femoral prosthesis in hip replacement and considered that its relatively high strength warranted study and development. He interpreted the opinion of the 'top-level British metallurgists' at the meeting as satisfaction with EN58J, and the emphasis was that its mechanical strength should not be reduced in an attempt to increase its corrosive resistance. He, therefore, felt no

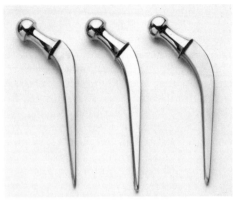

*Types of the earliest design of what came to be called the 'first-generation flat-back' femoral prosthesis.*

reason for not continuing to use stainless steel; he was, of course, attracted by its cheapness compared with chrome cobalt alloys and titanium which were being advocated by some surgeons and metallurgists because of their improved corrosion resistance. Charnley was always concerned that the cost of the operation should be kept within reasonable limits so that it could be readily available to patients through the National Health Service.

From July 1971, En58J was replaced by another double vacuum remelt stainless steel, 316LVM, which was more corrosion resistant but weaker in resistance to bending. He recognised the difficulties which lay ahead:

> While I strongly support the use of stainless steel . . . evidence is beginning to accumulate that there will be considerable resistance in different parts of the world in favour of chrome–cobalt. The pressure is coming from commercial interests . . . and also from perfectionist engineers who are interested in metals, but have no experience of surgical applications.
>
> . . . it might well be that Thackrays would be advised to start considering the possibility of offering a chrome–cobalt prosthesis as well as the stainless steel . . . (9.6.71)

The matter continued to rankle and a rival firm was 'sweeping the board' in the United States with their chrome–cobalt Charnley-type prosthesis. He considered that the failure to sell his prosthesis 'is purely because it is in stainless steel, and the Americans just do not like stainless steel'.

He also thought that there might be problems with the global supply of chrome–cobalt within a decade; and, in case there ever was a shortage, Thackrays would be wise to maintain their expertise in steel:

> The working of chrome–cobalt by casting employs large numbers of relatively unskilled female labour and the working of stainless steel requires men who are true engineering craftsmen, and such a workforce could not very easily be mobilised again [if they ever were disbanded]. (7.7.72)

In spite of this, and perhaps because they were not able to achieve a franchise with another firm, Thackrays marketed chrome–cobalt Charnley implants during the middle to late 1970s, but this failed to improve their sales in the United States and the project was abandoned. Charnley, of course, never deserted stainless steel himself.

But there was a cloud on the horizon which threatened to bring more than a passing shower – fractures of the stem of the femoral prosthesis began to occur some years after operation: in the Wrightington cases there was one in 1968 and one in 1971; but then the numbers increased, two in 1972, five in 1973, ten in 1974 and eighteen in 1975. This looked alarming; but the figures need to be seen in perspective. The actual incidence in 6500 operations was only 0.23%, and indeed there had been no fractures in the first 2500 operations. The small numbers in the early years is understandable because the first patients were all elderly and relatively inactive. When the results were analysed, it was clear that nearly all the fractures had occurred in heavy men, and rarely in women.

Specimens of fractured stems were sent to Wrightington from all over the world. One, for example, from New Zealand was a narrow stem which had been put into a man weighing $17\frac{1}{2}$ stone. Charnley remarked:

> It is quite unreasonable to put this [a narrow stem] into a $17\frac{1}{2}$ stone [about 250 kg] man and I am quite astonished that it should last nearly four years under these conditions having given such service under such loading. (14.5.73)

Litigation was threatened in North America and Charnley wrote apropos of a possible court case:

> I have been giving a lot of thought to this matter of legal action arising out of fractures of femoral prostheses and I feel that a trial case must be won in favour of the surgeons and as a precedent for all time . . . the failure in the body is the result more of the surgical manner in which it is inserted than the metallurgy of the implant.
>
> It is an irony of fate that the fracture of the prosthesis in a heavy patient indicates that the result of the operation was practically 100% because a poor result, with a load-sparing limp, is unlikely to result in a fatigue fracture. (5.3.74)

Although he was prepared to go into the witness-box to give evidence, he was never called to do so (and it is appropriate to mention here that he was never sued during the whole course of his surgical career).

The legal side was not, however, his main problem, and he immediately set about investigating the cause of the fractures, publishing his findings in 1975.[2] He believed that the method of insertion and pressurisation of cement was of prime importance, and he had already improved his technique (Chapter 11). It was now easier to insert the prosthesis correctly in the neutral position, and to ensure good support from cement on the medial side of the neck of the femur.

The problem of the heavy man remained. A second generation of round-back prostheses (in contrast to the first flat-backs) already had been produced, and this was now superseded by the third generation of flanged designs called, because of its appearance, the 'cobra'. The stem was a heavier calibre and the flanges on the shoulder retained the cement while the prosthesis was being pushed in. There were five different versions: heavy and extra-heavy, with two different off-sets and one with a taper-tip. The new design was introduced in 1975 and was patented in the United Kingdom and other countries.

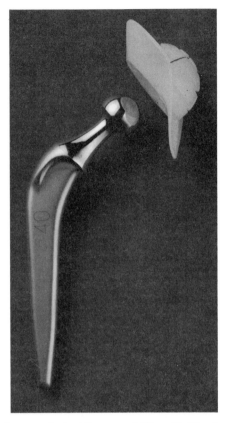

*The cobra prosthesis. (Courtesy of Chas. F. Thackray Ltd.)*

Charnley's response to the problem had been rapid and effective; meanwhile he encouraged Thackray's plans to improve the strength of the material for the femoral prosthesis. Boyd had built a testing rig in their research laboratory which was the first of its kind, able to fatigue a captive prosthesis in both bending and torsion. He suggested, in 1975, the use of Rex 734, a type of steel produced by Firth–Brown for oil-rigs in the North Sea. Boyd then set up an accelerated fatigue testing rig to evaluate Rex, and also to find out whether cold-working would improve the material's resistance to fatigue. These were complicated metallurgical matters, but Charnley did not hesitate to express his opinions, which sometimes caused a little irritation. He justified his incursion into a field which was not his own:

> Nevertheless the a priori approach is often quite a good stimulus to thinking. One has always to remember that a High Court Judge is trained to take decisions on evidence . . . in subjects which may originally be completely unfamiliar to him and in which he has absolutely no training. (29.9.75)

Charnley professed to have 'true humility' in his field, but his argument produced a spasm of irritation in the engineers he was dealing with.

The difficulties in the United States did not go away and he expressed his frustration:

> I have indicated from time to time that Thackrays will be overtaken in the United States by the build-up of publicity against stainless steel in favour of very sophisticated and expensive alloys . . . many of my loyal pupils [there] can no longer risk using stainless steel . . . a number of surgeons who are on the bio-engineering bandwagon are teaching that stainless steel is no longer acceptable . . . (3.3.79)

He was concerned that the firms with whom Thackrays were associated in the United States had been unable to change this unfortunate situation. Various schemes were suggested, and Charnley wanted the results of the fatigue testing carried out at Thackrays, and the 'general philosophy about the cold-worked prosthesis', to be promoted urgently. Six months later he tried to persuade the company to 'split off a division for implants where the personnel would not be distracted with other problems'.

Thackrays introduced Ortron 90, a new stainless steel derived from the development work on Rex 734, which was marketed in 1980, although it had been available at Wrightington during the previous two years. It was not only stronger than cold-worked 316LVM stainless steel, but was also stronger than chrome–cobalt alloys (whether case or wrought) and titanium alloy. The stronger material made it possible to reduce the diameter of the neck of the prosthesis so that impingement between the neck and the socket would be delayed when wear occurred. Theoretical calculations inferred that the life of the cup would be prolonged by as much as fifteen years. Of more immediate importance is the fact that fracture of an Ortron 90 femoral stem has not been reported during its first ten years' use at Wrightington.[8]

Charnley believed that it was important to investigate the possibility of finding a polyethylene with a much higher molecular weight than the RCH 1000 which he was using for the socket. He had approached the Shell Corporation in Manchester and although they had helped him in the past they were not now able to do so:

> This would appear to be the end of any hope of doing this research in this field in Britain . . . It would seem to me that only an organisation like the North American Rockwell Corporation would be big enough to tackle this. (2.12.68)

He went on to suggest that Thackrays should try 'to work out something ' with Rockwell. At the end of the same letter, he returned to more mundane affairs:

> I am wondering whether the time is near when we shall be hearing how much you will be able to pay into my research fund for implants sold since the last payment was made. We have a number of projects in hand and my research funds are running low.

Direct wear testing of sockets was carried out in the laboratory at Wrightington, and a machine had been in use since 1971 which could test four specimens simultaneously, often running day and night for three months. This was superseded by a new instrument in 1972 which could test ten specimens so that wear resistance could be assessed over a much shorter period. Any variation in quality of polyethylene, most of which was produced by Hoechst or Ruhr Chemie

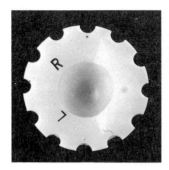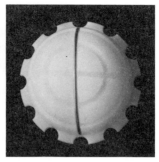

*The standard type of socket.* (LFA)

in Germany, could be detected by this type of sophisticated testing. A long letter was written to Boyd in October 1971:

> You can well imagine my anger at the defamatory statement you showed me from one American manufacturer suggesting that Thackrays were using a plastic only suitable for milk bottle tops!
>
> . . . I am probably the first writer to have talked freely about any relationship between molecular weight and wear resistance. My information on this was derived from original work by Pratt, Director of Research at the Glacier Metal Company . . .
>
> I think the Americans ought to be told that they are not teaching us anything here . . . (5.10.71)

He also took up the question of toxicity testing, which was a statutory requirement in the United States, and pointed out that he now had 500 hips in the human body for from five to eight years without any evidence of toxicity, and this was better than any laboratory testing.

Charnley was sent a specimen of HMWP, called Hi-Fax, from New York which he thought might be more resistant to wear. But research carried out by Professor Howard of the department of industrial chemistry, Birmingham University, who collaborated with Charnley in the 1970s, failed to find a better material – and the same high molecular weight polyethylene which Charnley first introduced is still used by Thackrays and other manufacturers.

Although the material remained the same, alterations were made to the design. A socket with a long posterior wall for added stability was introduced in 1971 to satisfy those surgeons who were worried about the risk of dislocation. The pressure injection socket was devised to produce pressurisation of cement during insertion on the basis that better cement technique would reduce the incidence of loosening. There were also sockets which were used for old congenital dislocation of the hip: small; extra-small and off-set bore.

The idea for the Ogee socket occurred to Charnley when he was in Australia in 1980. He telephoned Marsh in the workshop at Wrightington, and described it so clearly that Marsh had produced a prototype for him by the time he returned. This was an elegant design made possible by the use of cross-linked polyethylene which could be injection moulded. The wide flange could be fitted to the irregularities and different sizes of acetabulum. The results of experiments

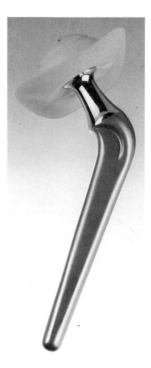

*The Ogee socket and cobra femoral prosthesis. (From Mr N. W. Nisbet, Orthopaedic Hospital, Oswestry.)*

carried out in Wrightington and published in 1988 have shown that this model gave consistently high injection pressure.[7]

Charnley's final piece of research concerned the question of whether changes in the sockets, which had been in patients for a long time, was due to wear or creep. D. Ludbrook, of Thackrays, had volunteered to make profiles of four sockets which Charnley was examining from his series of post-mortem specimens. Charnley wrote one month before he died:

> The ultimate object of this research is, of course, to try to find out if there has been any distortion, by creep or plastic flow which might make a significant contribution to the shape of the cast [which he had made] of the interior. It is my belief that the shape of the interior is 99% the result of wear, and not creep . . . (5.7.82)

He pointed out that the loss of weight of the worn sockets was very much in favour of wear rather than creep. He ended his letter:

> Thank you very much for this interesting co-operation and I hope we might get it together as a publication under our two names.

Why Charnley decided to invent a knee replacement is not altogether certain. But J. C. M. Murphy, who had been a registrar at Wrightington and became a consultant there in 1971, believes that because many new knee joints were being produced in other centres, Charnley decided to invent one himself. Undoubtedly many of his patients who were having their hips operated on for rheumatoid arthritis also needed to have their knees replaced. His interest may have been stimulated by work that was done at Wrightington by F. H. Gunston from Canada while he was a registrar there in 1967. Gunston designed a four-part replacement in which runners were cemented into the femur and ariculated with plastic tracks similarly cemented into the tibia.[6] It was difficult to align the components correctly and the operation took rather a long time to carry out, at least in the early cases. This did not appeal to Charnley, and so in 1970 he designed his own model, which was entirely original and unorthodox: the convex femoral components were plastic and the flat tibial plates were stainless steel (every other knee replacement devised has had the opposite arrangement – the femoral component is metal and the tibial plastic). One of the main advantages of Charnley's design was that it was very small and could be inserted without removing any significant amount of the patient's bone.

An application to obtain a patent for his implant in the United States was unsuccessful; none the less, the device was marketed in 1974 with the name Load Angle Inlay. The following year, Murphy and Charnley reported the results of 126 knees (all with rheumatoid arthritis) and the longest follow up was three years.[3] The conclusion was that 'the operation was valuable in rheumatoid arthritis and because it was a relatively small procedure it was justifiable to undertake it early in the disease'. But there were problems, and the Load Angle Inlay never became generally accepted and is no longer manufactured by Thackrays.

For knees which were more severely damaged by arthritis, Charnley devised another replacement which had a ball-and-socket articulation with stems which were cemented into the shaft of the femur and tibia for better fixation. This was inserted in only three patients.

Charnley's failure to pursue his ideas on knee replacement may seem surprising – after all he had solved the major problems of the hip. The knee was certainly a more difficult joint to replace than the hip, but this can hardly have been the reason. It is perhaps significant that from 1972 onwards, when the knee was being developed, fractures of the stem of the femoral prosthesis in the low friction arthroplasty began to be seen as an important complication. Murphy thinks that Charnley turned back to the hip, almost with relief, now that he had a new problem to overcome. He lost interest in the knee; and by the time he had designed the cobra range of femoral stems for the hip, he was totally involved in teaching the technique of his hip operation.

Correspondence to and from Thackrays continued over the years, and sometimes on a single day Charnley would write two or three letters. There is much material which reflects his character, and selection is difficult. He dealt with major issues of policy alongside minute details of his instruments. Admonition and criticism were almost unending; it was not until 1979 that he wrote 'I hope this is going to be the last of my belly-aching letters to you'. It was not, but his aim was always the same: to improve the efficiency of the manufacture and marketing of the prostheses and instruments. An example of his attention to detail was in a minor alteration to his self-ejecting socket holder:

> . . . I forgot to mention when you were here . . . the handle used to turn the screw should be a simple transverse bar . . . If this bar is about 2″

long . . . it is easy to turn quickly with the tip of one finger spinning it
round. The small knurled knob that you have is very slow to turn and
requires a number of quarter-turns each of which requires the knob to be
gripped between finger and thumb . . . whereas it is possible to spin a
cross-bar with the finger tip with minimal movement since the turning
action is continuous. (9.11.73)

Small financial matters did not escape his notice:

The local engineering firm who made these stampings quoted £350 for 250
including the cost of the dies. If you consider the dies worth £300 this
means that each stamping, passing through two dies, would cost 20p each,
or 40p a pair. We are paying you £14 per pair for polishing . . . these
implants [the tibial components of his knee replacement] (14.11.73)

Quotations from two letters indicate the broad issues which he wrote to
Tod Thackray about. He had been asked to visit Australia and did not feel able
to go:

. . . but I am doing all I can to dedicate 1976 to research and writing.

In that year the second edition of his book on cement had to be revised; he had
to give the Listerian Oration at the Royal College of Surgeons in May; in
September he had to mount an historical exhibition on total hip replacement at
the combined meeting of the English-speaking Associations at the Festival Hall
in London, and at the same meeting he had to deliver the Robert Jones lecture.
The letter continues:

Moreover during this year I shall have to face up to publishing experiences
on the not-so-glamorous aspects of total hip replacement. There are examples
of tissue damage resulting from particles of high density polyethylene and
it is my duty, as soon as possible, to publish examples of this. If not
carefully handled this subject could produce an hysterical level of excitement
among many surgeons. I have always attempted to promote an extremely
conservative attitude to this operation and have never been happy [about
doing it] in young patients . . . In America I feel that they are putting
these implants into quite young people without the same strict selection we
have employed here. I think there is going to be a harvest of very bad
results in the young people.
   It is not impossible that dangers of malignant transformation may be
alleged when the operation is done for patients who will have the material
in their bodies for thirty or forty years . . . I am absolutely confident of
the permanent place of this type of operation in patients of 60 years of age
and over, and possibly of 55 and over, but the time has come when I shall
have to issue a warning, supported by evidence, about its light-hearted use
in young patients. (12.12.75)

His attitude makes understandable an anecdote often repeated about him. After
a successful lecture at a meeting of the American Academy of Orthopaedic
Surgeons at Las Vegas, he was approached by a physician who insisted on
showing him the radiographs of the hips of a young woman. Charnley's response
to the request for advice was one word only – 'aspirin'. The questions were
repeated at greater length as the physician thought Charnley might not have

understood, but the reply was the same – 'aspirin'; and with that the discussion ended. Some might think that Charnley was being boorish and rude in not giving a fuller explanation; but he felt very strongly that young people should not be operated on. His response was definite and absolutely clear.

He was, in fact, correct in his anxiety about the 'harvest of bad results' in young patients as judged by some reports[5], but there have not been the cases of malignant transformation (with one or two possible exceptions) that he had feared. Charnley had given up the osteotomy operation because of its unpredictable results, although in the young person with only one hip affected, he was prepared to consider arthrodesis with the idea of converting this to an arthroplasty fifteen or twenty years later.

In 1980, P. D. Curwen-Walker, an orthopaedic surgeon in Australia who had worked at Wrightington in 1968/69, wrote about the relatively high cost of prostheses in his country. Charnley explained that there were a number of reasons for this, but the main factor was the expensive research and development programme which Thackrays (unlike some of their competitors) had undertaken during the previous five years. He listed a number of points that indicate the work which had been going on:

(1) A metallurgical section has been started with a whole-time PhD

(2) Fatigue testing rigs have been designed and built for actual implants under simulated conditions . . .

(3) The decision to produce the prostheses by "cold-forming" has necessitated the purchase of very expensive hydraulic presses from Germany . . .

(4) For over three years work has been going on in developing a new stainless steel by Firth–Brown . . .

(5) To complete the perfection of the modelling a new programme of electrochemical machining is under way which involves an expensive capital outlay . . .

(6) The range of some 18 different designs of femoral prosthesis, which eventually will all be in these expensive-to-make metals, inevitably has to be reflected in the price of the standard range . . .

(7) The inevitable marking up of prices . . . has been further complicated by the rise in freight costs . . .

. . . if Australian surgeons want these products they will have to approach their government to request that the allowance for these implants should be raised . . . (23.7.80)

As far as the United States was concerned, Thackrays were unable to overcome the commercial difficulties, and although about 70% of the replacements used in that country in the 1980s were of the cemented metal-on-plastic type, probably only about 2% to 3% were *Charnleys*. But in other parts of the world the proportion of *Charnleys* used rose to about 20%, and in the United Kingdom Thackrays now have about a half-share of the market.

The correspondence has thrown a fascinating light on Charnley and his relationship with Thackrays. Although criticisms were mainly in one direction, it should not be thought that the company did not reply with vigour from time to time. Despite his continued strictures, Charnley was respected by all the men he dealt with, and in some cases genuine and lasting friendship developed. Both sides deserve great credit for their perseverence. Loyalty was one of Charnley's qualities; this, and the fact that the company remained faithful to him, was of advantage to both sides. Charnley did a great deal for Thackrays in the early days, but as the company developed, he began to benefit more and more from what they had to offer. And their contribution, from 1966 onwards, to his research fund, which later extended to their paying the salaries of his workshop technicians, should not be forgotten. There can be few instances of such close and lasting collaboration between an orthopaedic surgeon (who sought so little financial reward for himself) and a commercial company.

Charnley had always taken a great deal of interest in the details of the Thackrays catalogue which described his prostheses and instruments. He made critical comments on each new edition, wishing everything to be absolutely correct. Indeed his last letter in the file, dated July 8, 1982, was to Tod Thackray about the draft Charnley was preparing for the forthcoming catalogue. This was not published until after his unexpected death, and there is no better way of closing this chapter than by quoting some words of the introduction:

> Chas. F. Thackray, and myself in particular, feel honoured that we were allowed to participate in the development and manufacture of his instruments and prostheses, used and proven by Sir John in the twenty-six years applied to the perfection of this very successful operation.
>
> Perhaps only once in a lifetime does one come across a man prepared to devote so much time in one direction . . . Most of the text was written for me by Sir John himself, to whom I was deeply indebted.
>
> W. P. Thackray, Chairman

*Chapter 14*

# SPREADING THE WORD

## 1967–1982

*If a man write a better book . . . or make a better mouse-trap than
his neighbour, tho' he build in the woods, the world will make a
beaten path to his door.*

R.W. Emerson 1803–1882

ON TAKING UP his appointment at the Manchester Medical School after the war,
Charnley soon found that routine teaching of medical students was frustrating
and kept him from the work he really wanted to do; although he remained an
enthusiastic and popular postgraduate teacher. From 1959 onwards, when he was
concentrating his efforts at Wrightington, he determined never to undertake
undergraduate teaching again. Sir Harry Platt wrote to him in 1967 about plans
for 'teaching orthopaedics in the Manchester of the future'. Charnley explained
his attitude:

> Ever since my own student days I have believed that the idea of a Teaching
> Hospital trying to cope with teaching medical students, carrying-out first-
> class clinical work . . . and doing research, all simultaneously, is futile.
> The teaching of undergraduates should be raised to a high professional level
> by doctors paid well enough to study teaching techniques . . .
>
> I have proved to myself that immense progress in the quality of services
> to patients in a Welfare State and immense contributions to basic science
> and surgery, can only be made by breaking out from the conventional
> atmosphere of the Teaching Hospital. The only form of planned teaching
> I am prepared to do is: (1) to teach the teachers of undergraduates, and
> (2) postgraduate teaching, and even this very selective. (5.12.67)

By this time he was fully engaged by his work on the hip, and when he wrote
that his postgraduate teaching would be 'selective', he meant that he was only
going to teach about the low friction arthroplasty and his related research. He
did this for the rest of his life with unflagging enthusiasm and without remission.

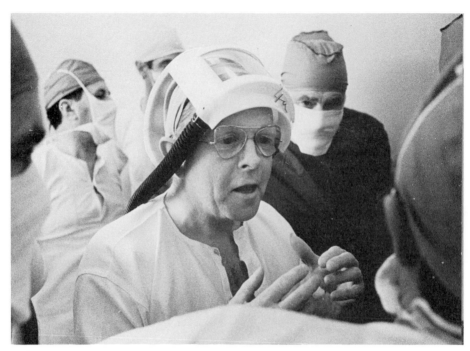

*Charnley teaching after an operating session. The helmet of the body exhaust is tilted back over his head.*

Once he was satisfied that the operation was successful, he determined to ensure that the procedure would only be carried out by those who understood the principles on which it was based; and he made certain, as far as he was able, that the technique would be carried out to the highest possible standards. This chapter will describe the ways in which he spread his message to the rest of the orthopaedic world.

First and foremost, he went to great trouble to teach his assistants about every aspect of the operation. Each resident was taken through the surgical steps, and they all gained practical experience commensurate with their skill. Once the decision to operate was made, each patient was classified into one of three groups depending on the predicted degree of operative difficulty: (1) those which were expected to be straightforward were assigned to a relatively junior member of the staff; (2) those which were more difficult and should be done by a senior registrar, and (3) those presenting special technical problems which Charnley would undertake himself. More than this, he conveyed to his staff an understanding of the indications for the operation and the care of the patients afterwards. It normally took about three months for a resident to carry out about thirty arthroplasties which Charnley held was the time needed to become 'comfortable with this type of surgery'. Those staying at the hospital for six months were able to perform about 100 operations, and also take part in a research project. These men (and they were all men) came from all over the world and were the nucleus of the Low Friction Society which was formed in 1974 (Chapter 10).

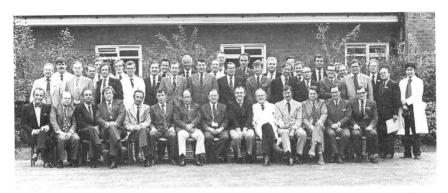

*Charnley with members of the Low Friction Society at their first meeting, 1974. (From Dr Henry Hamilton, archivist, The Low Friction Society.)*

Orthopaedic surgeons everywhere were becoming aware of the advances in hip replacement being made at Wrightington, and many came to visit the Centre for Hip Surgery. What had begun as a trickle rapidly became a deluge, and it is difficult to give a measure of the numbers. Signatures in the visitors' book provide a rough guide, and for each of the five years from 1969 to 1973, the count was: 320, 570, 540, 380 and 218. The book also gives an indication of where the visitors came from. Taking, at random, the two months of September and October 1971, there were 36 from North America, 7 from the United Kingdom, 7 from other parts of Europe, 4 from Australia and New Zealand, 3 from South Africa, 2 from Mexico, 2 from India and one each from Israel and Brazil. The preponderance of North Americans was typical, making it all the more surprising that the operation was not adopted on a large scale in those countries. The reasons for this have been discussed in Chapter 13, but it should be emphasised that most of the arthroplasties used in North America in the late 1960s and early 1970s could be fairly described as 'Charnley-type' – that is, they incorporated his low friction principle and the use of acrylic cement.

The visiting orthopaedic surgeons had to be dealt with efficiently if their time was to be as rewarding as possible. Charnley was good at this sort of organisation, and after a few years a routine was established. His policy of not allowing surgeons to buy the prostheses unless they had been to Wrightington (Chapter 10), meant that a visit was obligatory for those who seriously wanted to do the operation. However, by the early 1970s, purchase was no longer restricted, and yet the numbers reached their highest in 1970 and 1971. So surgeons continued to come to Wrightington, not because they were obliged to, but because they recognised the importance of seeing the operation for themselves and the way Charnley was managing the whole problem.

An American orthopaedic surgeon, Dr Lou Brady, first visited Charnley in 1970 with his colleague, Dr W. H. Enneking, and has written his impressions:

We found there were three types . . . who came to Wrightington: the visionary who, as a registrar would devote six months; the scientifically interested who would spend several weeks, and the curious who would

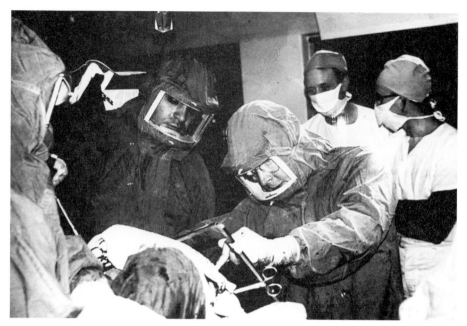

*Charnley operating. The spectators behind him are outside the perspex walls of the enclosure.* (*With acknowledgements to* Clinical Orthopaedics and Related Research.)

spend one or two days. All who came were exposed to a unique orthopaedic experience . . . Here they were seeing hundreds of patients being operated on by a team of surgeons using techniques literally unknown to the orthopaedic community . . . an operation . . . was being performed with such speed and skill that it literally trapped us . . . into thinking that it was a simple procedure . . . We saw clinics of enormous size . . . All of this with a . . . prospective study the magnitude of which boggled our minds, particularly so [because] so little had been published so far.

. . . disaster could follow when the principles were not understood and followed. On the spot innovation does not work with this procedure. I can well remember Bill Enneking's remark when I fell into the same trap, with such a suggestion. I quote his comment as I recall it. "Lou, don't you suppose that after 3000 low friction arthroplasties that John hasn't made just about every mistake one can imagine and, with his genius, already corrected it?" I withheld further comments after that.

Brady visited Wrightington once a year becoming a devoted follower and personal friend of Charnley.

The routine established for visitors was that formal 'middle-of-the-week' teaching sessions were held on alternate weeks at the busiest times, but observers could come to watch operations throughout the week. The programme was structured to allow the visitors to get the most out of the two days they spent at Wrightington:

Wednesday    0900h   Hip Centre. Clinical conference – 18 to 24 patients, who were going to be operated on during the following week, would be discussed.

                  1130h   Major weekly ward round – patients who had been operated on during the previous week were reviewed, as were those who were going to be discharged.

                  1300h   Lunch

                  1400h   Hip Centre. Long-term follow up clinic – this was related to the first 500 hips, usually 4 or 5 attended each clinic, together with other patients who presented problems of special interest.

                  1600h   Biomechanical workshop. Demonstrations of:
(1) forces acting on the hip,
(2) frictional torque in different types of arthroplasty, and
(3) wear testing of plastics.

                  1630h   Museum. Demonstration of different types of hip implants, the infection rate chart, histology of the bone-cement interface, followed by a general discussion.

                  1700h   Hip Centre. Slide-tape of the operation.

Thursday      0845h   Operating theatre.

Charnley usually performed two or three operations himself on the Thursday morning, more often than not those with technical problems. He also operated on Monday mornings and saw new patients at a clinic on Fridays. The rest of his week was spent in research, administration or seeing private patients.

The visit to the workshop was an important event and he always liked to demonstrate the swing pendulum comparator which had been built at Wrightington. This was described in the internal publications[4] and also in his book.[35] The apparatus was set up so that the friction in different types of artificial joint could be directly compared. It always gave him great pleasure to show that his small femoral head in a plastic socket kept swinging for longer than those implants which had a larger head, or a metal-on-metal bearing. He was aware of the criticisms of the method, but he excelled at this kind of visual demonstration. To understand his opinion of the value of the comparator, we need to go forward and see what he wrote in his journal in 1981:

When this was first started (and to me, of course, it was merely a dramatic demonstration of known simple engineering fact, and never a quantitative experiment) . . . I started with the most dramatic comparison to arrest attention . . . This was the 41 mm diameter McKee ball against the metal

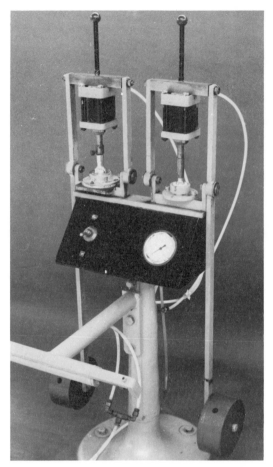

*The pendulum comparator developed by Charnley at Wrightington.* (LFA)

socket, lubricated with bovine synovial fluid. Thereafter we ran down a
scale of different implant combinations compared with the 22 mm control.

He never could suppress his delight when the metal-on-metal McKee prosthesis
'petered out' first, as it always did.

In order to remind, and further inform, his residents and visitors to
Wrightington of his teaching, Charnley began a series of internal publications in
1966, at first producing them on a small offset printing machine which he had
bought for the purpose. Many of these were papers which he had published
elsewhere; but others, often on important subjects have, for one reason or
another, not been published in scientific journals. These often give valuable
information and references are given to some of them at the end of this chapter.
Charnley also used the internal publications to give instructions about practical
matters. 'Remarks for the guidance of residents in the presenting of cases at the

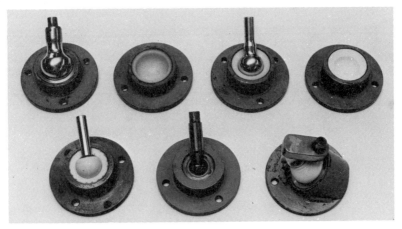

*Different sockets and femoral prostheses to be tested in the pendulum comparator. (LFA)*

Wednesday conference' is a good example of the latter type.[2] A few extracts indicate Charnley's style:

> The mental discipline in making a good clinical presentation of a patient . . . is an important element in the training of the resident surgical staff in the hip centre.
>
> Residents should adjust the length of their presentations to the ease or difficulty of the problem. This is the area which demonstrates that hip surgery is more than just a small, highly specialised technology but that it is part of the whole corpus of orthopaedic surgery . . .
>
> Although this centre is dedicated to research . . . it is, first and foremost, a surgical clinic . . . geared to handling large numbers of patients at the highest standard . . . Short and quick presentations can also be profound . . . Woolly and long-winded presentations do not help the patient . . .

This, of course, was a parochial matter; of more value to visitors was the detailed description of the 141 steps of the operation – an invaluable aide-memoire to take home.[1] To those learning the technique for the first time, the operation was a complicated technical procedure which had to be followed correctly. The passage of time has brought familiarity so that the operation is now a routine procedure; it is easy to forget the difficulties which could arise in mastering a completely new technique, and these instructions were a great help. Any modifications, such as the details of wound closure[3], were described (often with helpful diagrams) in later numbers.

One of the purposes of these publications was to record changes in technique, and so meet the criticisms of those who found they could not keep up with his innovations. It was difficult for a surgeon who was evolving a new operation to be in communication with all his followers, and there was no easy answer to this problem.

There were 78 internal publications, the last being in 1980, and they form a valuable corpus of knowledge dealing with all aspects, major and minor, of low friction arthroplasty. As the number of papers increased they were presented to visitors in a large ring-binder provided by Thackrays.

Charnley made films and videos of the low friction arthroplasty in his efforts to ensure that the operation would be carried out by others using his precise technique. In 1982, when he was introducing a new method for re-attaching the trochanter (Chapter 16), he made drawings which were to be printed and placed in 'double wraps' which could be sterilised be γ-radiation. The idea was that they could be referred to by a surgeon while he was actually carrying out the procedure. Charnley had discussed this with orthopaedic surgeons in the United States and wrote to Thackrays:

> They all agree that if you are not doing an operation very frequently any means of helping would be very valuable. The analogy of a world renowned pianist who has not played a certain concerto for six weeks and does so with the aid of music is a good one and we all agree that the pianist does not lose face in this way nor does he impair the quality of his music, in fact very much the other way. (3.2.82)

Publications in orthopaedic journals were Charnley's most effective method of communicating his research, and, later, his results to surgeons in the United Kingdom and overseas. These are listed at the end of the chapter, but this is an appropriate place to review them briefly in order to give an idea of the scope of his work. His papers, which have not already been considered in earlier chapters, can conveniently be described under four main headings: biomechanical research; research on wear of plastic; the results of the operations, and venous thrombosis and pulmonary embolism.

The first paper which Charnley gave on the biomechanical aspects of his new artificial hip joint was published in the proceedings of the Institution of Mechanical Engineers in 1966.[5] Although he emphasised the engineering considerations and the importance of wear testing in the laboratory, he concluded:

> It is clear . . . that only by judicious testing in the human body is it likely that we can get further with this research . . . It is impossible to do this work in a large quadruped . . . It cannot be too strongly emphasised, however, that these surgical techniques still have not reached a stage when they can be used light-heartedly as an alternative to less spectacular methods in younger patients . . .

He published five papers between 1967 and 1972 which dealt with basic observations which, although of importance to orthopaedic surgeons, were probably of greater interest to engineers and so, with one exception, they are to be found in journals of medical and biological engineering, and biomechanics. The first, written with an Australian registrar Dr B. T. Hammond, followed his work on joint lubrication (Chapter 9) and set out to determine the shape of the normal femoral head.[6] Ten specimens were examined by seven different methods and the findings showed that the head was spherical, which differed from the only previously published work on the subject.

The next paper was based on the material from the failed PTFE arthroplasties (Chapter 10). The direction of the resultant force on the hip, which was relevant to the design of future hip replacements, was deduced from the pattern of wear in 37 sockets which had been removed from patients.[7] His co-author was

Mr R. A. Elson, then a senior registrar at Wrightington and later a consultant orthopaedic surgeon in Sheffield.

Charnley had been trying to develop an instrument for recording the way patients walked (gait analysis) since 1961, and he designed a prototype which was made at Wrightington. There were some difficulties, and he went to the department of mechanical engineering at UMIST for advice. The head of the department, Professor W. Johnson, allocated one of his lecturers to help Charnley. Dr Jan Skorecki made many visits to Wrightington, and built a new walkway about eleven feet long which was mounted in five tons of concrete embedded in the floor.[43] Graphic recordings could be made of patients' gait before and after operation which allowed any resulting changes to be assessed objectively. Useful information was obtained over a number of years, but once the pattern had been established, gait analysis was no longer needed in routine clinical practice. Charnley described the apparatus and its use in 1968 in a paper written with Dr R. Pusso, an assistant from Buenos Aires.[8] A product of this research on gait was published in 1972[10] by Charnley, Skorecki and Jacobs (also from UMIST). The vertical component of force exerted during walking, in normal and abnormal gaits, was analysed into harmonic components in order to classify the different wave forms recorded by the machine.

Dr R. D. McLeish was another lecturer at UMIST with whom Charnley collaborated closely at this period, and in 1970 they published a paper analysing the abduction forces at the hip.[9]

McLeish and Skorecki both enjoyed working with Charnley although they found he sometimes had difficulty in understanding engineering concepts. He would always listen to advice, but discussions were one-sided and, more often than not, he would end up doing what he wanted. Some of his early schemes, such as making a walking robot, proved to be impractical. He acted quickly and always wanted results as soon as possible. All in all, they accepted him as a 'marvellous leader of a research team'. Skorecki's acknowledgement of Charnley's help in a published paper refers to an 'inspiring and invigorating collaboration at all stages'[43] which does justice to the relation between Charnley and his engineering colleagues. His association with these two men led to his involvement with the Manchester Medical Engineering Club which was founded in 1967; he was on the committee and spoke at meetings from time to time. Charnley was made an honorary lecturer at UMIST and also helped with project work on the MSc course in medical engineering; the students would occasionally visit him at Wrightington.

One of the first investigations that Charnley asked McLeish and Skorecki to undertake was on the wear of the plastic socket in a spherical joint and they published a mathematical analysis on the subject in 1969.[45] After the failure of PTFE, this matter was of the greatest importance and Charnley was determined to learn as much as possible from the experience. He cast his net widely wherever he felt help would be available, and another paper was published in the same year with Dr M. D. Longfield from the department of mechanical engineering in the University of Leeds (Dr A. Kamangar, a registrar at the hip centre, was also a co-author).[11] The aim was to find the optimal size for the head of the femoral prosthesis in order to produce the minimum volume of wear debris over a given period. The conclusion, based on a study of the PTFE sockets, was that the best size of the head would be half that of the external diameter of the socket, which was further support for Charnley's concept of the small (22 mm) femoral head. What was almost an addendum to the paper gave cause for optimism: one HMWP socket, from a patient who had led a normal life for three and a half years after the operation (and who had died from an unrelated cause), had been examined; the total linear wear over this period was only 0.5 mm.

Charnley continued testing the wear of HMWP against stainless steel in the biomechanical laboratory at Wrightington and in September 1975 he gave a paper to a symposium on plastics in medicine and surgery which was organised by the Plastics and Rubber Institute at Strathclyde University, Glasgow – this was included as an internal publication.[14] He described his method of laboratory testing using reciprocal movement between discs for periods up to ten days. The rate of wear of HMWP was 250 times better than PTFE in these circumstances. When this was compared with clinical wear in patients, the result was not so favourable; a rate of wear of 1.5 mm in ten years was only 15 times better than PTFE. Charnley's explanation of the paradox was that in the laboratory a 'protective layer of a changed plastics substance' formed over the surface of the socket, and he thought that biological conditions might prevent this from forming in the human body. Descriptions of the work on laboratory wear testing and the results were published in the internal publications.[12]

Estimation of wear in sockets, which were in patients, was made from the radiographs by measuring the distance between the metal head and the wire marker in the radiolucent plastic. Technical problems in making this measurement arise because of the difficulty in obtaining films which are exactly comparable at different times and in different patients. Much work was done by Charnley on the subject and papers on the method he devised were published in 1975 and 1978 in the American journal, *Clinical Orthopaedics and Related Research*.[13,15] In the second paper, measurements had been made in 547 low friction arthroplasties after an average period of 8.3 years. The average rate of wear in operations carried out in 1967 and 1968 was 0.07 mm a year.

In an attempt to elucidate further the different rates of wear of HMWP in the laboratory and in the human body, the appearance of the sockets was studied by optical and electron microscopy in collaboration with the departments of mechanical engineering and metallurgy at Leeds.[16] It was found that after an initial running-in period in the body, most wear takes place in the superior part of the socket. The question of whether this was due to corrosion fatigue, fretting fatigue, third-body wear (due to the inclusion of abrasive particles) or creep, was discussed. It was thought that these four mechanisms probably all occurred together, in addition to true wear. The subject is complicated and of scientific interest, but in practical terms HMWP serves as a lasting material in the socket in operations carried out after the age of, say, fifty years.

Charnley first spoke at a formal meeting about his low friction arthroplasty (using HMWP) in 1966 when he gave a paper at the International Congress of Orthopaedics and Traumatology in Paris.[17] He described his method and reported that approximately 1100 operations had been performed at Wrightington between November 1962 and April 1966. His conclusions were that: (1) the operation should be carried out in centres equipped for the purpose; (2) the results should be recorded in a standard manner; (3) special aseptic precautions in the operating theatre ought to be taken; (4) the facilities of a biomechanical workshop were needed, and so was (5) co-operation with university departments of engineering.

Two papers in 1968 and 1969, which described the operation, were published in Swiss journals[18,19] in which he recognised the surgeon's dilemma. Was the surgeon to wait another five years before submitting patients to the operation in the hope that animal experiments might bring reassuring information? Or use his clinical judgement and balance the patient's disability against the worst that could happen should the replacement fail? Charnley stressed that the position should be fully discussed with each patient.

From 1970 onwards, publications from Charnley appeared regularly and more were in the American journal *Clinical Orthopaedics* than in the British volume of the *Journal of Bone and Joint Surgery*. Perhaps this demonstrated innate British conservatism in not wanting to publish results of a new operation too soon. Or maybe it was just a case of 'a prophet is not without honour, save in his own country . . .'. There was possibly another factor. Reading his writing leads to the conclusion that his use of the English language was of a higher standard in the 1950s than it was in the 1970s. This may be because many of his later papers were written by assistants and, as he became increasingly busy, he simply did not have time for the repeated revisions which he would have carried out in his earlier days. None the less his message was always clear.

The results of his first group of patients with a follow up of six to seven years was published in *Clinical Orthopaedics* in 1970[20] and a series of 379 operations with a follow up of four to seven years was published in the British *Journal of Bone and Joint Surgery* in 1972.[23] As Charnley had kept accurate records, these were prospective studies using the numerical system of grading the condition of the patient and the state of their hip, before and after operation (the data being stored on punch-cards). The following year, he reported nine and ten year results of 185 low friction arthroplasties (in 170 patients, some of whom had both hips operated on) which were carried out from November 1962 to December 1963.[25] The results were encouraging: 92% were considered to be completely successful and the incidence of loosening was less than 1.6%. Late dislocation also occurred in a different 1.6%, and Charnley recognised that this might be a 'blessing in disguise' which correlated with the low rate of loosening. He had earlier made the point that 'the ability to subluxate provides a very valuable safety device to safeguard the cemented bonds . . . in the event of a patient sustaining accidental violence which forces the joint beyond its normal range'.

Over subsequent years Charnley wrote about the application of the operation to special conditions, for example: after failures of previous operations;[24] after fracture dislocation of the hip;[31] following infection in the opposite hip;[33] after healed septic and tuberculous arthritis,[36] and many other situations[21,22,26,27,34]. The use of the operation for hips in which the head and neck of the femur had been removed previously[29] and those which had been arthrodesed[30] indicated special, and technically difficult, applications of the procedure. He also dealt with such complications as ectopic bone formation[28] and dislocation occurring after operation.[32] A number of other publications not mentioned here are listed (without numbers) at the end of the book.

His book, *Low Friction Arthroplasty of the Hip*,[35] was published in 1979 (Chapter 16) and dealt with all aspects of the operation, including the 12 to 15 year follow up which he carried out in 1977. It was then possible to review 77 arthroplasties out of the original group of 396 (164 of the patients had died). The rate of loosening was 1.5% which was much higher than in the 10 000 LFA operations performed subsequent to this prospective series. The total failure rate,

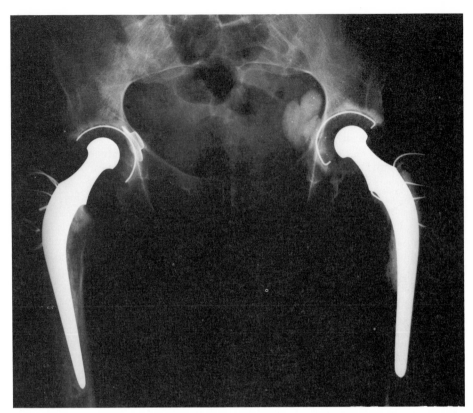

*Radiograph of a patient who had both hips operated on by Charnley: the left hip 22 years previously (note that a cement restrictor was not in use at that time), and the right 15 years previously. He has no pain or disability apart from that associated with ankylosing spondylitis. There appears to be a little wear of the sockets on both sides. (Radiograph from Mr B.J. Holdsworth.)*

which includes death, infection, dislocation and so on, was estimated to be in the region of 2%. Presentation of the results is complicated and all the problems are discussed in the book.

Blood clots form in the veins of the legs after many operations, and may produce chronic swelling of the leg. Sometimes the clots become detached and lodge in the lungs causing sudden death. This complication occurred more often after hip operations than other types of surgery. The causes are uncertain and many factors are involved; it has been suggested that the position in which the leg is held during low friction arthroplasty may twist the femoral vein, and so predispose to thrombosis.[44] To put the matter in perspective, the mortality from pulmonary embolism in almost 8000 arthroplasties (in some of whom special methods of prevention were used, in others they were not) at Wrightington was 1.04%.[37] If the causes are many, so are the methods of prevention. The whole subject is complex and can only be considered superficially here.

Charnley certainly never liked giving anticoagulant drugs to his patients because of the risk of bleeding into the wound, and at other sites. He devoted a great deal of time to studying the problem. His first investigation was recorded in an internal publication (and not elsewhere) in 1968[37]. Pheniodone (an anticoagulant) was given to alternate patients in 999 arthroplasties and there was a reduction in fatal emboli in the group who were treated, but no decrease in venous thrombosis (as judged clinically). This was, however, balanced by the number of deaths from bleeding; the infection rate was also greater in the treated group because there were more haematomas. In 1972, he wrote to *The Lancet*[38] reporting his experience of subcutaneous injections of heparin used as prophylaxis. He had given it up after a trial in 48 consecutive patients because one patient had died from bleeding from the lungs and another had a fatal pulmonary embolism. A statistical study was undertaken to elicit the factors which predisposed to thromboembolism[39] and it was suggested that anticoagulation should only be used in those especially at risk.

Charnley decided to test the effect of the drug Plaquenil (hydroxychloroquine sulphate) in the hope that it would prove as effective as other agents and have fewer complications. In many ways Wrightington was the ideal place to carry out this sort of investigation because of the large numbers of patients undergoing the same operation in standard conditions. Papers were published in *Clinical Orthopaedics* in 1977 and 1978[40,41,42] with the conclusion that when Plaquenil was given the incidence of fatal pulmonary embolism in 2144 patients was reduced to 0.28% with no serious bleeding complications. In spite of this, the drug did not gain general acceptance as a preventive measure. Some limitations of Charnley's research were criticised because he had not carried out prospective randomised controlled trials. His attitude towards this difficult type of clinical investigation has been discussed in relation to clean air and infection (Chapter 12).

Reading papers at orthopaedic meetings and taking part in discussions is probably the best way of convincing colleagues, and Charnley continued to go to meetings of the British Orthopaedic Association at least once a year. He had always travelled abroad, but before the development of the low friction arthroplasty was stabilised he regarded any absence from his unit as an intrusion into the time he needed for research and writing. But by the middle 1970s he was much in demand and he began to accept more invitations. He went to meetings of orthopaedic associations in the United States, Australia and South Africa and particularly to the American Academy of Orthopaedic Surgeons. He also went to Japan, and in Europe the countries he most often visited were Spain and Sweden. After he retired from the National Health Service he began to travel more. Unfortunately, there is no complete record of his overseas visits, except for the year 1980; this in itself illustrates the pressures of his international travel and will be presented in Chapter 16.

# Chapter 15

# AN OUTPOST IN THE SOUTH: MIDHURST

1969–1982

*Once the operation is completed there is nowadays almost nothing that can go mechanically wrong . . .*

Instructions for Professor Charnley's patients

CHARNLEY'S FRIENDS were surprised when they learnt in 1969 that he had set up a centre for hip surgery at King Edward VII Hospital, Midhurst, West Sussex, and many must have wondered what had prompted him to take this step. The hospital was well known as a first-class private sanatorium for the treatment of pulmonary tuberculosis in the south of England. Why did he do it? And why Midhurst? There are a number of reasons, but the answer lies, at least to some extent, in the background of this unique institution. What follows in the next few paragraphs comes from an excellent history of the hospital written by Dr S.E. Large and published in 1986.[1]

King Edward VII was keenly interested in hospitals and when his financial adviser, Sir Ernest Cassel, put £200,000 at his disposal 'for charitable or utilitarian purposes', he decided that the money should be used for the benefit of sufferers from tuberculosis. Open-air treatment had only recently been introduced and the King had been very impressed by a sanatorium which he had visited in the Taunus mountains near Frankfurt.

'What we require', the King said to one of his medical advisers, 'is a sanatorium for the poorer middle classes. Rich people can avail themselves of private sanatoria; the really poor are provided for by municipalities and through public benevolence; but between these there is a stratum of educated yet indigent patients such as teachers, clergymen, clerks, governesses, young officers, etc,

199

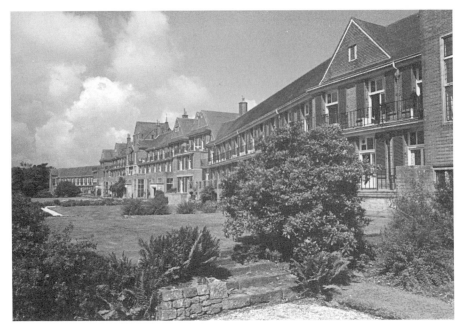

*Midhurst Hospital. (From the administrative secretary, Mr W.H. Mitchell.)*

who cannot afford the costs of a private sanatorium, whilst they are too bashful to avail themselves of public charity. My sanatorium is principally to take care of them.'

A committee of eminent doctors, three of whom were royal physicians and three experts in the treatment of tuberculosis, was formed. A site was chosen: 150 acres of wooded land on a south-facing slope on Easebourne Hill, above the small town of Midhurst, and about 60 miles south of London. The sanatorium, with 100 beds, was opened in 1906 by the King who became its first president (an office held by the reigning monarch up to the present time). The executive committee met at St James's Place, London, and continued to do so until 1969.

The reputation of the sanatorium grew over the years, and was further strengthened by Dr G. S. Todd (later Sir Geoffrey) who was medical superintendent from 1933 to 1970. Todd was an outspoken Australian, and a firm disciplinarian, who devoted his life to the institution – in Dr Large's words 'For thirty-seven years Midhurst was Todd and Todd was Midhurst'.

After the Second World War an increasing amount of major surgery was carried out in the management of pulmonary tuberculosis; but by the 1960s Midhurst had to face similar problems to those faced by Wrightington as the incidence of tuberculosis declined, and hospital beds were no longer needed for long-term treatment. Various steps were taken, and in 1964 the name was changed to King Edward VII Hospital, instead of Sanatorium, so that patients with nontuberculous chest diseases, or any other condition, could be treated in beds which might be unoccupied (107 were now available). The medical committee wanted the hospital to remain a national institution with its traditional interests upheld, but at the same time its ambit was widened so that all types of medical and surgical conditions could be treated. To this end, twelve new consultants were invited to join the staff; they mostly came from London, but some were from the local district hospitals.

A number of schemes were discussed and Colonel Miles Reid, a member of the council, suggested that consideration should be given to the possibility of carrying out hip replacements in the hospital. An interesting coincidence determined what happened next, and justifies a digression. In 1912 the committee at Midhurst had asked the advice of Mr Isodore Salmon, who was a director of Lyons Company Limited, about the finances and administration of the sanatorium, and he advised various economies. Lyons was then a successful company with large hotels, restaurants and tea-shops in London. The Midhurst connection was continued when Mr B.A. Salmon became a member of the council in 1935. He died in 1965 and was succeeded by Sir Norman Joseph, also a director of Lyons. The point of digression arises from the coincidence that Jill Charnley had been Sir Norman's personal assistant before her marriage, and now he proposed that Professor Charnley (as he was then) should be approached and his advice sought about the prospects of setting up a centre for hip surgery at Midhurst. Sir Norman Joseph arranged for Charnley to meet the Duke of Norfolk, who was chairman of the council, and they lunched together in London. Sir Geoffrey Todd and his deputy, Dr Douglas Teare, then went to Wrightington to continue discussions, and Charnley visited Midhurst. He was impressed, although he thought the scheme might not be practical in view of the travelling which it would involve for him.

These negotiations took place in 1969. In the previous year Charnley had given up the idea of creating a research institute at Wrightington (Chapter 10). It could well be that this undoubted disappointment made him more receptive to the Midhurst proposal. The only written evidence about his attitude at the time is in a letter he wrote to Howorth (Chapter 12):

. . . I have just spent a recent Saturday at the King Edward VII Hospital, Midhurst, where they were asking my advice about starting a centre for hip surgery in a hospital which originally was devoted to tuberculosis, but which now has the capacity to develop . . . hip surgery.

This hospital . . . is not part of the Health Service and concentrates largely on private patients. The Duke of Norfolk . . . is extremely interested in keeping the hospital going . . . I had two hours of discussion with him, and I was very impressed by the determination shown in planning the new role for the hospital. (20.3.69)

The King Edward VII Hospital had recently installed what Charnley considered to be 'a very good ventilation plant' for the operating theatre, but he advised that they should also have a clean air enclosure. His letter to Howorth continued:

. . . this would form an attraction for them getting the appropriate surgeons interested in the unit. They [Midhurst] do have problems because of the remoteness of the hospital . . . but only by providing a sterile enclosure do I think that they are likely to get surgeons interested . . . my point was that they were in a position to get [it] into operation long before any of the

National Health Service hospitals in the vicinity and this would help their staffing problems.

The final paragraph of this letter reveals the attention which Charnley paid to the structure of the enclosure, and adds an unexpected domestic touch:

> At our last meeting I think one of the details which had to be settled was the design of the mobile side walls because I had failed to find any aluminium extrusions which were suitable . . . Since then I have been to the Ideal Homes Exhibition at Olympia and there were quite a number of firms exhibiting anodised aluminium sliding windows for houses. One firm in particular . . . was using extruded sections which I thought could be very easily adapted for our purpose. (20.3.69)

Once Charnley had made up his mind, rapid progress followed and on December 23, 1969, he told Howorth in a letter that 'he had operated on two patients in the new installation and everything was satisfactory'. This was no doubt true, but he omitted to tell him that his first patient had died after the operation from a pulmonary embolism. Surgeons know that such a disaster can happen at any time, but it was nevertheless an unfortunate start. Charnley was resilient, and his work at Midhurst became enormously successful. So much so, that although his original intention was merely to get the hip centre established and leave others to continue, his visits became a very important part of his life.

It is not the case that he went to Midhurst to increase his private practice, nor did he choose it because it was a convenient place to operate on his wealthy patients who lived in the south of England. Midhurst was a very special hospital which maintained old-fashioned standards which were entirely admirable as far as the medical staff were concerned. It was policy to attract the best men and to provide them with the best facilities. In this respect, Charnley was looked after well and in turn he appreciated the atmosphere of the place.

The operating theatre had been upgraded and the clean air enclosure installed before he started, and he had arranged for ward and theatre staff to go to Wrightington for training. A specially designed ward unit with two groups of three beds was made for his patients (a further three beds were added later). Charnley was not prepared to have men and women patients in the same recovery wards; so to make observation easy, a large window was inserted into the wall between each room which was covered by a picture when the patients had recovered. The ward was later appropriately named the Miles Reid ward.

The journey from Knutsford to Midhurst presented a problem to which Charnley devoted a great deal of thought. At first, he went by air from Manchester to Heathrow, usually arriving at about ten o'clock at night. He was met by a chauffeur-driven Austin Princess car from Midhurst and taken to the hospital where he stayed at Uppershaw, Sir Geoffrey Todd's house in the grounds. Being met in this style was a considerable bonus, and he was fortunate always to have the same chauffeur, Mr Alfie Purdew. In fact, he was able to call on Purdew whenever he came to or left Midhurst; and, if he had to go to London for a meeting or a dinner while he was at the hospital, Purdew would drive him. The two men got on well: Charnley would sit in the front of the car and talk freely about his home and family. Occasionally, when the time was right, they might stop and have a drink together. After a few months, Charnley was provided with a room in the doctors' quarters at the hospital, and when he arrived Purdew would lay out his pyjamas and make tea for him. Charnley enjoyed Purdew's company and would often ask his advice about domestic matters. An example, which arose some years later, was – how to get rid of the rabbits which were damaging the roses at Birchwood? Purdew, a Sussex countryman, taught Charnley how to make snares, but the family cat was the first and only thing that was trapped.

He tried various ways of travelling; using for a while a private aircraft to Goodwood, where there was a small airfield close to Midhurst, but this was unreliable. In the end, he chose British Rail and had a more restful journey. On the train, he attempted to isolate himself by listening to classical music on a Walkman tape-player. It was not so much that he did not like his fellow-passengers, but he found extraneous noise distracting. When he was on his own in a compartment, he dictated letters into a pocket dictaphone and read orthopaedic papers. The journeys were pleasant enough, but there were times when he was upset by the inefficiencies of the service, and he protested furiously about the dirt and filth of the trains on many occasions. Purdew met him at Euston, but if there was a rail strike, or some other reason, Jill Charnley would drive him to a hotel at a roundabout north of Oxford, where Purdew with the Austin Princess would be waiting for him.

Having arrived on a Thursday night, he did a ward round at half past eight the next morning, after which he would carry out two or three low friction arthroplasties. Out-patients were seen in the afternoon and on Saturday morning. During 1970, he came every three weeks, but from then onwards he increased his visits to every two weeks whenever possible.

On balance, the inconvenience of the journey was acceptable in view of the advantages gained from being able to operate at Midhurst. Furthermore, he intended to go on operating after he retired from the National Health Service, and he was able to do so at Midhurst, more or less on his own terms. From 1975 onwards, his pattern of work altered: he now arrived on a Wednesday; operated on Thursday morning, and then again all day on Friday, with the result that he was able to do five or six hip replacements at each visit.

Charnley described what he called his 'bits of luck' at Wrightington which made possible the development of the Centre for Hip Surgery there; and there is no doubt that he had similar good fortune at Midhurst. Purdew, of course, was a 'bit of luck', but so also was the doctor who assisted him and looked after his patients. Dr Paddy Doyle came from a naval family and served himself, reaching the rank of Lieutenant-Commander, before qualifying as a doctor in 1954. He developed pulmonary tuberculosis and was a patient at Midhurst, after which he was appointed as a senior medical officer there in 1957. He worked with Charnley from 1969 and they combined perfectly. Doyle, who retired in 1983 and died in 1988, is said to have been able to 'accept the way Charnley ruled the world'. Neither man could tolerate compromise, or put up with second best, and a strong bond developed between them. Good liaison was essential in the circumstances and someone had to take responsibility for the medical care of the patients after operation. When Doyle was not available, there were always physicians in the hospital, some of whom lived in houses in the grounds. Patients who were ill would find themselves being looked after by a senior doctor at any time of the day or night, rather than by a junior house physician. Charnley explained the situation to his patients, each of whom were given a printed pamphlet written by him. He was meticulous in addressing this personally to each patient and he signed it himself. The opening paragraphs were:

> I have prepared these notes to help you to understand your role in rehabilitation under the guidance of a member of the physiotherapy staff (who will visit you twice daily).
>
> First of all I would like to reassure you in the early days after your operation, when sometimes you might feel rather isolated from the surgeon who is totally responsible for your welfare. Once the operation is completed there is nowadays almost nothing that can go mechanically wrong . . . Medical complications can follow any type of surgery . . . The medical and nursing staff at Midhurst are experienced in handling complications after operations of much greater magnitude than hip surgery (serious operations on the chest and lungs, for instance). There is, therefore, no need to feel that my absence in the early days . . . will affect this aspect of the problem.
>
> You are free at any time to speak on the telephone [and he gave his home and hospital numbers].

The pamphlet continues with a description of the after-treatment, and the following paragraphs are characteristic extracts which illustrate his approach to patients and the operation:

> **General psychological matters**. Try to avoid developing an apprehensive attitude by fearing that the slightest 'incorrect' movement on your part might wreck the whole procedure and 'undo all the good work'. This particular surgical operation is a very sound engineering job and can survive quite remarkable violence (even falling out of bed!) . . .
>
> **Returning home**. A robust patient can usually return home two weeks (plus one or two days) after the operation for one hip. If two hips have been operated on then about three weeks is necessary. On returning home no special nursing and no physiotherapy is required. Rehabilitation at home is by a common-sense extension of the activities you will have been practising during the last days of your hospital stay. Emphasis is on rehabilitation by attempts to carry out daily chores . . . graded by a common-sense appreciation of what you find you can do without forcing yourself . . . A stick MUST be used (in the hand opposite the hip operated on) for four weeks after leaving hospital EVEN THOUGH YOU MAY BE ABLE TO WALK WITHOUT IT . . .
>
> **Do's and Don'ts**. In the early years while the operation was being developed patients were told to sleep on their backs, with a pillow between their knees and for the first two months they were warned against sitting in very low chairs . . . Since those early years experience has shown that these fears were without foundation and recent technical developments in the operation now make dislocation even less likely than formerly. There is now no longer any need to prohibit particular movements . . . [this version was written in 1976 or thereabouts].

Things did occasionally go wrong and one patient had a dislocation in 1978 (at the time when he was writing *Low Friction Arthroplasty of the Hip*). Mrs Cock, the senior physiotherapist, wrote to tell him what had happened and he sent her this brief handwritten note:

Dear Ros,

Don't worry! . . . There will always be an occasional failure – I suppose it is the nature of surgery.

There are other dislocations – he was not the only one in 800!

. . . There was one old boy, years ago, who used to take a bottle of gin (without a label so his wife might not see) down to the bottom of the garden.

I think perhaps low chairs might be prohibited for some weeks – but nothing else.

I am lucky this should happen before I am too "cocky" in the book – talking about *never*.

> Yours,
>
> John Charnley

This spontaneous response throws an interesting light on Charnley's character, and explains why people appreciated working for him. His ward sister, Miss Norton, was at Midhurst when he arrived and stayed till after his death. There were times when she found the manner in which he spoke to some patients difficult to accept. For his part, he was no respecter of persons and if he thought that a patient was not cooperating, or was behaving in a way he considered incorrect, he told them so without hesitation and in no uncertain terms. Once he had a patient who claimed that her new hip was coming out of joint, but he wrote to her doctor that 'he could not make head or tail of her' as she would not let him examine her hip under anaesthesia. He admitted that he would not want to operate on her again even if he was able to demonstrate that the joint subluxated; but if this was the case, then 'at least I would be sympathetic with her'. He found it difficult to deal with those patients who did not live up to his expectations.

Charnley sometimes made harsh judgements about people because he was a man for whom white was white, and black, black. There was no grey, and he was never able to suffer gladly those whom he considered fools. Fortunately, his outbursts did not occur very often. On the other hand, he was good to his staff in small, but thoughtful, ways; for instance, he would arrange for Miss Norton to attend lectures he gave in London, and always introduced her to 'the right poeple'. His theatre staff were equally loyal and long-serving, and they liked and respected him. It is said that he mellowed and became easier to work with in the theatre as he grew older; occasional episodes of bad temper were momentary and quickly forgotten.

Anyone in serious trouble received consideration and help; and Charnley was known to have driven from Knutsford to Midhurst especially to see a patient with a problem. The great majority of his patients regarded him with affection and respect, and were fully aware of the work he had done to make their operations successful.

His appreciation of the staff was indicated clearly when he chose them to help him on the rare occasions when he agreed to operate away from Wrightington or Midhurst. He never could be called a peripatetic surgeon and he preferred to operate in his own theatre; surgeons had to come to watch him operate rather than him going to them. In 1981, he did perform a demonstration operation in the United States, but it was on a cadaver; latterly he preferred to use models

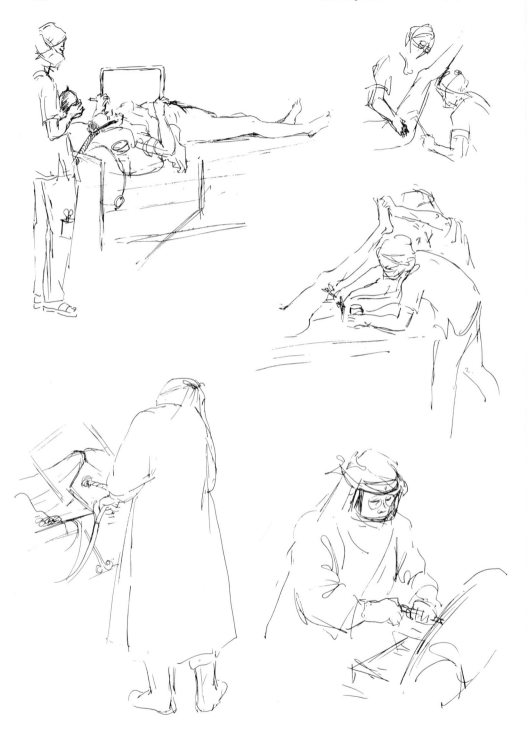

*Part of a series of sketches of Charnley operating at Midhurst by Mrs Juliet Pannett.*

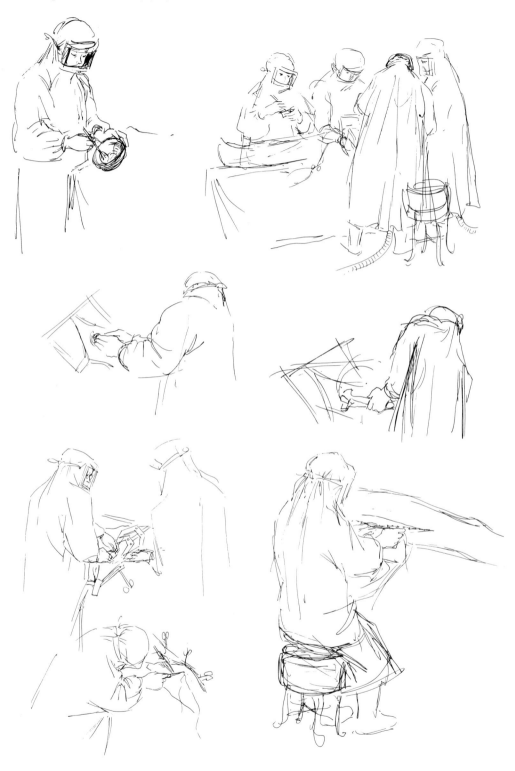

to demonstrate his technique of trochanteric wiring. There were, however, three special occasions when he took his team from Midhurst with him.

The first was the inaugural meeting of the International Hip Society which was held in Bern, Switzerland, in March 1977. Charnley's friend, Professor Müller, was the host and it was arranged that they each would demonstrate their own operations on closed circuit television. Charnley wrote to Thackrays:

> I have provisionally arranged for three of the hospital staff from Midhurst to come with me but . . . we shall have to get together to discuss the best way of moving the quite heavy equipment.
>
> I think this could be an exceedingly important occasion because the spectators will be probably not more than 25 and will be the founder members of this Society representing total hip replacement throughout the world.

The whole exercise was planned by Charnley with military precision.

Later in the year, Charnley was invited to treat King Khaled of Saudi Arabia who had a painful hip. He flew to Riyadh and advised a low friction arthroplasty, preceded by a biopsy. He had hoped to arrange for the King to be admitted to Midhurst, but 'it was found impossible to provide accommodation for the King's entourage locally'. Charnley is said to have been under some pressure from the Foreign Office for diplomatic reasons, and he reluctantly agreed to carry out the operation at a large private clinic in London. He took the precaution of asking Müller to help him and all went well. Charnley stayed for six weeks in a penthouse suite at the Dorchester Hotel and his team at the Swiss Cottage Holiday Inn. The staff from Midhurst were: Dr J.R. Bennett (anaesthetist); Dr T. Guthrie (physician); Miss Norton (ward sister); Miss Pring (theatre sister); Mrs Taylor, Mr Lejasmeiers and Mr Martin (theatre assistants); and Mrs Cock (physiotherapist). Charnley was rewarded by a gift of £25,000 to buy an MTS (Materials Testing System) machine which was set up in his research laboratory at Wrightington. This proved to be a considerable frustration to him; he always wanted to know exactly how everything he used worked, and he never was able to understand the electronics of the machine. He wrote to Thackrays: 'I don't think I shall ever master it' (5.8.80) and eventually sold it to them.

Patients from overseas might provoke a chauvinistic response, and he sometimes refused to operate on a foreign patient while he still had British patients on his waiting list. He was, of course, in a position to pick and choose and he did not hesitate to turn down patients for whatever reason.

On one occasion a present of a silver coffee-pot from the Middle East produced some indignation when he unwrapped it at Midhurst – 'shoddy rubbish', he said. He attacked it with the physiotherapist's scissors to find out how thick the silver was. He was persuaded to desist, so he took it to the operating theatre where he asked for a drill. His efforts had to be re-directed from drilling a hole at the bottom, so making the pot totally useless. He eventually penetrated the metal near the lid and was triumphant ('I told you so') when he demonstrated that the silver was only paper thin. The coffee-pot never reached Birchwood.

To return to more serious matters. The whole set-up at King Edward VII Hospital pleased him for understandable reasons. The staff provided a first class service for him and his patients – and in turn he added to the reputation of the hospital. No doubt he found the atmosphere a welcome change from the frustrations and pressures of the National Health Service. He liked bringing visitors to the hospital and did so often and in quite large numbers; 15 Japanese surgeons in 1979, for example. During his twelve and a half years at Midhurst he carried out over 1300 low friction arthroplasties. He frequently tried out new ideas and inventions there, and would make notes in the margin of the operation register such as:

5.1.77 started neck length jig
2.6.77 started prophylactic antibiotics
25.8.77 stopped iodine in socket – $H_2O_2$ [hydrogen peroxide] now

When he was not operating, he was able to read and write in his room without distraction. The satisfaction that his work at Midhurst gave him must have been sufficient to overcome the inconvenience of being away from home for two or three days every two weeks.

His last visit was in 1982 and Purdew thought Charnley looked ill when he met him at Euston station. But he carried out a revision operation the next day (July 28), just two weeks before he died. The patient had had an arthroplasty by a local orthopaedic surgeon, who referred her to Charnley after she had developed a late infection. The procedure was difficult and took about three hours. He filled in his standard operative pro forma by hand and was delighted with the way the operation had gone. One member of the staff who saw him as he left the theatre remembers that 'he was as happy as a schoolboy'.

Mr John Older, who is a consultant orthopaedic surgeon at Guildford, came to work with Charnley and assisted him at operations in the later years. He developed great respect and friendship for Charnley, and gave an address at the memorial service which was held at the hospital. A few sentences from it, in which he remembered Charnley at Midhurst, provide a appropriate epilogue to this chapter:

. . . the youthful . . . figure of Sir John bustling through this hospital, goading himself and those around him with energy and enthusiasm.
. . . sitting at the head of table for breakfast giving his forthright views on the state of the nation.
. . . hunched over the desk in the surgeons' room writing up his operation notes or sitting back in the armchair . . . discussing what is right or wrong with X-rays of the hip he has just replaced.

*Chapter 16*

---

# ACTIVE RETIREMENT
## 1975–1982

---

*I think it is now a matter of coasting home, with judicious lectures
and demonstrations from now on.*

John Charnley 1981

CHARNLEY CAN NEVER have had any intention of taking a conventional retirement, but he knew that he would be obliged to retire from the National Health Service on his sixty-fifth birthday in August 1976. In fact, he retired officially on August 29, 1975, not because he wanted to give up work, but because he wanted the freedom to do the work he wanted. His aims were to continue his research, particularly on the bone–cement interface, to write his book on the operation, and also to travel and lecture abroad. He was allowed to continue to use the workshop and laboratory at Wrightington, and also to operate there. Five years later he wrote to Thackray:

> We have to remember that this August [1980] I start the last year of my Honorary Consultantship with the NHS and it is possible that I may not be sanctioned to operate in the NHS after this, even though I understand I shall be permitted to carry on my research activities here as long as I wish. (18.8.80)

Although he clearly valued the privilege of being able to operate at Wrightington, he only did so very occasionally, and then on patients in whom he had a special interest. Charnley increased his visits to Midhurst, which gave him as much operating as he wanted (Chapter 15).

Work at the hip centre was continued by the two consultants who had been appointed in previous years: Mr J.C.H. Murphy in 1971 and Mr B.M. Wroblewski in 1973; and by Mr K. Hardinge who was appointed in 1976 (after Charnley's retirement). The post of director of the hip centre lapsed.

Charnley had never given a great deal of thought to income tax until he was faced with a really large demand from the Inland Revenue, and then (like everybody else) he reacted with some alarm. When he was considering retiring from the National Health Service, marginal rates of income tax had reached 90% or more, and he realised that he should take some steps to limit his liability by judicious tax planning. An opinion was sought from a barrister who was an expert in these matters. Advice that the family should move to a tax haven like the Channel Islands was completely unacceptable. Charnley discussed the possibilities with Ron Frank, with whom he had close contact through Thackrays and with whom he had become friendly outwith their professional connection. The two men met regularly from 1974 onwards, usually at Birchwood. Frank suggested a solution which would be tax-efficient and provide a satisfactory pension for Charnley, as well as making proper provision for his wife and young family (in 1975 Tristram was fifteen years old and Henrietta was fourteen, and they were both at boarding-schools). A company was bought 'off the shelf' for a nominal sum in 1976 and re-named Charnley Surgical Inventions Limited (CSI), which is correctly described as 'a property-holding company relating to patents which it licences to manufacturers'. In this case, the manufacturers were mainly Thackrays who paid royalties on instruments and prostheses specific to Charnley's design; there were, of course, no royalties on the original prosthesis which had never been patented, and Thackrays stopped paying the £1 per prosthesis to the Wrightington research fund in 1975. Royalties were also received from Howorth Engineering Limited, and other companies including Codman and Shurtleff Inc (USA) who were agents in the United States.

The initial capital of CSI was 100 £1 shares, most of which were held by Charnley himself. He had wanted Frank to become the full-time company secretary, but the work did not justify this. Thackray generously allowed Frank to devote one day a week to the company, and Jill Charnley became its first secretary. Frank's principal function was to ensure that the best possible agreements were made, and maintained, with Thackrays and other companies. The new flanged femoral prosthesis and the long posterior wall socket had been patented in the United Kingdom in 1974, and the pressure injection socket in 1976. In the same year, exclusivity for the Charnley design of the femoral prosthesis was given to Thackrays. Patents were also subsequently taken out in Australia, Canada, France, Germany, Ireland, Japan, South Africa, Sweden, Switzerland and the United States. Royalties on the various devices grew to be substantial. The office of the company is now in Winckley Square, Preston, and Miss Margaret Green (who was Charnley's secretary) is the secretary.

CSI did not really become an important part of Charnley's life and often he appeared to be bored at the company meetings. Frank believes that he never really appreciated how beneficial the company became to him and, more particularly, his family. Apart from their regular discussions, Charnley and Frank also travelled together to orthopaedic meetings, particularly to the United States and Japan. Charnley was somewhat sensitive and felt that they should not be seen together too much as he would be thought by his orthopaedic colleagues as being 'too commercial'. Frank resented this attitude on one trip, but the episode was quickly forgotten (as was often the case with Charnley) and they remained the best of friends.

Charnley's first aim when he retired from the National Health Service was to write his book on low friction arthroplasty and indeed this was probably the prime reason why he wanted to reduce his clinical work at Wrightington. He became totally absorbed in producing what he referred to as his 'magnum opus'. This was a complete account of the operation, its rationale and technique. The book, titled *Low Friction Arthroplasty of the Hip. Theory and Practice* was superbly illustrated with 440 figures (205 in colour), and published by Springer-Verlag in 1979.[3] He chose this publisher because he recognised that they would achieve the very high standard which he wanted. His step-by-step illustration of the operative technique has not been equalled and in acknowledgement he wrote:

> Dr Heinz Götze [Springer's managing partner and managing director] has taken the responsible step (for a publishing house so dedicated to perfection as Springer-Verlag) of permitting my own drawings to be used to illustrate the steps of the operation, (professionally 'touched up' where necessary) in order not to lose those surgeon's details which professional artists can miss.

As in his earlier books (Chapter 6) Charnley succinctly puts forwards his basic philosophy in the introduction:

> The challenge comes when patients between 45 and 50 years of age are to be considered for the operation, because then every advance must be used if there is to be a reasonable chance of 20 and more years of trouble-free activity. It is not in a young patient's interest to count on a successful 'revision' . . . The best time to use acrylic cement is the first time; this is when the gritty surface of cancellous bone can best accept cement.
>
> Strictly speaking the operation described in this book should not be regarded as a surgical operation at all. It should be seen as an exercise in practical mechanical engineering . . .
>
> Surgeons who are diffident about embarking on new and apparently complicated procedures can take heart in the knowledge that mechanical aptitude is a cerebral process. Aptitude which resides in the fingers is a dangerous talent, though some hours of instruction at a fitter's bench can work wonders in boosting any postgraduate's self-confidence.

The book begins with a description of the low friction principle and its evolution, but then departs from the expected pattern. The second and third chapters deal with the organisation of the follow up and the numerical grading of the results. After a very important review of the bone–cement interface, the long-term clinical results follow. Subsequent chapters discuss the design of the socket and the femoral prosthesis and practical aspects of their use. The superb description of operative technique is reached in Chapter 15 and runs to 100 pages; with three paragraphs of text on the left hand page and corresponding diagrams on the right. The last two chapters (21 and 22) concern biomechanics and the selection of patients. This somewhat idiosyncratic approach gives the book a welcome originality which is typical of Charnley and makes it an authoritative and unique personal record of his work. The book is still in print with four thousand copies sold in the decade after its publication.

Writing his book had been a commitment which Charnley had put before almost everything else; so after he had delivered it to the publishers he was able to accept some of the many invitations he had received to lecture in other countries. There is no detailed record of his travels except for the year 1980. He had resolved to keep a journal that year, but when he began again on January 5, 1981, he admitted that 'I must have left it in a hotel in Minneapolis'. But he

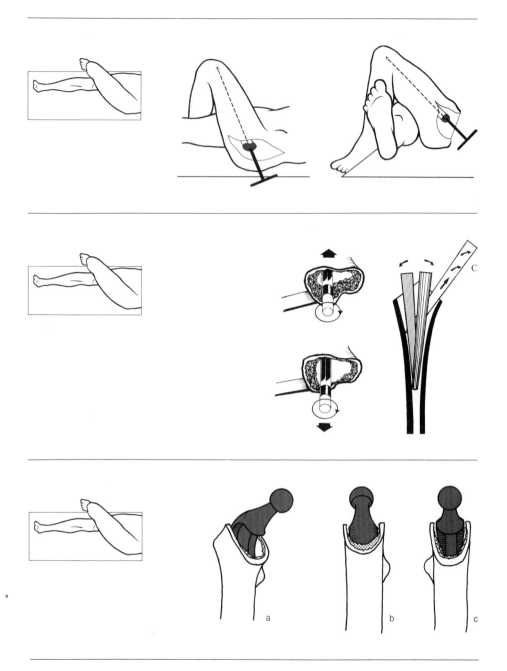

*A page of operative drawings from Low Friction Arthroplasty of the Hip*

went on to list where he had been in the previous year (although he did not always give the purpose of each visit):

| | | |
|---|---|---|
| 11–19.1.80 | Honolulu | Western Orthopaedic Association |
| 5–10.2.80 | Atlanta | American Academy of Orthopaedic Surgeons |
| 18.2–14.3.80 | Australia and New Zealand | |
| 15–16.3.80 | Florence | |
| 23–28.3.80 | Bern | International Hip Society |
| 1–3.10.80 | Amsterdam | British Orthopaedic Association |
| 23–25.10.80 | Minneapolis | |
| 11–19.11.80 | New York | Hospital for Special Surgery Jubilee meeting. American Academy Hip Course |
| 21–24.11.80 | Montevideo | Annual Orthopaedic meeting |
| 24.11–4.12.80 | Buenos Aires | |
| 6–9.12.80 | Nice and Lyon | |

More often than not, Jill Charnley went with him on these trips. He concluded this page of his journal with the remarks:

> All this time getting Thursday, Friday and Saturday at Midhurst whenever I could. Altogether a very stimulating year and 1981 looks as though it might be the same.

The only engagements in this country which he had noted were at the University of Hull where he received an honorary doctorate of science in July, and at the hip course at Oswestry 'which I enjoyed'. He refused many invitations to address local medical societies, which is not surprising in view of his overseas travels, but an abrupt refusal occasionally upset the organisers. However, he gave an interesting explanation to a friend and colleague:

> I get more averse to social contacts as I get older, and I loathe after-dinner speeches, finding myself totally devoid of humour, and being haunted by the thought of the forthcoming event to the detriment of my concentration on present work. It is quite otherwise with groups of postgraduates who are knowledgeable in total hip replacement and interested in technical minutiae. Americans are much easier to talk to after dinner than the British!
> (1981)

Concentration on his work was intense, and behind it was the feeling that he had not sufficient time left to complete the contribution which he believed he was capable of making, and which indeed he believed he was destined to make.

Although in 1981 he was in his seventieth year, he could scarcely be said to have retired, or even be semi-retired. Although much of his lecturing must have been repetitive (to him, at least), he continued to be inventive, and it was in 1980 that he had telephoned from Australia to his workshop technician describing his idea for the new Ogee socket. He also produced his adjustable test prosthesis at about this time. He regarded it as 'a lovely job, but it will be pricey and one does not know how it will catch on'. He wrote:

> It is curious how my ideas often clarify themselves when I leave my unit for a few days and have enforced idleness in hotel bedrooms or in aeroplanes.
> (1981)

This was an entry in his new journal; but his good intentions were short-lived because the last entry is in March, 1981. None the less, during these three months he revealed personal opinions on history and politics, as well as on orthopaedics. He had become a voracious reader of fiction in his few moments of relaxation, mainly thrillers which Jill Charnley used to collect for him in batches of half a dozen from the public library in Knutsford. But he also found time for more serious reading:

> This brings me to my reading again (several times over the last two years) of standard text books of English history: Trevelyan's 'History of England' and H.A.L. Fisher's 'History of Europe'. I am now, for the first time in my life, beginning to understand . . . the Stuart period from James I to William and Mary. The theory of Parliament and the nature of the American colonies is . . . clearer to me . . . I think that perhaps this Island of Britain might indeed have had some divine spark, not vouchsafed to other European countries, who are much harder working than us. (1.2.81)

His political views, patriotic and right-wing, were expressed in an intense admiration for the Prime Minister, Mrs Margaret Thatcher:

> I think she has more *guts* and more true realism and purity than any politician I have ever known in the flesh.

He wrote to her on at least two occasions: once to congratulate her on the way she was dealing with strikers in the car industry, and once to advise her to 'get rid of' a minister whom he did not like. Charnley had been invited to one of her luncheon parties at 10 Downing Street, and on another occasion she presented him with the Harding Award at the Action Research's annual meeting in November 1981. Sir Harry Platt wrote afterwards: 'Mrs Thatcher completely ignored her typescript and obviously sensed that here was a very great man'. Charnley had also attended a luncheon given by HM the Queen at Buckingham Palace. Conversation naturally turned to hip replacement and Charnley was much impressed by how quickly HRH Prince Philip grasped the principle of the way cement worked in the body – that it acted as a grout and not as glue.

When he began his short-lived journal, Charnley indicated that he intended to write 'for posterity', and he said what he thought in no uncertain terms, especially with regard to his fellow countrymen:

> Anyone who has travelled as much as Jill and myself recognises the crass ignorance and stupidity of the people of Britain . . . It used to be impossible to imagine 'peasants' in Britain . . . But [now] we have 'peasants' earning £8000 a year, well-dressed, driving cars, and going for package deal holidays to Costa Brava and Miami. The average American makes a Brit look a country bumpkin or a lout . . . The tragedy for Margaret Thatcher and Geoffrey Howe is the poor quality of the British workforce [which] I think could be traced to thirty years of emigration from the UK, under the effects of socialism and the Welfare State, of those working men who would have provided a powerful catalyst for good in our factories . . . Their loss has left an unleavened lump of stupidity behind . . . (10.3.81)

His adulation for Mrs Thatcher received a severe blow when Britain went to war with Argentina over the Falkland Islands in 1982. His patriotism did not stretch

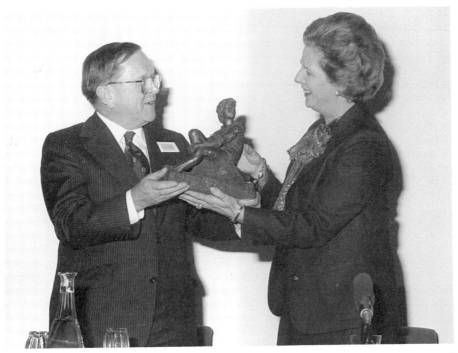

*Charnley receiving the Harding award from Mrs Thatcher. (By courtesy of Action Research for the Crippled Child)*

to being able to accept what he regarded as a totally unnecessary military operation, and he was deeply affected by the loss of life which occurred.

It would not be right to give the impression that much of his brief journal was taken up with the expression of his political opinions. He devoted far more space, and this should be no surprise, to orthopaedic matters. One technical point in the operation had become an overwhelming concern to him. This occupied so much of his thoughts that it needs to be considered in some detail because of the light it throws on his character. Some explanation is needed of the background to Charnley's problem.

When he returned to Manchester after the war, he had been taught an operative approach to the hip joint by Harry Platt. The greater trochanter (with its muscles) was detached and reflected upwards to improve the exposure. He then used it for the central dislocation technique of arthrodesis which he had devised in the 1950s (Chapter 6). Replacing and fixing the trochanter in position at the end of the operation was no problem; the hip was stiff afterwards, and therefore there was no tendency for the muscles attached to the trochanter to pull it out of place. Although Charnley gave up this operation after he had devised his low friction arthroplasty, he continued to employ what had become a familiar approach to the hip.

Certainly, detachment of the greater trochanter gave a very wide exposure and, having adopted the method for this reason, Charnley sought to use it to 're-

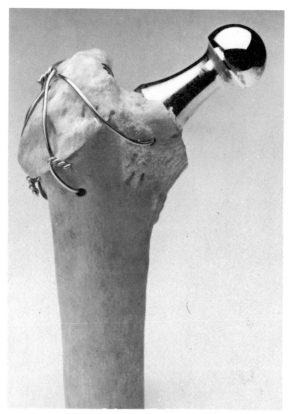

*Photograph of a model showing the cruciate wiring method of re-attaching the greater trochanter.*
(LFA)

structure' the hip. He displaced the detached bony fragment downwards and outwards, fixing it in a more distal position on the shaft of the femur, so that the power of the gluteal muscles would be enhanced. This now brought its own problems because the bony fragment did not always unite to the femur, and sometimes became separated from it. This did not matter after arthrodesis; and it seemed to matter remarkably little after arthroplasty, but it could cause symptoms and the postoperative radiographs were aesthetically displeasing to him. Even when he gave up transposing the bony fragment, and returned it to its original site; bony union did not always occur and detachment remained a problem.

Rather than use another approach, his next move was to devise the surest way of soundly re-attaching the trochanter. Various ingenious techniques of fixation were tried, but none achieved the perfection (100% bony union no less) that he demanded.

Many surgeons found the re-attachment of the trochanter a tedious manoeuvre at the end of the operation, and it was not long before some began to insert hip prostheses without detaching the trochanter. The orthopaedic world now divided

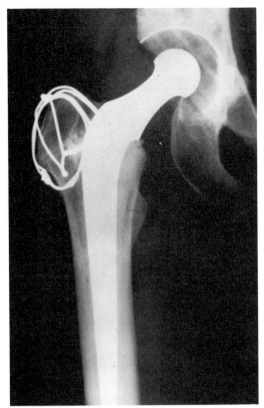

*Radiograph showing cruciate wiring.* (LFA)

into two camps on the issue: those who detached the trochanter and those who did not. Arguments and counter-arguments were discussed to the point of tedium.

Charnley believed that the very wide exposure was essential in order to be able to carry out the operation properly. He was determined to eliminate totally the risk of postoperative detachment and to produce radiographs which were technically perfect. He wrote in 1979 that he had delayed publication of the operative technique for ten years until he had solved the problem of re-attaching the trochanter, which he considered he had done (or almost done) at that time.

Many surgeons had by now given up detaching the greater trochanter in straightforward cases, and in 1977 Charnley acknowledged at a meeting of the British Orthopaedic Association in Liverpool that the operation could be done satisfactorily without taking this step. Nevertheless, he maintained that all surgeons in training should learn his method which would always be needed for 'difficult' hips and for revision operations, which was perfectly true. But he never gave up his search for the perfect method of re-attachment. When one of the surgeons at Wrightington published the description of a direct lateral approach to the hip (without detaching the trochanter),[5] he regarded this as a personal affront – 'the very end of all my teaching'.

The matter needs to be seen in perspective: in 1978, failure of radiological union of the trochanteric fragment at Wrightington was reported at 5%.[2] One of the men trained by Charnley reviewed his own experience in 500 operations and found that bony union occurred in 97.2%.[1] In those failing to reunite, there was 'surprisingly little ill-effect or loss of function'. This was published in 1986 and the method of wiring was one which Charnley would have regarded as 'old-fashioned'. The problem might not appear to be too serious as only a few patients had discomfort over the trochanter. Many of Charnley's followers were prepared to accept this situation in order to have the benefits of the really excellent exposure. In 1979, Charnley considered that his personal failure rate was negligible, certainly under 1%. But this was still not good enough and he especially wanted to teach a method which would be as good in every surgeon's hands, as it was in his own. He wrote in his journal when referring to his plans for travel:

> The idea is to put over re-attachment [of the trochanter] as I believe that this is the central feature of all hip replacement and I shall continuously be referring to it. At the moment not one surgeon in ten has any concept of how very important this subject is going to be.(6.1.81)

And in another entry:

> Still the greater trochanter! I have long desired to apply powerful spring-loaded compression and during the last year have been working on this more or less continuously in the workshop.
> The acid-test was [and he gave the name of a patient] . . .(24.1.81)

He then related the trials and tribulations which he had at Midhurst with this patient and his displaced trochanter. The second operation was difficult, but he managed to insert his new device:

> I wondered whether, being in my seventieth year . . . I might be older than I felt and possibly becoming incompetent. However I stuck at it, despite my waves of horror and panic, and did achieve a very powerful fixation. No other method could possibly have succeeded . . .
> So that is the situation. I feel sure that the mechanics are sound, and I feel that the biological stimulus to rapid union is present. But am I right? It is truly an agonising thought to have to wait for proof. And if I am wrong and some totally unexpected source of failure occurs – what shall I do then?
> I think my extreme anxiety here is partly because I become more anxious and less keen to take risks as I get older. On the other hand to anticipate and suffer the agonies of every conceivable source of failure is the only way to anticipate and prevent failure.

It may seem unnecessary to reveal Charnley's innermost anxieties, but many surgeons will recognise these sorts of feeling which often trouble them as they grow older. Caution is better than the alternative, and the over-confidence which can come with increasing experience and age can be alarming. Charnley was always a highly skilled operator with vast experience and he might well have become afflicted with a sense of superiority which would have allowed him to ignore surgical difficulties, but happily this was not the case.

To return to his patient at Midhurst:

> A specially inventive day – despite still being haunted by the patient whom
> I shall see in two days from now and whose X-rays I intend to have taken
> tomorrow and put on my bed [at Midhurst] for my arrival at 11 pm.
> (3.2.81)

And a few days later:

> Well the worst has happened and the compression device has failed
> . . .(9.2.81)

He always learnt from his failures and he goes on to analyse in detail exactly
what went wrong and how it could be overcome:

> Always optimistic in this type of research I tell myself that it is a good job
> that this did not work (!) or it could have concealed a defective design till
> another time. I have a better design already finished in the workshop
> together with instrumentation for its insertion.
>
> The fiasco of this my most private hope has been offset by a very
> unexpected improvement in the 'standard' cruciate wiring system on which
> I have expended so much thought . . . The detail is extremely simple and
> almost eliminates the need for 'spikes' to fix the trochanter . . . Strange I
> have not thought of this before . . . [it] may make it unnecessary to press
> on with the staple-clamp which very few surgeons like.
>
> Jill and I talked together last night on my return from Midhurst on the
> question of whether I might not be becoming obsessive about the trochanter!
> I mean insane and unnecessarily obsessive. I don't think so. I still believe
> it is the most important part of hip replacement and that it must be my
> mission to make it realised by all to be so. (9.2.81)

There are surgeons who feel that during the last years of his life Charnley wasted
his talent on this small facet of his operation. This view is counter-balanced by
entries in his journal on the following days. These show that he was dealing with
other matters as well as the trochanter:

> 10th Feb. Had a good day in the lab today.
>
> Finalised PMMA [acrylic cement] model to line socket of standard half
> pelvis to convert the normal acetabulum into an osteoarthritic acetabulum
> . . . [This was to be used for 'hands-on' teaching of the technique of the
> operation].
>
> Appears possible that the dilatometer to measure acrylic cement volumetric
> changes during setting may be within an inch or two of being perfected.
> This has occupied me for over six months and my patience has quite
> surprised myself . . .
>
> Have been feeling very well these last two days . . .
>
> I have just remembered that I started the day by X-raying and dissecting
> the . . . hip specimen from Mansfield [this is recorded in Chapter 11].
>
> 12th Feb. Interesting day today – all day in the workshop. Broke up
> volumetric PMMA apparatus and by the end of the day had 75% of new
> design 'on test'. It still amazes me how the failure of something I have

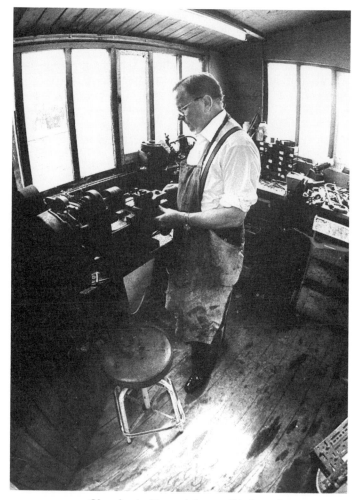

*Charnley in his workshop at Birchwood.*

worked on intensely for a year or so leaves me thrilled when the phoenix rises out of the ashes.

The designing and making of these things is one thing – using them is now something I must have the residents do – though I must continue to make observations and make up my own mind about the sensitivity and reliability of the experimental method. Too many immature young men cannot distinguish between the common-sense behaviour (of an experimental result) and something which is the purely fictitious result of some mechanical error. It must be the instinct for spotting mechanical errors which puts the true experimentalist streets ahead of the transient who tries his hand purely to produce a 'paper' for his own glorification – true or false being not specially important.

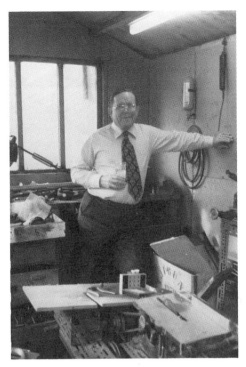

*Charnley relaxing with a gin and tonic. (From Mr M.A.R. Freeman.)*

Charnley's travels in the first six months of 1981 show his prediction that the year was going to be as busy as 1980 to be correct. He spent two days (January 29 and 30) in Münster where he did a practical teaching session with special emphasis on re-attachment of the trochanter. The next entry in his journal is for February 22, 1981:

We are off this morning for two weeks in the USA and Canada . . .

But he had noted just before he left:

I find forced absences from work very productive though I hate the thought of going away.

They first went to Burlington University, Vermont and then the meeting of the American Academy of Orthopaedic Surgeons in Las Vegas. Writing in his journal later, Charnley said:

. . . it is now quite clear that the double-cup is failing and that the Müller 32 mm head is also not doing well in the long term results. This I am sure now marks the watershed. I do not intend to adopt the 'I told you so' attitude. I think it is now a matter of coasting home, with judicious lectures and demonstrations from now on. (10.3.81)

Next he gave the Bruce lecture at the Wellesley Hospital, Toronto, to an audience of 550. Finally, on this trip the Charnleys visited Thunder Bay to stay with his old pupil and friend, Dr Henry Hamilton.

A symposium was held at St Thomas' Hospital, London in March 1981, when three exponents of the operation of the double-cup resurfacing arthroplasty were going to speak. It will be remembered that Charnley had used this technique in his very earliest experiments with PTFE (Teflon). Now, even when better materials were available, he believed that the method would fail because of the high torque created by the large femoral head. He was invited informally to take part in the discussion and he decided to show a cine-film of his comparator experiment. This was his version of what happened:

> Thus we started with the 32 mm Müller ball and got a pleasant mild gasp of surprise when the 22 mm control went on swinging twice as long as the Müller. When we ended on the 41 mm diameter metal against polyethylene [HMWP] (which was only just approaching the rather larger head used in the resurfacing femoral component) the film ended dramatically with a real gasp. Michael Freeman [an orthopaedic surgeon at the London Hospital and one of the principal speakers], who is impelled by a deeply sensitive scientific spirit said outright that this demonstration was "incontrovertible".

Unfortunately, he gave up writing his journal and his last entry notes a visit to Barcelona later in March which was one of the rare occasions when he operated away from home. There is other correspondence which shows that his travels over the next two months included three trips to the United States. He was at Emory University, Atlanta, Georgia, for three days at the beginning of April. A month later he was away for about ten days: first to Washington, Williamsburg and Charlottesville (his wife and daughter were with him), and then to Chicago where he was Visiting Professor at the University of Illinois. At the end of May, he was at the meeting of the American Orthopaedic Association in Boston.

And so his extraordinarily active life continued almost until the day he died.

As early as 1963, Sir Harry Platt had persuaded Charnley to submit his published work for the degree of Doctor of Science in the University of Manchester. Although Charnley had published a great deal by then, he had possibly not written as many papers as would be expected from an academic scientist. But the University recognised the importance of his contribution to knowledge and he was awarded the degree in 1964.

On 5 August 1966, Charnley wrote to Sir Harry:

> I have taken seriously your suggestion that I should seek election as FRS [Fellow of the Royal Society]. Since the suggestion that I should put in for the DSc was your idea, and it was successful, I have decided to think about the Royal Society.

He goes on to ask advice about the six Fellows who were needed to sign the proposal, 'of whom three at least should certify their recommendation by personal knowledge'. The Royal Society – its full name is The Royal Society of London for Improving Natural Knowledge – is the oldest scientific society in Great Britain, and its royal charter was granted in 1660. It was not until 1848 that the control of the society's affairs passed wholly into the hands of scientists, and election to the Fellowship became a recognition of high achievement. The number of Fellows is in the order of 500, each of whom is elected by the council of the Society. There are two main types of candidate: those who are selected either 'primarily for their contributions to scientific knowledge'; or 'on the basis of their major contributions being not so much to providing new scientific knowledge or understanding as to the application of existing scientific or technical knowledge in an innovative way'. Charnley was judged to fulfil one or other of these criteria and was elected FRS in 1975. This honour had never before been awarded to a practising orthopaedic surgeon.

A list of Charnley's numerous honours and awards is appended at the end of the book; they cannot be discussed in detail, but the number of honorary degrees from various universities is particularly impressive. Two awards, and his public honours, deserve special mention.

The Lister Medal was awarded to Charnley in 1975 for 'his original and distinguished contribution to the development of total joint replacement'. This prestigious award is made every three years by a committee comprising representatives of the Royal Society, the Royal Colleges of Surgeons of England and Ireland, and the Universities of Edinburgh and Glasgow. The citation summarised his achievement:

> In a period of some fifteen years totally concentrated on this difficult problem, by a combination of engineering, biological science, and superb technique, he has resolved these problems to the immense benefit of tens of thousands of patients. His investigation of the mechanical, material, and surgical problems of total replacement have helped to advance joint replacement in the knee, elbow and elsewhere.

This medal was given 'subject to the acceptance of the condition of delivering an address in London under the auspices of the Royal College of Surgeons of England'. Charnley duly gave the oration on 'Aspects of total asepsis in the operating room with special reference to clean air systems'. This was particularly appropriate in view of Lord Lister's contribution to surgery, but unfortunately the address was not published.

In 1981 the British Orthopaedic Association made Charnley an honorary Fellow which is the Association's highest distinction. Although it is only given rarely to British orthopaedic surgeons (most of the honorary Fellows today are from overseas), many wondered why the award to Charnley was so long delayed. Perhaps once more it was simply a case of 'a prophet is not without honour . . .'. Charnley had, of course, opted out of the Association's affairs when he was being considered for the vice-presidency in 1971 (Chapter 8); and, although he went regularly to the scientific meetings, he never became involved with any committee work. Furthermore, he had never sought favour from the orthopaedic establishment in London. It may not, however, be coincidental that in 1981 the president of the Association was Mr A.H.C. Ratliff who had worked with Charnley as a registrar at the Manchester Royal Infirmary just after the war (Chapter 4). It was a very great pleasure for him to make the award at a meeting in the Connaught Rooms, London. In introducing Charnley to the audience, he spoke of other surgeons, such as Percival Pott, John Hunter, Astley Cooper, Benjamin Brodie, James Paget and Joseph Lister, who had become Fellows of the Royal Society in the eighteenth and nineteenth centuries. He concluded that they, and John Charnley, were all characterised by four attributes: remarkable dedication; outstanding originality; their relative youth when they became successful, and their international reputation. Ratliff remembers that Charnley was extremely nervous and was 'thoroughly embarrassed by the whole business'. At this time of his life he had, as we have seen, come to dislike public speaking and sought to avoid it whenever possible. Talking about low friction arthroplasty was a different matter; he continued to lecture superbly well, his enthusiasm for his subject never flagging.

He had been appointed a Companion of the Most Excellent Order of the British Empire in 1970 and his highest public honour came in 1977 when he was made Knight Bachelor, receiving the accolade from Her Majesty the Queen Mother. On his retirement from the National Health Service in 1975 he had been made professor emeritus by the University of Manchester, and so he became Professor Sir John Charnley.

Charnley went to the meeting of the American Academy of Orthopaedic Surgeons in New Orleans in January 1982. He was, in his own words, 'committed to making a personal appearance each year for the Cintor Company'. The Academy has a very large exhibition for manufacturers of orthopaedic equipment and it is customary for surgeons to give talks or demonstrations on behalf of companies who are selling instruments, for example, which they have designed. As well as this, Charnley gave a major lecture to an open scientific meeting of the Hip Society with the title 'The future of total hip replacement'.[4]

Meetings of the American Academy were important to Charnley, and on one occasion he went unannounced to a session on hip problems. He was recognised by the chairman and introduced to the audience of several thousand surgeons. This was followed by a standing ovation which lasted five minutes; a remarkable spontaneous tribute and he was deeply touched by it.

A letter written in May 1982 summarises his views on the current status of hip replacement:

> Unfortunately for the patient . . . a primary operation for total hip replacement is deceptively easy to perform: even in the hands of beginners success of 80% can be expected when judged at one year . . . Compared with previous forms of hip surgery . . . this is a very high success rate indeed . . . the successful results, in popular assessment by the public, totally swamp the failures . . .
>
> The sad thing is that in the hands of surgeons who have dedicated their lives to this type of work, the success rate after a primary operation is certainly as high as 98 to 99% [presumably at one year].
>
> How difficult it is to guarantee a successful result after a secondary operation to repair the failure of a first operation . . .
>
> . . . I believe the time is now ripe, world-wide, for the public to be protected from those relatively inexperienced operators who, having produced a failure after a primary operation, are prepared to attempt a secondary operation . . . To recommend the public to have secondary, salvage, operations in a special centre would be a humanitarian measure of the first magnitude. . .

Charnley had developed a somewhat protective attitude towards his operation, and it is clear that he was determined to do his best to ensure that other surgeons should maintain the high standards which he set. He also affirmed his belief that difficult revision operations should only be carried out in special centres where the surgeons had both the experience and the facilities needed to give the patient the best chance of a successful result.

Sir Harry Platt was to be interviewed in a television programme recorded in April 1982, by the local BBC North-West network, called Home Ground, and Charnley was invited to take part. Sir Harry, who was in his ninety-seventh year, reminisced about his life-time in orthopaedics, and concluded by emphasising the great contribution which Charnley had made to surgery. He stressed that Charnley was a surgeon-biologist, rather than a surgeon-engineer, and that his work on the prevention of wound infection would place him alongside Lord Lister in the surgical hall of fame.

In the recording of the television programme, Charnley looked drawn and he appeared subdued. Colleagues at Wrightington remember that about this time he remarked 'the corridors [in the hospital] seemed to be getting longer', and occasionally he had asked a porter to carry his bag. Jill Charnley also became aware that he was getting breathless rather easily and was having difficulty in keeping up with her – she was a very fast walker. In spite of this, he worked hard in his laboratory at Birchwood making histological preparations from the autopsy specimens he had collected. He had certainly used up a great deal of energy getting the project under way and he believed that time was running out.

This was the year of their twenty-fifth wedding anniversary and for a special celebration Jill Charnley suggested that they might take the Orient Express to Venice in June and spend a few days there. He said he did not feel up to it and that he would find walking round the galleries too exhausting. This rather surprised her, but she was less surprised when he countered with the idea that they might spend 'a few days in the New Forest'. He had never been enthusiastic about foreign holidays and even two or three days in the south of England meant time from his work which he resented. They did manage to get away in the middle of June and travelled to the New Forest from Midhurst. Charnley benefited from the rest, and one of his moments of great pleasure was when the Falklands War ended on the very day of their anniversary. He celebrated the occasion by taking a photograph of his wife holding up a newspaper with its banner headlines.

A few days after his last operation at Midhurst on July 23 (Chapter 15), Jill Charnley found him sitting in their garden room at Birchwood in a state of complete exhaustion. He admitted that he had been fibrillating, saying 'I've had it for a bit'; presumably he had been suffering from paroxysmal atrial fibrillation for a few months. He agreed to see a medical colleague in Manchester and when he returned he was casual: 'there's no need to bother at all – I've just got to take it easy for a bit'.

His son, Tristram, had come home from London on his motor-cycle for the weekend; his efforts to repair it met with a typical response from his father – 'the boy is a fool, he'll never get it together again'. Charnley was more tetchy and irritable than usual that weekend.

On Monday morning, he woke very early with severe pain in his chest and was obviously ill. Jill Charnley telephoned immediately for an ambulance and he was taken straightway to the coronary care unit in Wythenshawe Hospital, Manchester. Tristram had planned to return to London that morning, but he was still at home when the crisis occurred, and he went to fetch Charnley's sister, Mary, and his daughter, Henrietta. Charnley seemed to improve a little initially;

his spirits were not low and to cheer up his wife he told her: 'I'll be better when I've had a gin and tonic'. That night he had a second massive myocardial infarct and became unconscious. He was put on a ventilator, but he remained in a coma and died on Thursday, August 5, 1982, four days after his admission to hospital.

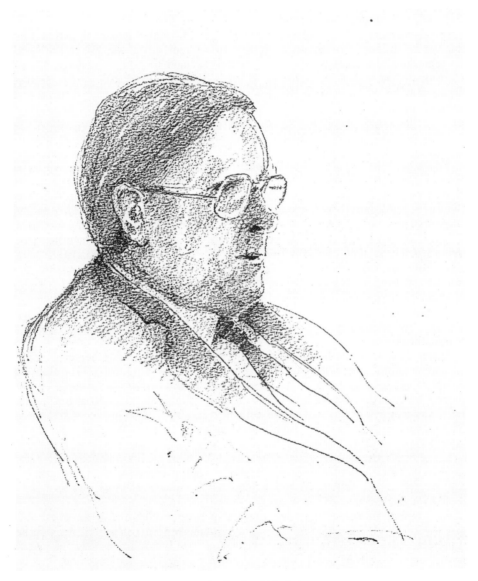

*Tristram's sketch of his father.*

# Chapter 17

# IN MEMORIAM

*If Sir Robert Jones is considered the father of modern orthopaedic surgery, then Sir John Charnley is the heir apparent – who even surpassed the father as Plato did Socrates.*

Dr F.E. Stinchfield,[4] New York, 1982

OBITUARIES were published in *The Times, British Medical Journal, The Lancet* and many orthopaedic journals, but the greatest personal tributes were paid at a thanksgiving service held in Manchester Cathedral on September 15, 1982. This was attended by a congregation of hundreds of Charnley's friends and orthopaedic colleagues. His old teacher, Sir Harry Platt, concluded his address with the words:

> And now, our own John Charnley has become part of surgical history, and has taken his place in the gallery of the great master surgeons who have gone before . . . The Charnley prosthesis is in essence a biological design by a man who was also an artist. It is something which a Leonardo da Vinci might have envisaged. But today we are thinking about the man, the human person we knew and held in affection. He had so much to give to the world of surgery, both in fundamental knowledge and to the relief of human suffering . . .[3]

The congregation was also addressed by Dr Mark Lazansky of New York and Henrietta, Charnley's daughter. Professor Maurice Müller of Bern read the lesson.

The service had been planned to coincide with a meeting of the British Orthopaedic Association which was taking place in Manchester on September 15, 16 and 17. Lady Charnley felt that this would make it easier for many of Charnley's friends to attend which was indeed the case, and the arrangement was much appreciated. On the following day, a visit to Wrightington was on the programme at which Professor Sir John Charnley was to have presented 'patients with acrylic cement that had been in situ for up to twenty-two years with excellent results'. It was Lady Charnley's express wish that this should not be cancelled.

Mr B.M. Wroblewski presented the cases; the demonstration was an outstanding success and an appropriate tribute to Sir John's life and work.

Before this, Lady Charnley had decided that one posthumous engagement, a trip to Japan to demonstrate the new technique of trochanteric wiring, should be undertaken by Tristram. He was not a doctor, but he had helped his father with various aspects of medical illustration. Together they had made an excellent 16 mm cine-film of the low friction arthroplasty at Midhurst. Tristram had learnt the latest wiring technique and was able to carry it out on model bones, exactly as devised by Charnley. He went to Japan within three weeks of his father's death and successfully fulfilled this commitment. Wroblewski and Dr Z. Cupic from Houston, Texas, who were pupils and old friends, were also there, and provided encouragement and support. Tristram subsequently became professionally involved in making videos for medical teaching and set up his own business.

Henrietta had trained at the Royal Academy of Dramatic Art in London, and had embarked on acting as a career. Brother and sister came to realise that their father was an exceptional man who had dedicated his life to perfecting an operation and that he had put this aim above everything else. Like many families, they had had difficulties and disagreements in their adolescent years, but as they came to understand what had been going on while they were children, they again grew closer to their father.

Lady Charnley was determined to ensure that the research, which Charnley already had begun on his collection of hip prostheses, should be completed (Chapter 11). She consulted Charnley's friends and colleagues and decided to form a charitable trust in his name. An appeal was launched, firstly to his former patients, and sponsorship was obtained from companies with whom he had worked on various aspects of total hip replacement. The initial sponsors were: Chas. F. Thackray Limited; Charnley Surgical Inventions Limited; Churchill Livingstone; Johnson and Johnson Inc; Kirby-Warrick Pharmaceuticals Limited; Springer-Verlag Gmbh, and the Royal Bank of Scotland.

The John Charnley Trust was set up in 1984 with Sir Reginald Murley as president, and a board of trustees, which included Lady Charnley, with Charnley's old friend, Mr Ronald Frank as chairman. The objectives of the Trust are:

1. Research into the field of human joint replacement and in particular that of Low Friction Arthroplasty of the Hip
2. The creation of Research Fellowships to enable young orthopaedic surgeons to visit centres of excellence in orthopaedic surgery
3. The sponsorship of lectures, seminars and conferences to further the technique of Low Friction Arthroplasty organised by orthopaedic surgeons trained by Sir John Charnley

The John Charnley Fellowship has been awarded each year and smaller grants have been given to a number of young orthopaedic surgeons to enable them to travel or to assist the funding of research projects. The annual John Charnley lecture is given under the auspices of the Universities of Manchester and Liverpool.

The Trust is now soundly established and will be able to continue its benefactions for many years to come. The success of the venture is largely due to Lady Charnley's enthusiasm and energy in fund-raising and promotion. She has travelled to orthopaedic meetings all over the world to talk to surgeons about the Trust and its work. The contribution, which she made to her husband's career during his life, and her subsequent efforts to ensure that his work would continue, cannot be overstated.

Certain fiscal difficulties arose in dealing with contributions from surgeons, and also patients in the United States whom Charnley had operated on in England. The solution was to set up a separate Trust, with the same aims, which has been very effectively administered by the Orthopaedic Research and Development Foundation in Chicago. Substantial donations have been received and the first Fellow in the United States has been appointed.

At Wrightington, the hospital created a memorial garden which was dedicated to Sir John Charnley by the Bishop of Lancaster on August 16, 1983. The Wrightington Hospital Education Centre Appeal has been set up with a committee of which Mr K. Hardinge is chairman.

There is no doubt that Charnley had been very highly regarded in the United States, ever since he had made such a favourable impression at his first visit in 1948. Most of his later papers were published in an American journal, *Clinical Orthopaedics and Related Research*, and in October 1986 that journal produced a symposium on low friction arthroplasty with the intention of paying tribute to his work.[2] Dr Nas Eftekhar, who worked closely with Charnley in 1967 and 1968 and who had followed his methods when he returned to New York, was the guest editor. He brought together 23 papers which, with one exception, were written by members of the Low Friction Society. Charnley's first paper on *A clean air operating enclosure*, originally published in the *British Journal of Surgery* in 1964, was selected as 'The Classic' and reprinted in full. Personal tributes to Charnley were paid by Eftekhar and Older. Next, Wroblewski reported the 15- to 21-year results of Charnley's cases which had been operated on at Wrightington. Experiences of the Charnley operation were reported from the United Kingdom, the United States, Canada, Republic of Ireland, South Africa, Japan and Korea. In all, the symposium covered many aspects of the operation and presented a truly international appraisal of the results. The penultimate paragraph of Eftekhar's editorial summarises the aim of the volume:

> John Charnley's life has marked an epoch in orthopaedic surgery. His name will remain with posterity for low friction arthroplasty of the hip, the surgical revolution that brought relief to countless patients crippled by arthritis. This volume of Clinical Orthopaedics is an appropriate and well deserved tribute.

Today we stand too close to Charnley to be able to evaluate his contribution in the total context of medical history. He did not invent the artificial hip joint, but he did develop it in an entirely original way. During this process, he explored and overcame many problems which arose with alarming frequency. Solving any one of these problems would, for any ordinary person, have proved to have been a life-time's task. Despite an initial failure, he established the low friction principle and the fixation of implants by acrylic cement (a story not yet complete); and proved the importance of a clean operating environment. Furthermore, he profoundly influenced concepts of rational documentation of operative procedures for the purposes of scientific evaluation in the future. Any one of these developments would have been sufficient to ensure lasting recognition, even leaving aside his earlier contributions to the understanding of bone healing and fracture management.

But what sets his work even farther above the ordinary was his total commitment to low friction arthroplasty, and the extraordinary amount of energy he expended on achieving his aims. His pupils, whom he trained at Wrightington, continue to develop his work in centres throughout the world. They know well the stresses to which he subjected himself in his search for perfection.

Furthermore, his concentration on the task of carrying out large numbers of operations and making prospective records allowed the outcome to be fully assessed. As a consequence he established that, if his technique was carefully followed, the operative results were consistent and predictable. Whatever advances occur in the future, and new and better materials may become available, his results provide a bench-mark against which any new operation should be tested.

The present position of hip replacement in the United Kingdom was summarised in an editorial in The *British Medical Journal* in 1986:[1]

> Despite the cemented Charnley hip being one of the first joints to be used in large numbers twenty-five years ago, it still reigns supreme as the gold standard. Not one of the dozens of "newer", "better", and more expensive implants being used by many surgeons in the Health Service can match the figures obtained with the Charnley hip in proper hands. Nor can they ever do so. A controlled trial of several hundreds of implants over at least fifteen years would be required to make valid comparisons . . .

In spite of the difficulties of evaluation, advances continue to be made: methods of improving further the technique of using cement are being introduced; on the other hand, many surgeons are exploring the possibilities of fixing the prosthesis without the use of cement. The low friction principle is, however, generally accepted.

The success of hip replacement has been accepted by the public at large, and the demand for the operation has increased. Rightly or wrongly the procedure is being undertaken in patients who are younger and less disabled than allowed by Charnley's strict criteria. About 35 000 hip replacements are now performed each year in the United Kingdom (perhaps about half of these are of the Charnley design and manufactured by Thackrays). The Department of Health has recognised the need for increasing the number of replacements as a result of popular outcry, often voiced in the media, and special funds have been allocated to enable more operations to be carried out. The increase in primary procedures inevitably leads in the long run to the need for more revisions: it was said in 1986[1] that one in five operations to replace hips at the Nuffield Orthopaedic Centre at Oxford were revisions.

Charnley's work played a very important part in this 'surgical revolution' and it may be asked what manner of man it was who was capable of making such a contribution. His family background provides no clue; his mother and father seemed to be not out of the ordinary, but they produced two gifted children. John Charnley showed early promise of his intellectual ability, but it was his single-minded determination and his belief that he had a contribution to make which put him head and shoulders above his contemporaries. By nature, he was genial and good company, but he could be irascible and demanding, although his sudden outbursts of rage were short-lived, and more often than not were followed by an apology. He never attempted to be all things to all men, but his personal qualities brought him many friends who remained loyal through thick and thin. He, and his devoted family, made sacrifices which allowed him to dedicate so much of his time to his work; sacrifices that would not be accepted by many families today.

The story of the evolution of the low friction arthroplasty has been one of the themes of this book. Charnley began with basic research from which he formed an hypothesis; but his first attempts to carry out an arthroplasty ended in disaster. Determination, with serendipity playing a part, led to his climb out of the slough of despond and to ultimate success, which fulfilled his first hypothesis. Even so he continued the search for surgical perfection until the end of his life. Certainly, the results of his painstaking efforts have deserved the gratitude of the many thousands of people throughout the world whose suffering has been relieved and, as they so often say, whose lives have been 'transformed' by total hip replacement.

# APPENDIX: HONOURS AND AWARDS CONFERRED ON JOHN CHARNLEY

## Honours

1970 Companion of the Order of the British Empire
1974 Freeman of the Borough of Bury
1975 Fellow of the Royal Society
1977 Knight Bachelor
1977 Emeritus Professor of Orthopaedic Surgery, University of Manchester

## Honorary Degrees and Fellowships

1972 Honorary Fellow, American College of Surgeons
1976 Honorary MD, University of Liverpool
1977 Honorary MD, University of Uppsala, Sweden
1978 Honorary DSc, University of Leeds
1978 Honorary MD, Queen's University, Belfast
1978 Honorary Fellow, American Academy of Orthopaedic Surgery
1980 Honorary DSc, University of Hull
1981 Honorary Fellow, British Orthopaedic Association

## Medals, Prizes and Special Lectures

1969 Olaf Af Acrel Medal of the Swedish Surgical Society
1971 Prix Mondial Nessim Habif of the University of Geneva
1971 Gold Medal of the Society of Apothecaries of London
1971 Lawrence Poole Prize of the University of Edinburgh
1972 Cecil Joll Prize, Royal College of Surgeons of England

1973 Wade Professor, Royal College of Surgeons of Edinburgh
1973 Gairdiner Foundation Award, Canada
1974 Albert Lasker Medical Research Award
1975 Cameron Prize, University of Edinburgh
1975 Lister Medal and Oration, Royal College of Surgeons of England
1975 John Scott Prize, City of Philadelphia, USA
1976 Robert Jones Lecturer, British Orthopaedic Association
1976 Prince Philip Gold Medal Award of the Plastics and Rubber Institute
1976 Prize Buccheri La Ferla
1978 Albert Medal, Royal Society of Arts
1981 Harding Award, Action Research for the Crippled Child
1981 Faltin Lecture, Helsinki
1981 Bruce Lecture, Toronto


## Honorary and Foreign Memberships

American Orthopaedic Association
Belgian Orthopaedic Association
Brazilian Orthopaedic Association
Canadian Orthopaedic Association
Finnish Orthopaedic Association
French Orthopaedic Association
Scandinavian Orthopaedic Association

This list has been compiled, with permission, from that given in *Biographical Memoirs of Fellows of the Royal Society*, volume 30, November 1984, with a few additions. The lectures recorded here have been selected from the very large number given by Charnley; it is not possible to include them all.

# ACKNOWLEDGEMENTS

## 1 Growing up in Bury 1911–1929

Miss M. Bentley; Mrs E. Byrom; Mr Fred Campbell, writer; Professor P. Fentem; Mrs R. Hirst, librarian, Bury; Mr D.S. Hodgkiss, Second Master, Bury Grammar School; Mr L. Hyde; Mr Frank Ibbotson, physics teacher; Mrs Barbara Vance, cousin; Mr Fred Taylor Monks, contemporary, Bury Grammar School; Mr E.W. Warburton at Bury Grammar School.

## 2 Training for Surgery 1929–1940

Mrs C. Beswick, curator, Manchester Medical School; Professor M.W. Bradbury, King's College, London; Mr Arthur Bullough, Mr Alan Nicholson and Mr W Weatherstone Wilson, general surgeons, colleagues; Mrs Stella Butler, Greater Manchester Museum of Science and Technology; Dr Harry Cohen, physician, Salford Royal Hospital; Miss P. Cummings, librarian, John Rylands Library, University of Manchester; Professor W.E. Kershaw and Dr Eric Greenhalgh, fellow medical students; Dr George Komrower, colleague, paediatrician; Mr D. Lloyd Griffiths, orthopaedic surgeon, colleague; Mr I.F. Lyle, librarian, Royal College of Surgeons; Mr Frank Nicholson, thoracic surgeon, colleague; Mr D.S. Poole-Wilson, Salford Royal Hospital; Mrs S.K. Reddy, Jefferson Library, Manchester Royal Infirmary.

## 3 War Service 1940–1946

Sir Reginald Murley, Mr Clifford Brewer, Mr Arthur Bullough, Mr Frank Nicholson, Mr L. Turner and Mr Bernard Williams, general surgeons; Major-General J.C. Coull, Director of Army Surgery; Mr A. Eyre-Brook and Mr P.H. Newman, orthopaedic surgeons; Professor G.A.G. Mitchell, surgeon, anatomist; Dr R. Stone, physician, Park Hospital, Davyhulme; Mrs Brian Thomas.

## 4  Back to Manchester 1946–1960

Dr F.B. Beswick, physician; Mr N.J. Blockey, Mr A.F. Bryson, Mr F.C. Durbin, Mr T.J. Fairbank, Mr K. Hume (Australia), Mr N. Laurence, Mr N.W. Nisbet, Mr K.I. Nissen, Professor B.T. O'Connor, Mr A.H.C. Ratliff, Professor J. del Sel (Argentina), Mr G.C. Slee, Mr E.W. Somerville and Dr J.J. Wiley (Canada), orthopaedic surgeons; Professor Sir Louis Matheson (Australia), Professor J. Diamond, Professor J. Edwards and Professor R.L. Tanner (Australia), engineers; Mr I.F. Lyle, librarian, Royal College of Surgeons; Mr R. Wall, administrator, Park Hospital, Davyhulme.

## 7  Turning Points 1957 & 1958

Professor J.H. Kellgren, rheumatologist; Miss J. Pass, Medical Research Council; Mrs S.K. Reddy, Jefferson Library, Manchester Royal Infirmary.

## 8  Personal Interlude 1957–1977

Lady Charnley; Tristram and Henrietta Charnley; Mr Arthur Bullough; Mr S.C. Chen (skiing); Mrs Harry Crossley; Dr George Komrower; Mr R.H. Maudsley (skiing); Mr Frank Nicholson.

## 10  The Plan Fulfilled 1959–1969

Dr L. Brady (USA), Dr W.J. Crawford (Australia), Dr N. Eftekhar (USA), Mr R.A. Elson, Dr H.W. Hamilton (Canada), Mr B.T. Hammond (Australia), Mr K. Hardinge, Mr J.C.M. Murphy, Mr P.H. Newman, Mr J.L. Read, Mr J. Watson-Farrar and Mr B.M. Wroblewski, orthopaedic surgeons; Mr F. Brown, Mr H.C. Craven, Mr K.S. Marsh and Mr G. Middleton, workshop technicians; Dr F.N. Marshall and Mr J.H. Nuttall, administrators; Mrs E. Mitchell, anaesthetist; Mr D.F. Nicholson, West Lancashire Health Authority; Miss J. Pass, Medical Research Council; Professor J.T. Scales, biomedical engineer; Mr R. Travis, hospital manager; Dr D.H. Vaughan, North Western Regional Health Authority; Mrs J. Walker, Action Research: the National Fund for Research into Crippling Diseases.

## 11  Bone Cement: Grout not Glue 1958–1982

Dr M. Coventry (USA), Professor J. Stevens and Mr B.M. Wroblewski, orthopaedic surgeons; Mr C.G.C. Hammond and Mr G.C. Thurman, CMW Laboratories; Dr A.J.C. Lee, engineer; Dr A.J. Malcolm, pathologist; Mr W.C. Mellor, dental surgeon; Professor D.C. Smith, Department of Biomaterials, Toronto University; Mrs M. Stringfellow, histology technician; Mr L.B. Ward, School of Dental Technology, Manchester.

## 12   Clean Air Against Infection 1960–1983

Mr H.C. Craven, workshop technician; Mr R.A. Elson and Mr J.L. Read, orthopaedic surgeons; Mr Hugh Howorth, Howorth Air Engineering Ltd.


## 13   The Charnley/Thackray Relationship 1947–1982

Mr W.P. Thackray (chairman), Mr J.D. Boyd and Mr J.P. Thackray (directors), Mr R. Frank (director, deceased), Mr P.D. Gossedge (product group manager), Chas. F. Thackray Ltd.


## 14   Spreading the Word 1967–1982

Dr L. Brady (USA), orthopaedic surgeon; Dr R.D. McLeish and Dr J. Skorecki, UMIST; Professor J.P. Paul, engineer.


## 15   An Outpost in the South 1969–1982

Dr J.R. Bennett, anaesthetist; Mr J.A. Boulton and Mr W.H. Mitchell, administrators; Mrs R. Cock, physiotherapist; Dr W.I. Gordon and Dr S.E. Large, physicians; Mr N. Martin, theatre assistant; Miss W. Norton, ward sister; Mr M.W.J. Older, orthopaedic surgeon; Mr A. Purdew, chauffeur; Mrs J. Pannett, artist.


## 16   Active Retirement 1975–1982

Lady Charnley; Mr Ronald Frank; Mr I.F. Lyle, Royal College of Surgeons; Mr A.H.C. Ratliff; Mr N.H. Robinson, librarian, The Royal Society, Mr G.C. Slee.

# GLOSSARY OF ORTHOPAEDIC TERMS

Some of the technical terms used in this book are listed here, but the difficulty for the general reader is not only in understanding the words themselves, but in appreciating that simple words are often used synonymously and interchangeably. For example, the socket of a hip prosthesis may be called the socket or the cup.

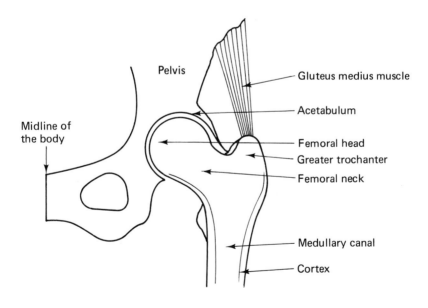

*Diagram of normal anatomy of the left hip joint*

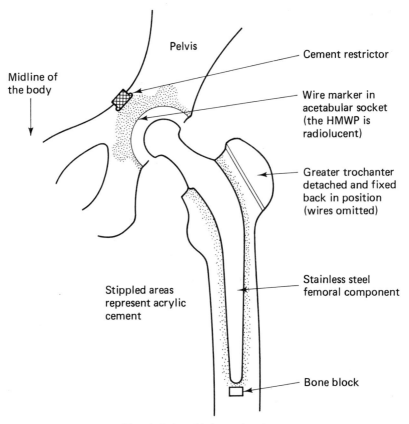

*Charnley's low friction arthroplasty*

**acetabulum:** the socket of the normal hip joint, made up of the pelvic bones.

**acrylic:** a plastic material, polymethylmethacrylate, e.g. perspex when in block form; was used as a *femoral head prosthesis*, but proved unsuitable.

**acrylic cement:** a form of self-curing polymethylmethacrylate which changes from a soft doughy material to a hard solid when powder and liquid are mixed together; used as grout to bond implants to bone.

**ankylosing spondylitis:** an inflammatory condition which affects the spine and hips.

**ankylosis:** the situation where a joint is destroyed by surgery (e.g. *arthrodesis*) or disease and the bone ends become fused together by bone or fibrous tissue.

**anticoagulant drugs:** drugs given to slow the coagulation of circulating blood and hence prevent clotting (*venous thrombosis*) after operation.

**appliance:** a device applied to the external surface of the body for support (see *calliper*).

**approach:** in surgery, incision and exposure of the part, for example the hip joint, to be operated on.

**arthritis:** inflammation of a joint which may be acute or chronic.

**arthrodesis**: an operation carried out to fix, or fuse, a joint. No movement is possible afterwards and pain is relieved (see *compression*).

**arthroplasty**: an operation to reconstruct a joint damaged by chronic arthritis (see *osteoarthritis, rheumatoid arthritis*). The aim is to restore movement and stability, and to relieve pain.

**articular**: adjective of articulation or joint, usually applied to cartilage which is the white slippery material which covers the ends of the bones within a joint.

**bacteria**: microscopic organisms, such as those responsible for wound infection.

**bilateral**: affecting both sides, e.g. both hips.

**bioengineer**: an engineer who is also concerned with biological problems in the body; sometimes biomedical or biomechanical engineer.

**biopsy**: removal of a small piece of tissue for examination under a microscope.

**bone cement**: see *acrylic cement*.

**bone–cement interface**: the junction between bone cement and the living bone.

**bone graft**: a piece of bone taken from one part of the body and transplanted to another part, usually to help to produce union of a fracture.

**bone plug**: a small piece of bone inserted into the *medullary canal* of the *femur* below the lower end of a *prosthesis* to limit the flow of cement.

**cadaver**: a dead body (adjective: cadaveric).

**calliper**: an appliance fitted to the leg to support the knee; extending from a padded ring in the groin to a socket in the heel of the shoe (may be spelt caliper).

**capsule**: the thick fibrous tissue which holds the two bones of a joint together; it is lined by synovial membrane (see *synovial fluid*).

**cartilage**: articular cartilage is the firm white tissue which covers the bone ends within a joint.

**cement**: see *acrylic cement*.

**cement restrictor**: a small piece of wire mesh, shaped like a Mexican hat, which is inserted into the hole made in the floor of the *acetabulum*, with the aim of limiting the flow of cement into the pelvis.

**central dislocation**: a technique of *arthrodesis* or stabilisation of the hip devised by Charnley.

**chrome–cobalt**: a metallic alloy made of chrome, cobalt, molybdenum and other elements and used for surgical implants, known as vinertia or vitallium.

**clean air**: air from which dust particles (and thus bacteria) have been removed by filtration in order to achieve sterile conditions in an operating theatre.

**collagen**: the important constituent of tough fibrous tissue.

**Colles' fracture**: a fracture of the wrist.

**components**: used to describe the parts, or *prostheses*, used in a hip replacement. Hence the *femoral prosthesis* is one component, the other is the acetabular *cup* or socket.

**compression arthrodesis**: the operative technique where two bones, the ends of which have been removed, are held together under pressure which is exerted by screw-clamps attached to nails passing through the bones above and below the joint.

**cortex**: the thick outer layer of a long bone.

**cup**: in the context of a joint replacement this refers to the artificial socket inserted to replace the arthritic *acetabulum*. Thus interchangeable with socket or acetabular component.

**dislocation**: displacement of one part of a joint out of the other part, e.g. the *femoral head* out of the *acetabulum*. This can follow an injury, but there are other causes. It can also occur after a joint replacement.

**epiphysis**:  the growing end of a bone in childhood.

**exchange operation**:  the components of an *arthroplasty* are replaced, usually carried out for loosening or infection.

**FRCS**:  Fellow of the Royal College of Surgeons.

**femoral head**:  the round upper end of the *femur* which forms the ball of the ball-and-socket joint.

**femur**:  the thigh bone (adjective: femoral; e.g. the femoral head).

**Fluon**:  see *PTFE*.

**formaldehyde**:  formic aldehyde used for sterilisation.

**fusion**:  the result of an operation to fix (stiffen) a joint. A spinal fusion is an operation designed to fuse a joint (or joints) in the spine.

**gamma ($\gamma$) radiation**:  high energy radiation resembling X-rays, used for sterilising powders etc.

**gluteus medius**:  a powerful muscle which plays an important part in controlling the stability of the hip and which passes from the side of the pelvis to the *greater trochanter*.

**greater trochanter**:  a bony protuberance on the outer side of the upper end of the *femur* to which the powerful muscles (especially *gluteus medius*) are attached.

**haematoma**:  a collection of blood in a wound.

**hemiarthroplasty**:  an *arthroplasty* which replaces only one half of a joint, e.g. the *femoral head* and not the *acetabulum*.

**herniation**:  bulging through a covering; hence a disc herniation occurs when the soft centre (nucleus pulposus) of a lumbar intervertebral disc bulges through its outer fibrous covering (annulus fibrosus); synonymous with protrusion, prolapse (see *intervertebral disc protrusion*).

**hindquarter amputation**:  amputation of the whole of the lower limb and half the pelvis, usually carried out for malignant bone tumours.

**hip joint**:  the ball-and-socket joint between the *acetabulum* and the *femoral head*; it lies deeply between the middle of the groin and the buttock.

**histology**:  study of tissues by the microscope.

**imbibition**:  taking up of fluid.

**implant**:  a general term for material implanted into the body, so a *femoral prosthesis* is an implant.

**intervertebral disc**:  the soft tissue between the vertebral bodies.

**intervertebral disc protrusion**:  when a lumbar intervertebral disc swells and ruptures producing pressure on a spinal nerve and causing lumbago and sciatica; sometimes called a prolapse, and incorrectly, a 'slipped' disc.

**intramedullary**:  within the *medullary canal*.

**ligament**:  tough fibrous tissue which supports and protects a joint.

**MB,ChB**:  Bachelor of Medicine, Bachelor of Surgery.

**medullary canal**:  the natural canal, filled with marrow, in the shaft of a long bone. This is reamed to insert the femoral prosthesis.

**meniscus**:  the wedges of fibrocartilage within the knee joint, often incorrectly referred to as 'cartilages'. Meniscectomy is the operation to remove a meniscus.

**neck of the femur**:  between the *femoral head* and *greater trochanter*.

**neurosurgeon**:  a surgeon specialising in disorders of the brain and spinal cord.

**nucleus pulposus**:  the soft centre of an intervertebral disc.

**orthopaedics**:  the surgery of bones and joints (including fractures).

**osseous**: bony (or boney).

**osteoarthritis**: a degenerative condition, usually affecting weight-bearing joints in the lower limb.

**osteoarthrosis**: a synonym for *osteoarthritis*, possibly a more correct usage, but the more familiar osteoarthritis is used throughout this book.

**osteogenesis**: bone formation by new growth.

**osteomyelitis**: infection of bone.

**osteotome**: a chisel for dividing bone.

**osteotomy**: an operation in which a bone is divided; this can be carried out through the upper end of the femur to relieve pain in *osteoarthritis*.

**periosteum**: fibrous tissue covering the outer surface of a bone.

**physical medicine**: treatment by physical measures (heat, exercises etc.); the same as physiotherapy.

**plate**: metal plate with screws used to fix a fracture.

**polyethylene**: high molecular weight polyethylene (HMWP) used for the socket in Charnley's arthroplasty of the hip.

**Pott's fracture**: a fracture of the ankle.

**prosthesis**: a substitute for part of the body; e.g. an artificial limb. Also used for internal replacement when endoprosthesis becomes the correct term. Prosthesis alone is however used for convenience and by custom throughout this book to indicate internal prostheses, such as the replacement of the head of the *femur*.

**pseudarthrosis**: a false joint such as may form when a fracture fails to unite.

**PTFE**: polytetrafluorethylene (also *Teflon*, *Fluon*), the plastic which Charnley used initially for the socket of his *arthroplasty*.

**pulmonary embolism**: occurs when a clot from a vein becomes detached and lodges in the lungs.

**radiograph**: the correct name for an X-ray plate.

**radiolucent**: not visible in *radiographs*.

**radio-opaque**: visible in *radiographs*.

**randomised trials**: trials in which the participants are randomly selected.

**revision operation**: the operation is done again and usually new components are inserted (in the case of joint replacements).

**rheumatoid arthritis**: an inflammatory condition which affects many joints in the upper and lower limbs.

**sacrum**: the solid bone at the very bottom of the spine (adjective: sacral).

**settle plates**: dishes filled with agar on which bacteria will grow, and exposed in an operating theatre.

**slit sampler**: apparatus for sampling air by collecting dust particles and bacteria.

**Steinmann's nail**: an eponymous term for a nail used to transfix a bone.

**subluxation**: partial displacement of a joint where the two bones remain in contact, although displaced.

**supracondylar fracture of the femur**: a fracture just above the knee.

**surface replacement**: replacement of the articular cartilage of the *femoral head* and the *acetabulum* by two cups made of foreign material (e.g. plastic or metal); also called a double cup *arthroplasty*.

**synovial fluid**: the fluid which lubricates normal joints, produced by the synovial membrane (or synovium) which lines the capsule of a joint.

**Teflon**: see *PTFE*.

**Thomas' splint**: a metal splint used to immobilise the leg after fractures.

**tibia**:  the main bone below the knee.

**total replacement**:  an *arthroplasty* which replaces both parts of a joint, e.g. the *acetabulum* and the *femoral head*.

**trephine**:  a cylindrical instrument with a circular cutting edge often used for taking a *biopsy*.

**unilateral**:  affecting one side, e.g. one hip only.

**vascular**:  adjective describing blood vessels.

**venous thrombosis**:  clotting of blood in the veins of the leg which may occur after operation.

# REFERENCES

References are listed by chapter, but the method of presentation is somewhat unconventional.

References to Charnley's papers are always given first, and in date order, so that the reader can easily appreciate the scope of his work.

If other authors are named before him in the title, the reference has been changed to the form: 'Charnley J. with . . .' followed by the other authors' names.

Those papers referred to in the text are numbered, those without a number are listed for completeness, although they are not specifically mentioned in the body of the chapter.

When work of other authors is mentioned, it is listed and numbered after Charnley's references.

## 1 Growing up in Bury 1911–1929

1. Brockbank W. (1965) The Honorary Medical Staff of the Manchester Royal Infirmary. Manchester University Press, Manchester
2. Campbell Fred (1968) Bury in the Nineteen-Twenties. Published by Neil Richardson, 375 Chorley Road, Swinton, Manchester
3. Nisbet N.W., Woodruff M.F.A. (1984) John Charnley. Biographical Memoirs of Fellows of the Royal Society, London, 30:119–37
4. Pevsner N. (1969) The Buildings of England: South Lancashire. Penguin Books, London

## 2 Training for Surgery 1929–1940

1. Briggs A. (1963) Victorian Cities. Odhams Press 1963 (Penguin edition, 1977)
2. Brockbank W. (1952) Portrait of a Hospital. William Heinemann, London
3. Charnley J. (1944) Experimental Shock. Br Med J i:716–18
4. Platt H. (1985) John Charnley. In: Elwood W.J., Tuxford A.F. (eds) Some Manchester Doctors. Manchester University Press, Manchester

## 3   War Service 1940–1946

1. Jack E.A., Charnley J. (1943) The two-stage amputation. Br Med J ii:131–2
2. Charnley J. (1944) Fractures of the femoral shaft. Lancet I:235–9
3. Charnley J. (1945) Adjustable Army Calliper. J Bone Joint Surg (Br) 27:348

## 4   Back to Manchester 1946–1960

### Charnley references

1. Charnley J. (1948) Proceedings of British Orthopaedic Association, Oct 1947. J Bone Joint Surg (Br) 30:208
2. Charnley J. (1950) Method of inserting the Smith-Petersen guide wire. J Bone Joint Surg (Br) 32:271–72
3. Charnley J. (1952) Fluid imbibition as a cause of herniation of the nucleus pulposus. Société Internationale de Chirurgie Orthopédique et de Traumatologie meeting, Stockholm, May, 1951. J Bone Joint Surg (Br) 33:472
4. Charnley J., with Blockey N.J., Purser D.W. (1957) The treatment of displaced fractures of the neck of the femur by compression. J Bone Joint Surg (Br) 39:45–65

### Other references

5. Editorial (1948) Nuffield and Travelling Fellows to US and Canada. J Bone Joint Surg (Br) 30:405–407
6. Hardinge K.H. (1988) The development of the Charnley low friction arthroplasty. In Galasko C.S.B., Noble J. (eds) Current Trends in Orthopaedic Surgery. Manchester University Press, Manchester, pp 242–5
7. Honours to Orthopaedic Surgeons (1948) Sir Harry Platt. J Bone Joint Surg (Br) 30:205
8. Jones R., Girdlestone G.R. (1919) The cure of crippled children. Br Med J ii:457–60
9. Proceedings & reports (1952) Time-tables of clinical programmes: Manchester. J Bone Joint Surg (Br) 34:144

## 5   An Exact Man 1946–1960

### Charnley references

#### Papers

1. Charnley J. (1945) Exposure of the posterior horn of the medial meniscus. Lancet II:771
2. Charnley J. (1947) The walking calliper. Lancet I:464–7
3. Charnley J. (1947) Knee movement following fractures of the femoral shaft. J Bone Joint Surg (Am) 29:679–86
4. Charnley J. (1948) Amputations. Practitioner 160:206–11

5. Charnley J. (1948) Positive pressure in arthrodesis of the knee joint. J Bone Joint Surg (Br) 30:478–86
6. Charnley J. (1948) Horizontal approach to the medial semi-lunar cartilage. J Bone Joint Surg (Br) 30:659–63
7. Charnley J. (1949) Biomechanicalorthopaedicengineeringung. Manchester Univ Med School Gazette, pp 97–105
8. Charnley J. (1950) Method of inserting the Smith-Petersen guide wire. J Bone Joint Surg (Br) 32:271–2
9. Charnley J. (1950) Sprains and dislocations. Practitioner 164:314–19
10. Charnley J. (1951) Orthopaedic signs in the diagnosis of disc protrusion, with special reference to the straight-leg-raising test. Lancet I:186–92
    Charnley J. (1951) Compression arthrodesis of the ankle and shoulder. J Bone Joint Surg (Br) 33:180–91
    Charnley J., Baker S.L. (1952) Compression arthrodesis of the knee – a clinical and histological study. J Bone Joint Surg (Br) 34:187–99
11. Charnley J. (1952) Imbibition of fluid as a cause of herniation of the nucleus pulposus. Lancet I:124–7
12. Charnley J. (1953) Injuries of the spine and pelvis. Practitioner 170:142–9
13. Charnley J. (1955) Acute lumbago and sciatica. Br Med J i:344–6
14. Charnley J. (1956) Congenital pseudarthrosis of the tibia treated by intramedullary nail. J Bone Joint Surg (Am) 38:283–90
    Charnley J., Ollerenshaw R. (1956) Investigation of cancellous bone. Med Biol Illust 6:205–8
    Charnley J. (1956) Technique of compression arthrodesis. Iconographia Chirurgia 64:116
    Charnley J. (1956) Just what is a slipped disc? Family Doctor 8:586
15. Charnley J. (1957) Contribution to symposium on the use of metal in bone surgery. Proc R Soc Med 50:837–42
16. Charnley J., with Blockey N.J., Purser D.W. (1957) The treatment of displaced fractures of the neck of the femur by compression. J Bone Joint Surg (Br) 39:45–65
17. Charnley J., Lowe H.G. (1958) A study of the end-results of compression arthrodesis of the knee. J Bone Joint Surg (Br) 40:633–5
18. Charnley J. (1959) Contribution to symposium on the treatment of fractures of the shafts of long bones. Proc R Soc Med 52:291–5
    Charnley J. (1959) The lubrication of animal joints. In: Symposium on Biomechanics. Institution of Mechanical Engineers, London, pp 12–22
19. Charnley J. (1959) Peri-arthritis of the shoulder. Postgrad Med J 35:384–8
20. Charnley J. (1960) Arthrodesis of the knee. Clin Orthop 18:37–42
    Charnley J. (1960) Arthrodesis of the hip in the treatment of osteoarthritis. Am J Orthop 2:169–71
21. Charnley J. (1960) Surgical treatment of un-united fractures. J Bone Joint Surg (Br) 42:3–4 (editorial)
22. Charnley J. (1960) The treatment of fractures of the neck of the femur by compression. Acta Orthop Scand 30:29–48

*Papers written after 1960 on 'pre-hip' subjects*

23. Charnley J., Guindy J. (1961) Delayed operation in the open reduction of fractures of long bones. J Bone Joint Surg (Br) 43:664–71
    Charnley J. (1964) Le traitement des fractures ouvertes des os longs. Acta Orthop Belg 28:432–43
24. Charnley J., Houston J. (1964) Compression arthrodesis of the shoulder. J Bone Joint Surg (Br) 46:614–20

## New instruments and apparatus

25. Charnley J. (1945) New dissecting forceps for no-touch technique. Br Med J i:702
26. Charnley J. (1947) Retractor for operation on the nucleus pulposus. Lancet II:274
27. Charnley J. (1951) New walking aid for spastic paralysis. J Bone Joint Surg (Br) 33:122–3
28. Charnley J., Wright J.K. (1951) A spring exerciser for arthroplasty of the hip joint. J Bone Joint Surg (Br) 33:634–5
29. Charnley J. (1953) A new pattern of bone-holding forceps. J Bone Joint Surg (Br) 35:288–9
30. Charnley J. (1965) A drilling jig for intertrochanteric osteotomy of the femur. Lancet I:360
31. Charnley J. (1965) Improved short hip spica cast. Lancet II:275

## Letters to medical journals

    1945 Penicillin-sulphonamide mixture. Lancet I:772
32. 1947 Appearance of protruded discs. Lancet I:295
33. 1949 Osteopathy. Lancet I:41
34. 1950 Prolapsed intervertebral disc. Lancet I:276
35. 1951 Intramedullary nailing of fractures after fifty years. J Bone Joint Surg (Br) 33:291–2
36. 1952 Intramedullary nailing of fractures. J Bone Joint Surg (Br) 34:162
37. 1954 Arthroplasty v arthrodesis. Lancet I:1346
38. 1955 Low backache. Br Med J i:344
39. 1958 Physical changes in the prolapsed disc. Lancet I:1277
40. 1959 Sore over the sacrum. Lancet II:914–5

## Recorded contributions at meetings (by date of publication)

This list contains Charnley's contributions to various meetings which were recorded in the *Journal of Bone and Joint Surgery* and the *British Medical Journal*. The nature of the meeting and the reference summarising the proceedings is given in each case. The subjects indicate the range of Charnley's orthopaedic interests and his regular attendance at meetings during this period.

1945

    The army adjustable walking caliper. British Orthopaedic Association meeting, London, December 1944. J Bone Joint Surg 27:348

1946

41. Fractures of the femoral shaft (symposium). British Orthopaedic Association meeting, London, October 1945. J Bone Joint Surg 28:195

1948

    The three-point action of splints. Compression arthrodesis and primary spinal fusion after laminectomy and foraminotomy (demonstration). British Orthopaedic Association meeting, Manchester, October 1947. J Bone Joint Surg (Br) (1948) 30:208
42. The backache and sciatica syndrome (discussion). Joint meeting of Liverpool Medical Institution and Manchester Medical Society. J Bone Joint Surg (Br) 30:395
    Compression arthrodesis. Combined meeting of the American, British and Canadian Orthopaedic Associations. J Bone Joint Surg (Br) 30:573

## 1949

43. Compression arthrodesis. British Orthopaedic Association meeting. Belfast, October 1948. J Bone Joint Surg (Br) 31:134
    The healing of fractures. Manchester regional orthopaedic meeting. J Bone Joint Surg (Br) 31:141

## 1950

Compression arthrodesis. Manchester regional orthopaedic meeting, July, 1949. J Bone Joint Surg (Br) 32:134
Histology of bone union after compression arthrodesis. British Orthopaedic Association meeting, Cardiff, July, 1949. J Bone Joint Surg (Br) 32:283

## 1951

Osteoarthritis of the hip. Section of Surgery, Manchester Medical Society. Br Med J i:296
Late results from disc operations (discussion). British Orthopaedic Association meeting, Cambridge. J Bone Joint Surg (Br) 33:286
44. Fluid imbibition as a cause of herniation of the nucleus pulposus. Société Internationale de Chirurgie Orthopédique et de Traumatologie meeting, Stockholm, May, 1951. J Bone Joint Surg (Br) 33:472

## 1952

Experience in the evolution of a new operation for osteoarthritis of the hip. British Orthopaedic Association meeting, BOA, Edinburgh, July 1952. J Bone Joint Surg (Br) 34:506
Paraplegia in Pott's disease (discussion). Manchester regional orthopaedic clinical meeting with Liverpool Orthopaedic Association. April, 1951. J Bone Joint Surg (Br) 34:525
45. Modern advances in internal fixation will render obsolete the use of splints in the treatment of fractured bones (debate). Orthopaedic day, University of Liverpool, July 1952. J Bone Joint Surg (Br) 34:712

## 1953

Treatment of lumbar intervertebral derangements by traction (discussion). British Orthopaedic Association meeting. Sheffield, October 1952. J Bone Joint Surg (Br) 35:145

## 1954

Acromioclavicular dislocation (discussion). British Orthopaedic Association meeting, Birmingham, October 1953. J Bone Joint Surg (Br) 36:148
All methods of arthroplasty of the hip have failed to achieve their purpose (debate). British Orthopaedic Association meeting, Buxton, May 1954. J Bone Joint Surg (Br) 36:509
46. Stabilisation of the hip by a technique of central dislocation. Société Internationale de Chirurgie Orthopédique et de Traumatologie meeting, Bern, September 1954. J Bone Joint Surg (Br) 36:692
Monarticular osteoarthritis of the hip. Clinical forum at the CIBA Foundation, 1954. Br Med J ii:408

## 1955

Slipperiness of articular cartilage. British Orthopaedic Association meeting, London, October 1954. J Bone Joint Surg (Br) 37:164
Lumbosacral fusion and low back pain (discussion). British Orthopaedic Association meeting, London, October 1954. J Bone Joint Surg (Br) 37:165

47. Stabilisation of the hip by central dislocation. Combined meeting – French Association of Orthopaedic Surgery and Traumatology and British Orthopaedic Association, Paris, May 1955. J Bone Joint Surg (Br) 37:514
    Repair of cancellous bone under high pressure. Bone & Tooth Society, Royal National Orthopaedic Hospital, London, March 1955. J Bone Joint Surg (Br)

48. That Lucas Championnière was right (debate). British Orthopaedic Association meeting, Liverpool, October 1955. J Bone Joint Surg (Br) 37:720

1956

49. Stabilisation of the hip by central dislocation. South African Orthopaedic Association, Pretoria, October 1955. J Bone Joint Surg (Br) 38:592
    Treatment of fractures of the femoral neck by compression. British Orthopaedic Association meeting, Gleneagles, May 1956. J Bone Joint Surg (Br) 38:772

1957

Cancellous strip grafting (discussion). British Orthopaedic Association meeting, Oswestry, May 1957. J Bone Joint Surg (Br) 39:585

1958

50. Surgical treatment of osteoarthritis of the hip – excluding arthroplasty (symposium). Société Internationale de Chirurgie Orthopédique et de Traumatologie meeting, Barcelona, September 1957. J Bone Joint Surg (Br) 40:156

1959

Experimental investigation of spinal injuries (discussion). British Orthopaedic Association meeting, London, October 1959. J Bone Joint Surg (Br) 41:855

1960

Replacement of skin loss (discussion). British Orthopaedic Association meeting, Glasgow, April 1960. J Bone Joint Surg (Br) 42:646

*Book reviews by Charnley in the British volume of the* Journal of Bone and Joint Surgery *(including some after 1960)*

*Kinesiology of the human body* by Arthur Steindler. J Bone Joint Surg (Br) 1955 37:736–7
*The proximal end of the femur* by Stig Backman. J Bone Joint Surg (Br) 1958 40:370–1
*Studies on weight distribution upon the lower extremities in individuals working in a standing position* by Axel Marsk. J Bone Joint Surg (Br) 1959 41:653
*Open reduction of common fractures* by O.P. Hampton, W.T. Fitts. J Bone Joint Surg (Br) 1960 42:168
*Metals and engineering in bone and joint surgery* by C.O. Bechtol, A.B. Ferguson, P.G. Laing. J Bone Joint Surg (Br) 1960 42:865
*Lumbar intradiscal pressure* by Alf Nachemson. J Bone Joint Surg (Br) 1961 43:414
*Disease of the intervertebral disc and its surrounding tissues* by R. Rabinovitch. J Bone Joint Surg (Br) 1962 44:251
*An experimental study of the rate of fracture healing* by J. Falkenberg. J Bone Joint Surg (Br) 1962 44:253

51. *Technique of internal fixation of fractures* by M.E. Müller and others. J Bone Joint Surg (Br) 1966 48:200–1

*La march et les boiteries* by Jean and Pierre Ducrocquet. J Bone Joint Surg (Br) 1966
48:403

Obituary: J. Albert Key (1890–1955). J Bone Joint Surg (Br) 1955 37:713

## *Other references*

52. Annotation (1958) Physical changes in the prolapsed disc. Lancet II:1214–15
53. Burns B.H., Young R.H. (1947) Backache. Lancet I:623–6
54. Calvert L.S. (1954) Low backache. Br Med J ii:1488
55. Disabilities 44 (1950) Prolapsed intravertebral disc. Lancet I:177–8
56. Editorial (1954) Osteoarthritis of the hip. Lancet I:1119–20
57. Jarry L., Uthoff H.K. (1960) Activation of osteogenesis by the petal technique.
    J Bone Joint Surg (Br) 42:126–36
58. Key J.A. (1932) Positive pressure in arthrodesis for tuberculosis of the knee joint.
    South Med J 25:909–15
59. Key J.A. (1937) Arthrodesis of the knee with a large central autogenous bone peg.
    South Med J 30:574–9
60. Turner L. (1988) John Charnley. Lives of the Fellows, Royal College of Surgeons,
    pp 71–3
61. Watson-Jones et al. (1950) Medullary nailing of fractures after 50 years. J Bone Joint
    Surg (Br) 32:694–729

## 6   Books to Instruct 1950 & 1953

### *Books by Charnley*

1. Charnley J. (1950) The Closed Treatment of Common Fractures. Churchill Livingstone,
   Edinburgh and London. Subsequent editions 1957, 1961 (reprinted 7 times)
2. Charnley J. (1953) Compression Arthrodesis. Churchill Livingstone, Edinburgh and
   London.

### *Chapters in textbooks*

3. Fracture Treatment. In: Modern Trends in Orthopaedics. Ed Sir Harry Platt.
   Butterworth, London, 1950
4. Epiphyses, Diseases and Injuries. In: Encyclopaedia of British Medical Practice,
   5:277–92. Butterworth, London, 1951
5. Orthopaedic Surgery. In: Bailey H., Love R.J.M. (eds) A Short Practice of Surgery,
   10th to 13th editions. H.K. Lewis & Co Ltd, London, 1956–1965

### *Book reviews of* The Closed Treatment of Common Fractures

6. Gissane W. (1950) J Bone Joint Surg (Br) 32:757
7. Gissane W. (1958) J Bone Joint Surg (Br) 40:612–13
8. Watson-Jones R. (1961) J Bone Joint Surg (Br) 43:869

## Book Review of Compression Arthrodesis

9. Newman P.H. (1953) J Bone Joint Surg (Br) 35:497–98

## 8  Personal Interlude 1957–1977

Hare E. (1988) Branestawm's disease (book review). Br Med J 297:1275

## 9  The Growth of an Idea 1951–1961

### Charnley references

1. Charnley J. (1951) Osteoarthritis of the hip. Report of a meeting of the section of surgery, Manchester Medical Society. Br Med J i:296
2. Charnley J. (1954) All methods of arthroplasty have failed to achieve their purpose (debate). British Orthopaedic Association. J Bone Joint Surg (Br) 36:509
3. Charnley J. (1955) The 'slipperiness' of articular cartilage. J Bone Joint Surg (Br) 37:164
4. Charnley J. (1956) Arthroplasty of the hip. Discussion. South African Orthopaedic Association (1955). J Bone Joint Surg (Br) 38:592
5. Charnley J. (1958) Surgical treatment of osteoarthritis of the hip. Société Internationale de Chirurgerie Orthopédique et de Traumatologie meeting, Barcelona, 1957. J Bone Joint Surg (Br) 40:156
6. Charnley J. (1959) The lubrication of animal joints. In: Symposium on Biomechanics, Institution of Mechanical Engineers, London, pp 12–22
7. Charnley J. (1959) The lubrication of animal joints. The New Scientist, 9 July, 60–61
8. Charnley J. (1960) The lubrication of animal joints in relation to surgical reconstruction by arthroplasty. Ann Rheum Dis 19:10–19
9. Charnley J. (1960) Surgery of the hip joint, present and future developments. Br Med J i:821–6
   Charnley J. (1960) How are joints lubricated? Triangle 4:175–9
   Charnley J. (1960) The future of hip surgery. Nursing Mirror 110:2190–2
10. Charnley J. (1961) Surgeon and engineer (letter). Lancet I:449
11. Charnley J. (1961) Arthroplasty of the hip – a new operation. Lancet I:1129–32
    Charnley J. (1962) L'arthroplastie de la hanche. Med et Hyg 21:367–9
12. Charnley J. (1962) An artificial bearing in the hip: implications in biological lubrication. Fed Proc 25:1079–81
    Charnley J. (1979) Low Friction Arthroplasty of the Hip. Theory and Practice. Springer, Berlin Heidelberg New York

### Other references

13. Annotation (1961) Surgeon and engineer. Lancet I:325–6
14. Armstrong C.G., Mow V.C. (1980) Friction, lubrication and wear in synovial joints. In: Goodfellow J.G., Owen R. (eds) Scientific Foundations of Orthopaedics and Traumatology. Wm Heinemann, London, pp 223–32
15. Brailsford J.L. (1960) Osteoarthritis of the hip (letters). Lancet I:1280 and I:1959
16. Editorial (1960) Surgery of osteoarthritis of the hip. Br Med J i:1261–2
17. Hardinge K. (1988) The development of the Charnley low friction arthroplasty. In: Current Trends in Orthopaedic Surgery. Manchester University Press, Manchester, pp 242–5

18. Jones E.S. (1934) Joint lubrication. Lancet I:1043–4
19. Jones E.S. (1936) Joint lubrication. Lancet I:1426–7
20. Judet J., Judet R., LaGrange J., Dunoyer J. (1954) Resection–reconstruction of the hip: arthroplasty with an acrylic prosthesis. E & S Livingstone, Edinburgh
21. MacConnaill M.A. (1932) The function of intra-articular cartilages. J Anat 66:210–27
22. McKee G.K. (1951) Artificial hip joint. J Bone Joint Surg (Br) 33:465
23. McKee G.K. (1970) Development of total prosthetic replacement of the hip. Clin Orthop 72:85–103
24. Moore A.T. (1952) Metal hip joint: a new self-locking vitallium prosthesis. S Med J 45:1015–19
25. Scales J. (1967) Arthroplasty of the hip using foreign materials: a history. In: Symposium on Lubrication and Wear in Living and Artificial Human Joints. Institution of Mechanical Engineers, London, paper 13, pp 1–22
26. Smith-Petersen M.N. (1939) Arthroplasty of the hip: a new method. J Bone Joint Surg 39:269–88
27. Thompson F.R. (1954) Two and a half years' experience with a vitallium hip prosthesis. J Bone Joint Surg (Am) 36:489–500
28. Wiles P.W. (1958) The surgery of the osteoarthritic hip. Br J Surg 45:488–97
29. Walton J. (1950) Progress in gastric surgery in the last half century. Br Med J i:206–10

## 10   The Plan Fulfilled 1959–1969

*Charnley references*

1. Charnley J. (1961) Arthroplasty of the hip by the low friction technique. J Bone Joint Surg (Br) 43:601
2. Charnley J. (1963) Tissue reactions to polytetrafluorethylene (letter). Lancet II:1379
3. Charnley J. (1964) Specialist qualifications (letters). Br Med J i:1249, 1506
4. Charnley J. (1965) Prosthetic replacement of arthritic hips by the McKee-Farrar artificial hip joint (discussion). J Bone Joint Surg (Br) 47:185
5. Charnley J. (1968) Total prosthetic replacement of the hip in relation to physiotherapy. Physiotherapy 54:406–11
6. Charnley J. (1970) Total hip replacement by low friction arthroplasty. Clin Orthop 72:7–21
7. Charnley J. (1970) Subspecialisation or superspecialisation in surgery. Br Med J ii:719–22
8. Charnley J. (1972) The long-term results of low friction arthroplasty of the hip performed as a primary intervention. J Bone Joint Surg (Br) 54:61–76
9. Charnley J. (1973) The organisation of a special centre for hip surgery. Br J Hosp Med 9:389–96
10. Charnley J. (1979) Low Friction Arthroplasty of the Hip. Theory and Practice. Springer, Berlin Heidelberg New York, p 376
11. Charnley J. (1983) The development of the centre for hip surgery at Wrightington hospital (written in 1982). In: Swinburn W.R. (ed) Wrightington Hospital, the story of the first 50 years. Wrightington Hospital

*Other references*

12. Hardinge K. (1983) Hip Replacement – the Facts. Oxford University Press, Oxford
13. McKee G.K., Farrar J.W. (1966) Replacement of arthritic hips by the McKee–Farrar prosthesis. J Bone Joint Surg (Br) 48:245–59

14. Müller M.E. (1970) Total hip prostheses. Clin Orthop 72:46–68
15. Ring P.A. (1970) Total replacement of the hip. Clin Orthop 72:161–8
16. Röttger J., Elson R.A. (1986) A modification of the Charnley low friction arthroplasty. Clin Orthop 211:154–63
17. Swinburn W.R. (1983) Wrightington Hospital, the story of the first 50 years. Wrightington Hospital

## 11  Bone Cement: Grout not Glue 1958–1982

### Charnley references

1. Charnley J. (1960) Anchorage of the femoral head prosthesis to the shaft of the femur. J Bone Joint Surg (Br) 42:28–30
2. Charnley J. (1964) The bonding of prostheses to bone by cement. J Bone Joint Surg (Br) 46:518–29
   Charnley J. (1964) L'adherence des prostheses a l'os vivant. Acta Belg Orthop 30:663–72
3. Charnley J. (1965) A biomechanical analysis of the use of cement to anchor the femoral head prosthesis. J Bone Joint Surg (Br) 47:354–63
   Charnley J. (1965) The elimination of slip between prosthesis and femur. J Bone Joint Surg (Br) 47:56–60
   Charnley J., Crawford W.J. (1968) Histology of bone in contact with self-curing acrylic cement. J Bone Joint Surg (Br) 50:228 (abstract)
4. Charnley J. (1969) The healing of human fractures in contact with self-curing cement. Clin Orthop 47:157–63
5. Charnley J., Follaci F.M., Hammond B.T. (1968) The long-term reaction of self-curing acrylic cement. J Bone Joint Surg (Br) 50:822–9
6. Charnley J. with Follaci F.M. (1969) A comparison of the results of femoral head prosthesis with and without cement. Clin Orthop 62:156–61
7. Charnley J. (1970) Acrylic cement in orthopaedic surgery. E & S Livingstone, Edinburgh and London
8. Charnley J. (1970) The reaction of bone to self-curing cement. J Bone Joint Surg (Br) 52:340–53
9. Charnley J. with Weber F.A. (1975) A radiological study of fractures of acrylic cement to the stem of a femoral head prosthesis. J Bone Joint Surg (Br) 57:297–301
10. Charnley J. (1975) Risks of total hip replacement (letters). Br Med J ii:498 and iv:101
11. Charnley J. with DeLee J.G. (1976) Radiological demarcation of cemented sockets in total hip replacement. Clin Orthop 121:20–32
12. Charnley J. with Bocco F., Langan J. (1977) Changes in the calcar femoris in relation to cement technology in total hip replacement. Clin Orthop 128:287–95
13. Charnley J. with Blacker G.J. (1978) Changes in the upper femur after low friction arthroplasty. Clin Orthop 137:15–23
14. Charnley J. with Griffiths J., Seidenstein M.K., Williams D. (1978) Eight-year results of Charnley arthroplasties with special reference to the behaviour of cement. Clin Orthop 137:24–36
15. Charnley J. with Loudon J.R. (1980) Subsidence of the femoral prosthesis in total hip replacement in relation to the design of the stem. J Bone Joint Surg (Br) 62:450–3

### Other references

16. Department of Health and Social Security (1974) Report of working party on acrylic cement in orthopaedic surgery. HMSO, London

17. Dutton J. (1956) Intracranial aneurysm – a new method of surgical treatment. Br Med J ii:585–6
18. Dutton J. (1959) Acrylic investment of intracranial aneurysms. Br Med J ii:597–602
19. Editorial (1975) The risks of total hip replacement. Br Med J i:296–7
20. Haboush E.J. (1953) Arthroplasty of the hip based on biomechanics, photo-elasticity, fast-setting dental acrylic, and other considerations. Bull Hosp Joint Dis 14:242–77
21. Harrod C.G.C. (1988) Personal communication
22. Kiaer S. (1953) Experimental investigation of the tissue reactions to acrylic plastics. Vth Congrès International de Chirurgie Orthopèdique, Stockholm 1951. Bruxelles: Imp Lielens
23. Ling R.S.M., Halawa M., Lee A.J.C., Vangala S.S. (1981) Total hip replacement with the Exeter prosthesis. J Bone Joint Surg (Br) 63:283 (abstract)
24. Malcolm A.J. (1988) Osseo-integration of bone and cement in long-standing hip joint replacements. J Pathol (abstract) 155:341
25. Robinson R.G., MacAlister A.D. (1954) Cranioplasty: a simple one-stage method. Br J Surg 42:312–5

## 12 Clean Air Against Infection 1960–1983

### Charnley references

1. Charnley J. (1964) A clean air operating enclosure. Br J Surg 51:195–202
2. Charnley J. (1964) A clean-air operating enclosure. Br J Surg 51:202–5
3. Charnley J. (1965) Operating-room conditions (letter). Lancet II:907–8
4. Charnley J. with Eftekhar N. (1969) Postoperative infection in total prosthetic replacement arthroplasty of the hip joint. Br J Surg 56:641–9
5. Charnley J. with Eftekhar N. (1969) Penetration of gown material by organisms from the surgeon's body. Lancet I: 172–3
   Charnley J. (1969) La 'serre' de Wrightington. Rev Chir Orthop 55:231–3
6. Charnley J. (1970) Operating theatre ventilation (letter). Lancet I:1054–5
   Charnley J. (1972) Postoperative infection after total hip replacement with special reference to air contamination in the operating room. Clin Orthop 87:167–87
   Charnley J. (1973) Clean air in the operating room. Cleve Clin Q 40:99–114
7. Charnley J. (1979) Low Friction Arthroplasty of the Hip. Theory and Practice. Springer, Berlin Heidelberg New York
   Charnley J. (1980) Theatre design. In: Karran S. (ed) Controversies in Surgical Sepsis. Praeger, New York, pp 3–13
8. Charnley J. (1982) The future of total hip replacement. In: The Hip (Proceedings of the 10th open scientific meeting of the Hip Society). C.V. Mosby, St Louis, pp 198–210
9. Charnley J. (1983) The development of the centre for hip surgery at Wrightington hospital (written in 1982). In: Swinburn W.R. (ed) Wrightington Hospital, the story of the first 50 years.

### Other references

10. Blowers R., McCluskey M. (1965) Design of operating room dress for surgeons. Lancet II:681–3
    Eftekhar N.S. (1984) Infection in Joint Replacement Surgery. C.V. Mosby, St Louis
    Howorth F.H. (1972) Air technology in medicine. Eng Med 1:2–5

11. Howorth F.H. (1984) The air in the operating theatre. In: Johnson I.D.A., Hunter A.R. (eds) The design and utilisation of operating theatres. Edward Arnold, London Howorth F.H. (1985) Prevention of airborne infection during surgery. Lancet I:306–8

12. Lidwell O.M. (1986) Clean air at operation and subsequent sepsis in the joint. Clin Orthop 211:91–102

13. Lidwell O.M. et al. (1987) Ultraclean air and antibiotics for the prevention of postoperative infection. Acta Orthop Scand 58:4–13

14. Petty W. (1978) The effect of methylmethacrylate on bacterial phagocytosis and killing by human polynuclear leucocytes. J Bone Joint Surg (Am) 60:752–7

## 13   The Charnley/Thackray Relationship 1947–1982

*Charnley references*

1. Charnley J. (1971) Stainless steel for femoral hip prosthesis in combination with a high density polythene socket. Report of forum on metallic surgical implants. J Bone Joint Surg (Br) 53:342–3

2. Charnley J. (1975) Fractures of femoral prostheses in total hip replacement. Clin Orthop 111:105–120

3. Charnley J. with Murphy J.C.M. (1976) The load-angle inlay knee arthroplasty. Proceedings British Orthopaedics Association. J Bone Joint Surg (Br) 58:58–9

4. Charnley J. (1979) Low Friction Arthroplasty of the Hip. Theory and Practice. Springer, Berlin Heidelberg New York

*Other references*

5. Chandler H.P., Reineck F.T., Wixson R.L., McCarthy J.C. (1981) Total hip replacement in patients younger than thirty years old. J Bone Joint Surg (Am) 63:1426

6. Gunston F.H. (1971) Polycentric knee arthroplasty. J Bone Joint Surg (Br) 53:272–7

7. Shelley P., Wroblewski B.M. (1988) Socket design and cement pressurisation in the Charnley low friction arthroplasty. J Bone Joint Surg (Br) 70:358–63

8. Wroblewski B.M. (1987) Stepping into the future. In: Symposium at King Edward VII Hospital, Midhurst.

## 14   Spreading the Word 1967–1982

*Charnley references*

<u>On teaching</u>

1. Charnley J. (1967) Operative technique of the low friction arthroplasty. Wrightington Internal Publications (6)

2. Charnley J. (1967) Remarks for the guidance of residents presenting cases at the Wednesday conference. Wrightington Internal Publications (7)

3. Charnley J. (1971) Wound closure. Wrightington Internal Publications (33)

4. Charnley J. (1971) Comparison of dynamic frictional torque in different total hip implants by a pendulum method. Wrightington Internal Publications (35)

## On biomechanics

5. Charnley J. (1966) Factors in the design of an artificial joint. Proc Inst Mech Eng 181:104–11
6. Charnley J. with Hammond B.T. (1967) The sphericity of the femoral head. Med Biol Eng 5:445–53
7. Charnley J. with Elson R.A. (1968) The direction of resultant force in total prosthetic replacement of the hip joint. Med Biol Eng 6:19–27
8. Charnley J., Pusso R. (1968) The recording and analysis of gait in relation to the surgery of the hip joint. Clin Orthop 58:153–64
   Charnley J. (1965) Biomechanics in orthopaedic surgery. In: Kenedi R.M. (ed) Biomechanics and Related Bio-engineering Topics. Pergamon Press, Oxford, pp 99–110
   Charnley J. (1970) The fixation of prostheses in living bone. In: Simpson D.C. (ed) Modern Trends in Biomechanics. Appleton-Century-Crofts, New York, pp 52–79
9. Charnley J. with McLeish R.D. (1971) Abduction forces in one-legged stance. J Biomech 3:191–209
10. Charnley J. with Jacobs N.A., Skorecki J. (1972) Analysis of the vertical component of force in normal and pathological gait. J Biomech 5:11–34
    Charnley J. (1973) Biomechanical considerations of total hip prosthetic design. In: The Hip (Proceedings of the Hip Society) C.V. Mosby, St Louis, pp 101–17

## On wear

11. Charnley J. with Kamangar A., Longfield M.D. (1969) The optimum size of femoral heads in relation to the wear of plastic sockets in total replacement of the hip. Med Biol Eng 7(1):31–9
    Charnley J. (1974) Clinical and laboratory observations on the rate of wear of different plastic materials in the sockets of artificial hip joints. Materials for use in Medicine and Biology. 55th meeting of Biological Engineering Society, Cambridge, July 1974
12. Charnley J. (1974) The status of research into the wear of high molecular weight polyethylene in total hip replacement. Wrightington Internal Publication (49)
13. Charnley J., Halley D.K. (1975) Rate of wear in total hip replacement. Clin Orthop 112:170–9
14. Charnley J. (1975) The wear of plastics materials in the hip joint. Paper presented at symposium at Strathclyde University, September 24, 1975. Wrightington Internal Publication (56)
15. Charnley J. with Griffith M.J., Seidenstein M.K., Williams D. (1978) Socket wear in Charnley low friction arthroplasty of the hip. Clin Orthop 137:37–47
16. Charnley J. with Dowling J.M., Atkinson J.R., Dowson D. (1978) The characteristics of acetabular cups worn in the human body. J Bone Joint Surg (Br) 60:375–82

## On results of the low friction arthroplasty and other related papers

17. Charnley J. (1965) Total replacement for advanced coxarthrosis. In SICOT Xc congrès, Paris, pp 311–19
18. Charnley J. (1968) Total prosthetic replacement of the hip. Triangle (Switzerland) 8 (6):211–16
    Charnley J. (1968) Total prosthetic replacement of the hip in relation to physiotherapy. Physiotherapy 54:406–11
19. Charnley J. (1969) Total prosthetic replacement of the hip. Reconstr Surg Traumatol (Switzerland) 11:9–19
20. Charnley J. (1970) Total hip replacement by low-friction arthroplasty. Clin Orthop 72:7–21

21. Charnley J. with Welch R.R. (1970) Low-friction arthroplasty of the hip in rheumatoid arthritis and ankylosing spondylitis. Clin Orthop 72:22–32
    Charnley J. (1971) Present status of total hip replacement. Ann Rheum Dis 30:560–4
    Charnley J. with Eftekhar N. (1971) Charnley 'low friction torque' arthroplasty. Clin Orthop 81:93–104
22. Charnley J. with Jaffe W.L. (1971) Bilateral low-friction arthroplasty as a single operative procedure. Bull Hosp Joint Dis 32:198–214
23. Charnley J. (1972) The long term results of low friction arthroplasty of the hip performed as a primary intervention. J Bone Joint Surg (Br) 54:61–76
24. Charnley J. with Dupont J.A. (1972) Low-friction arthroplasty of the hip for failures of previous operations. J Bone Joint Surg (Br) 54:77–87
25. Charnley J., Cupic Z. (1973) The nine and ten year results in low friction arthroplasty of the hip. Clin Orthop 95:9–25
26. Charnley J., Feagin J.A. (1973) Low friction arthroplasty in congenital subluxation of the hip. Clin Orthop 91:98–113
    Charnley J. (1973) The rationale of the low friction arthroplasty. The Hip (Proceedings of the Hip Society). C.V. Mosby, St Louis, pp 92–100
    Charnley J. (1974) Total hip replacement. JAMA 230:1025–8
27. Charnley J. with Halley D.K. (1975) Results of low friction arthroplasty in patients thirty years of age or younger. Clin Orthop 112:180–91
28. Charnley J. with DeLee J., Ferrari A. (1976) Ectopic bone formation following low friction arthroplasty of the hip. Clin Orthop 121:53–9
    Charnley J. (1976) Principles and practice in hip replacement. Proc R Soc Lond (B) 192:180–91
29. Charnley J. with Ferrari A. (1976) Conversion of hip joint pseudarthrosis to total hip replacement. Clin Orthop 121:12–9
30. Charnley J. with Hardinge K., Williams D., Etienne A., MacKenzie D. (1977) Conversion of fused hips to low friction arthroplasty. J Bone Joint Surg (Br) 59:385–95
    Charnley J., Boardman K.P., Bocco F. (1978) An evaluation of a method of trochanteric fixation using three wires in the Charnley low friction arthroplasty. Clin Orthop 132:31–8
31. Charnley J. with Boardman K.P. (1978) Low friction arthroplasty after fracture dislocation of the hip. J Bone Joint Surg (Br) 60:495–7
32. Charnley J. with Etienne J., Cupic Z. (1978) Postoperative dislocation after Charnley low friction arthroplasty. Clin Orthop 132:13–23
    Charnley J., Griffith M.J., Seidenstein M.K., Williams D. (1978) Eight-year results of Charnley arthroplasties of the hip with special reference to the behaviour of cement. Clin Orthop 137:24–36
33. Charnley J., Del Sel H.J. (1978) Total hip replacement following infection in the opposite hip. Clin Orthop 141:138–42
34. Charnley J., Sotelo-Garza A. (1978) The results of Charnley arthroplasty of the hip performed for protrusio acetabuli. Clin Orthop 132:12–8
35. Charnley J. (1979) Low Friction Arthroplasty of the Hip. Theory and Practice. Springer, Berlin Heidelberg New York
36. Charnley J. with Hardinge K., Cleary J. (1979) Low friction arthroplasty after healed septic and tuberculous arthritis. J Bone Joint Surg (Br) 61:144–7
    Charnley J. (1982) The future of total hip replacement. In: The Hip (Proceedings of the Hip Society) C.V. Mosby, St Louis, pp 198–210
    Charnley J. (1982) Evolution of total hip replacement. Ann Chir Gynecol 71:103–7

*On osteoarthritis*

Charnley J. with Batra H.C. (1969) Existence and incidence of osteoid in osteoarthritic femoral heads. J Bone Joint Surg (Br) 51:366–71

Charnley J. (1968) Osteoarthritis. Med Soc Trans (Lond) 85:89–91
Charnley J. with Wroblewski B.M. (1982) Radiographic morphology of the osteoarthritic hip. J Bone Joint Surg (Br) 64:568–9


## On thrombosis and pulmonary embolism

37. Charnley J. with Crawford W.J., Hillman F. (1968) A clinical trial of anticoagulant therapy in elective hip surgery. Wrightington Internal Publications (14)
38. Charnley J. (1972) Prophylaxis of postoperative thromboembolism (letter) Lancet II (768):134–5
    Charnley J. (1974) Deep vein thrombosis (letter). Br Med J ii:499
39. Charnley J. with Kelsey J.L., Wood P.H. (1976) Prediction of thromboembolism following total hip replacement. Clin Orthop 114:247–58
40. Charnley J., Johnson R. (1977) Treatment of pulmonary embolism in total hip replacement. Clin Orthop 128:149–54
41. Charnley J., Johnson R., Green J.R. (1977) Pulmonary embolism and its prophylaxis following the Charnley total hip replacement. Clin Orthop 127:123–32
42. Charnley J. with Johnson R. (1978) Hydroxyquinone in prophylaxis of pulmonary embolism following hip athroplasty. Clin Orthop 144:174–7


## Other references

43. Skorecki J. (1966) The design and construction of a new apparatus for measuring the vertical forces exerted in walking: a gait machine. J Strain Analysis 1:429–38
44. Stamatkis J.D., Kakkar K., Sagar S., Lawrence D., Nairn D., Bentley P.G. (1977) Femoral vein thrombosis and total hip replacement. Br Med J ii:223–5
45. McLeish R.D., Skorecki J. (1969) Analysis of wear in a spherical joint. Inst Mech Eng 183:1–4

## 15   An Outpost in the South 1969–1982

Large S.E. (1986) King Edward VII Hospital, Midhurst 1901–1986. Phillimore, Chichester, Sussex

## 16   Active Retirement 1975–1982

1. Browne A.O., Sheehan J.M. (1986) Trochanteric osteotomy. Clin Orthop 211:128–33
2. Charnley J. with Boardman K.P. and Bocco F. (1978) An evaluation of a method of trochanteric fixation using three wires in the Charnley low friction arthroplasty. Clin Orthop 132:31–8
3. Charnley J. (1979) Low Friction Arthroplasty of the Hip. Theory and Practice. Springer, Berlin Heidelberg New York
4. Charnley J. (1982) The future of total hip replacement. In: The Hip (Proceedings of the Hip Society) C.V. Mosby, St Louis, pp 198–210
5. Hardinge K. (1982) Direct lateral approach to the hip. J Bone Joint Surg (Br) 64:17–9
6. Nisbet N.W., Woodruffe M.F.A. (1984) John Charnley. Biographical memoirs of Fellows of the Royal Society, London 30:119–37

## 17  In Memoriam 1982

1. Bulstrode C. (1986) Keeping up with orthopaedic epidemics. Br Med J 295:514 (editorial)
2. Eftekhar N.S. (ed) (1986) Symposium on low friction arthroplasty. Clin Orthop Rel Res 211:2–179
3. Platt H.P. (1985) Sir John Charnley. In: Elwood W.J., Tuxford A.F. (eds) Some Manchester Doctors. Manchester University Press, Manchester
4. Stinchfield F.E. (1982) Obituary – Sir John Charnley. J Bone Joint Surg (Am) 64:1258

# INDEX

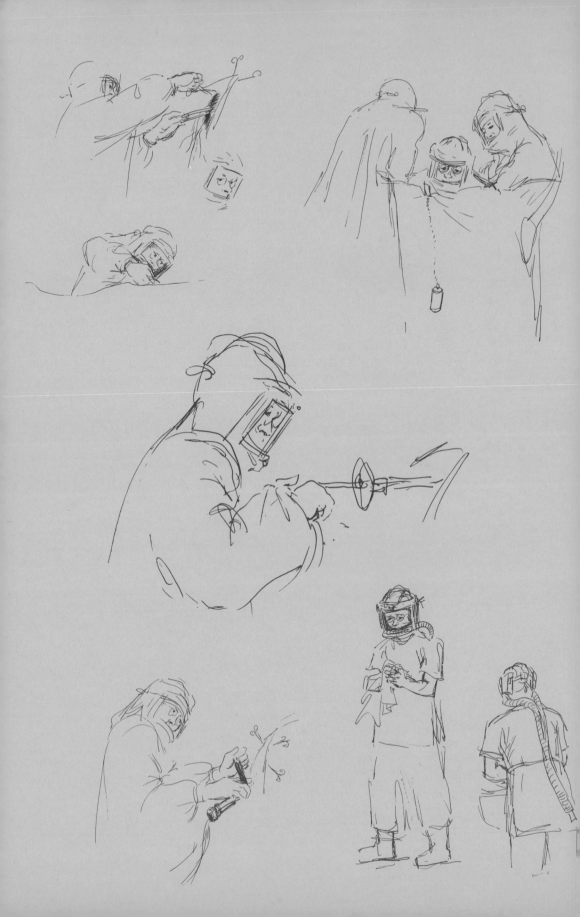